MORE 4U!

theclinics.com

This Clinics series is available online.

Here's what you get:

- Full text of EVERY issue from 2002 to NOW
- Figures, tables, drawings, references and more
- Searchable: find what you need fast

  Search [All Clinics ▼] for [ ] [GO]

- Linked to MEDLINE and Elsevier journals
- E-alerts

the**clinics**.com

DENTAL CLINICS
OF NORTH AMERICA

Periodontology: Present Status and Future Concepts

GUEST EDITOR
Frank A. Scannapieco, DMD, PhD

July 2005 • Volume 49 • Number 3

SAUNDERS

An Imprint of Elsevier, Inc.
PHILADELPHIA LONDON TORONTO MONTREAL SYDNEY TOKYO

W.B. SAUNDERS COMPANY
A Division of Elsevier Inc.

Elsevier, Inc. • 1600 John F. Kennedy Boulevard • Suite 1800 • Philadelphia, Pennsylvania 19103-2899

http://www.dental.theclinics.com

THE DENTAL CLINICS OF NORTH AMERICA	**Volume 49, Number 3**
July 2005	**ISSN 0011-8532**
Editor: John Vassallo	**ISBN 1-4160-2821-8**

The Dental Clinics of North America (ISSN 0011-8532) is published quarterly by W.B. Saunders Company. Corporate and Editorial Offices: Elsevier, Inc., 1600 John F. Kennedy Boulevard, Suite 1800, Philadelphia, PA 19103-2899. Accounting and circulation offices: 6277 Sea Harbor Drive, Orlando, FL 32887-4800. Periodicals postage paid at Orlando, FL 32862, and additional mailing offices. Subscription prices are $150.00 per year (US individuals), $242.00 per year (US institutions), $181.00 per year (Canadian individuals), $299.00 per year (Canadian institutions), $75.00 per year (US students/residents), $205.00 per year (foreign individuals), and $299.00 per year (foreign institutions) and $103.00 (Canadian and foreign students/residents). Foreign air speed delivery is included in all *Clinics* subscription prices. All prices are subject to change without notice. POSTMASTER: Send address changes to *The Dental Clinics of North America*, W.B. Saunders Company, Periodicals Fulfillment, Orlando, FL 32887-4800. **Customer Service: 1-800-654-2452 (US). From outside of the US, call 1-407-345-4000.**

The Dental Clinics of North America is covered in *Index Medicus, Current Contents/Clinical Medicine, ISI/BIOMED and Clinahl.*

Printed in the United States of America.

GUEST EDITOR

FRANK A. SCANNAPIECO, DMD, PhD, Professor and Chair, Department of Oral Biology, School of Dental Medicine, University at Buffalo, State University of New York, Buffalo, New York

CONTRIBUTORS

JASIM M. ALBANDAR, DDS, DMD, PhD, Professor of Periodontology, Department of Periodontology; Director, Periodontal Diagnostics Research Laboratory, Temple University School of Dentistry; and Professor of Oral Biology, Temple University Graduate School, Philadelphia, Pennsylvania

TORD BERGLUNDH, DDS, Odont Dr, Professor, Göteborg University, The Sahlgrenska Academy, Faculty of Odontology, Department of Periodontology, Göteborg, Sweden

JASON COOKE, DDS, Graduate Student, Department of Periodontics/Prevention/Geriatrics, School of Dentistry, University of Michigan, Ann Arbor, Michigan

ANDREW R. DENTINO, DDS, PhD, Associate Professor and Program Director of Periodontics, Department of Surgical Sciences, Marquette University School of Dentistry, Milwaukee, Wisconsin

WILLIAM V. GIANNOBILE, DDS, DMSc, Department of Periodontics/Prevention/Geriatrics, School of Dentistry; Michigan Center for Oral Health Research; and Department of Biomedical Engineering, College of Engineering, University of Michigan, Ann Arbor, Michigan

MARGARETA HULTIN, DDS, Odont Dr, Associate Professor, Karolinska Institutet, Institute of Odontology, Department of Periodontology, Huddinge, Sweden

MOAWIA M. KASSAB, DDS, MS, Assistant Professor of Periodontics, Department of Surgical Sciences, Marquette University School of Dentistry, Milwaukee, Wisconsin

AMY S. KIM, DDS, Michigan Center for Oral Health Research, University of Michigan, Ann Arbor, Michigan

JANET KINNEY, RDH, Department of Periodontics/Prevention/Geriatrics, School of Dentistry, University of Michigan, Ann Arbor, Michigan

BJÖRN KLINGE, DDS, Odont Dr, Professor, Karolinska Institutet, Institute of Odontology, Department of Periodontology, Huddinge, Sweden

PURNIMA S. KUMAR, BDS, MDS, Chief Resident, Advanced Education Program, Section of Periodontology, College of Dentistry, The Ohio State University, Columbus, Ohio

ERICA J. RENNER, RDH, MS, Assistant Clinical Professor of Periodontics, Department of Surgical Sciences, Marquette University School of Dentistry, Milwaukee, Wisconsin

MARIA EMANUEL RYAN, DDS, PhD, Professor and Director of Clinical Research, Department of Oral Biology and Pathology, School of Dental Medicine, Stony Brook University, State University of New York, South Campus, Stony Brook, New York

FRANK A. SCANNAPIECO, DMD, PhD, Professor and Chair, Department of Oral Biology, School of Dental Medicine, University at Buffalo, State University of New York, Buffalo, New York

ROBERT E. SCHIFFERLE, DDS, MMSc, PhD, Associate Professor, Departments of Periodontics & Endodontics and Oral Biology, School of Dental Medicine, University at Buffalo, State University of New York, Buffalo, New York

MARIO TABA, Jr, DDS, PhD, Department of Periodontics/Prevention/Geriatrics, School of Dentistry, University of Michigan, Ann Arbor, Michigan

DIMITRIS N. TATAKIS, DDS, PhD, Professor and Director, Advanced Education Program, Section of Periodontology, College of Dentistry, The Ohio State University, Columbus, Ohio

HENRI TENENBAUM, DDS, PhD, HDR(F), Professor and Chair, Department of Periodontology, Dental Faculty, University Louis Pasteur, Strasbourg, France

HOWARD C. TENENBAUM, DDS, PhD, FRCD(C), Associate Dean, Biological and Diagnostic Sciences; and Professor and Head, Discipline of Periodontology, Faculty of Dentistry, University of Toronto, Toronto, Ontario, Canada

HOM-LAY WANG, DDS, MSD, Professor and Director of Graduate Periodontics, Department of Periodontics/Prevention/Geriatrics, School of Dentistry, University of Michigan, Ann Arbor, Michigan

RON ZOHAR, DDS, PhD, FRCD(C), Disciplines of Periodontology and Biomaterials, Faculty of Dentistry, University of Toronto, Toronto, Ontario, Canada

CONTENTS

have been reported in certain populations. Chronic and aggressive periodontitis are multifactorial diseases caused primarily by dental plaque microorganisms, and with important modifying effects from other local and systemic factors. The study of the significance of demographic, environmental, and biologic variables is important for risk assessment and the control of periodontal diseases.

A number of studies suggest an association between periodontal disease and cardiovascular disease, pulmonary disease, diabetes, and pregnancy complications. Presently, the data must be regarded as preliminary. Additional large-scale longitudinal epidemiologic and interventional studies are necessary to validate these associations and to determine whether the associations are causal. The goal of this article is to review the history of this concept, describe the biologically plausible circumstances that may underlie these potential associations, and provide a summary of the published literature that supports or refutes them.

This article provides an overview of periodontal disease diagnosis that uses clinical parameters and biomarkers of the disease process. This article discusses the use of biomarkers of disease that can be identified at the tissue, cellular, and molecular levels and that are measurable in oral fluids such as saliva and gingival crevicular fluid. Biomarkers identified from these biologic fluids include microbial, host response, and connective tissue-related molecules that can target specific pathways of local alveolar bone resorption. Future prospects for oral fluid–based diagnostics that use microarray and microfluidic technologies are presented.

The ultimate goal of periodontal disease prevention is to maintain the dentition over a lifetime in a state of health, comfort, and function in an aesthetically pleasing presentation. This article focuses on primary and secondary periodontal disease prevention as they relate to gingivitis and periodontitis. Risk assessment, mechanical plaque control, chemical plaque control, current clinical recommendations for optimal prevention, and future preventive strategies are discussed.

with antimicrobial therapy, is the most successful concept. There is no reliable evidence that suggests which intervention is the most effective for treating peri-implantitis. This article includes background information on the biology of tissue-destructive periodontitis and peri-implantitis to help clinicians interpret the clinical manifestation of the risk for peri-implantitis.

FORTHCOMING ISSUES

October 2005
Incipient and Hidden Caries
Daniel W. Boston, DMD, *Guest Editor*

January 2006
Adolescent Oral Health
Deborah Studen-Pavlovich, DMD, and
Dennis N. Ranalli, DDS, MDS, *Guest Editors*

April 2006
Tissue Engineering
Franklin Garcia-Godoy, DDS, MS, and
Barbara Boyan, PhD, *Guest Editors*

RECENT ISSUES

April 2005
Geriatrics: Contemporary and Future Concerns
Roseann Mulligan, DDS, MS, *Guest Editor*

January 2005
Oral Soft Tissue Lesions
Thomas P. Sollecito, MD, *Guest Editor*

October 2004
Lasers in Clinical Dentistry
Donald J. Coluzzi, DDS, and
Robert A. Convissar, DDS, *Guest Editors*

THE CLINICS ARE NOW AVAILABLE ONLINE!

Access your subscription at:
http://www.theclinics.com

GOAL STATEMENT

The goal of the *Dental Clinics of North America* is to keep practicing dentists up to date with current clinical practice in dentistry by providing timely articles reviewing the state of the art in dental care.

ACCREDITATION

The *Dental Clinics of North America* are planned and implemented in accordance with the ADA CERP Recognition Standards and Procedures through the joint sponsorship of the University of Virginia School of Medicine and Elsevier.

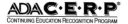

The University of Virginia School of Medicine is an ADA CERP Recognized Provider.

Dentists participating in this learning activity may earn up to 15 ADA CERP credits per issue or a maximum of 60 credits per year. Credits awarded may not apply toward license renewal in all states. It is the responsibility of each participant to verify the requirements of their state licensing board.

ADA CERP credit can be earned by reading the text material, taking the CME examination online at http://www.theclinics.com/home/cme, and completing the evaluation. After taking the test, you will be required to review any and all incorrect answers. Following completion of the test and evaluation, your credit will be awarded, and you may print your certificate.

FACULTY DISCLOSURE

The University of Virginia School of Medicine is accredited by the Accreditation Council for Continuing Medical Education (ACCME) to provide continuing medical education for physicians.

As a provider accredited by the Accreditation Council for Continuing Medical Education (ACCME), the Office of Continuing Medical Education of the University of Virginia School of Medicine must ensure balance, independence, objectivity, and scientific rigor in all its individually sponsored or jointly sponsored educational activities. All authors/editors participating in a sponsored activity are expected to disclose to the readers any significant financial interest or other relationship (1) with the manufacturer(s) of any commercial product(s) and/or provider(s) of commercial services discussed in an educational presentation and (2) with any commercial supporters of the activity (significant financial interest or other relationship can include such things as grants or research support, employee, consultant, stock holder, member of speakers bureau, etc.) The intent of this disclosure is not to prevent authors/editors with a significant financial or other relationship from writing an article, but rather to provide readers with information on which they can make their own judgments. It remains for the readers to determine whether the author's/editor's interest or relationships may influence the article with regard to exposition or conclusion.

The authors/editors listed below have identified no professional or financial affiliations related to the articles:
Jasim M. Albandar, DDS, DMD, PhD; Tord Berglundh, DDS, Odont Dr; Jason Cooke, DDS; William V. Giannobile, DDS, DMSc; Margareta Hultin, DDS, Odont Dr; Moawia M. Kassab, DDS, MS; Amy S. Kim, DDS; Janet Kinney, RDH; Björn Klinge, DDS, Odont Dr; Purnima S. Kumar, BDS, MDS; Erica J. Renner, RDH, MS; Frank A. Scannapieco, DMD, PhD; Robert E. Schifferle, DDS, MMSc, PhD; Mario Taba, Jr, DDS, PhD; Dimitris N. Tatakis, DDS, PhD; Henri Tenenbaum, DDS, PhD, HDR(F); Howard C. Tenenbaum, DDS, PhD, FRCD(C); John Vassallo, Acquisitions Editor; and Ron Zohar, DDS, PhD, FRCD(C).

The authors listed below have identified the following professional or financial affiliations related to the articles:
Andrew R. Dentino, DDS, PhD, has been a consultant for Pfizer and Braun Oral B.
Maria Emanuel Ryan, DDS, PhD, is a consultant, serves on a number of advisory boards, and is named on patents as an inventor of therapeutic applications of tetracyclines discussed. These patents are fully assigned to the research foundation of Stony Brook University and have been exclusively licensed to CallaGenex Pharmaceuticals.
Hom-Lay Wang, DDS, MSD, has received research grants for conducting research for the following companies: Zimmer Dental, BioHorizon, Inc., and Atrix Pharmaceutic Company.

Disclosure of discussion of non-FDA approved uses for pharmaceutical products and/or medical devices:
The University of Virginia School of Medicine, as an ACCME provider, requires that all authors/editors identify and disclose any "off label" uses for pharmaceutical products and/or medical devices. The University of Virginia School of Medicine recommends that each reader fully review all the available data on new products or procedures prior to instituting them with patients.

All authors/editors who provided disclosures will not be discussing any off-label uses except:
Andrew R. Dentino, DDS, PhD, will discuss the use of dilute povidone-iodine and dilute household bleach as antiseptic irrigants in the secondary prevention of periodontal disease.
Howard C. Tenenbaum, DDS, PhD, FRCD(C), will discuss the use of pulse dose high concentration HEBP to stimulate bone formation. These types of drugs (bisphosphonates) generally are used to inhibit bone resorption, but these authors have data to show that when used in a specific way, they actually stimulate bone formation in addition to their capacity to inhibit resorption. However, this is discussed within the context of potential future use and is not being recommended as a treatment approach now.

TO ENROLL

To enroll in the Dental Clinics of North America Continuing Medical Education program, call customer service at 1-800-654-2452 or sign up online at http://www.theclinics.com/home/cme. The CME program is available to subscribers for an additional annual fee of $79.95.

THE DENTAL
CLINICS
OF NORTH AMERICA

Dent Clin N Am 49 (2005) xi–xii

Preface

Periodontology: Present Status and Future Concepts

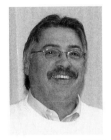

Frank A. Scannapieco, DMD, PhD
Guest Editor

Change is one thing, progress is another. "Change" is scientific, "progress" is ethical; change is indubitable, whereas progress is a matter of controversy. —Bertrand Russell

Because things are the way they are, things will not stay the way they are. —Bertolt Brecht

As seems to be the norm these days in most health care disciplines, periodontology is in a state of flux. The changing demographics of disease; significant disparities in oral health in racial and ethnic minorities; constant amendments to third-party insurance plans; the dwindling number of patients with access to insurance; the explosion of new research methodologies and findings; and even the rapid progress made in human genome-related areas now conspire and will continue to push the practice of periodontics in many, often divergent directions. Certainly, general practitioners are treating an ever-greater proportion of the periodontal cases that present to their practice. However, it is not always the case that the generalist is prepared to deal with the complexities that present in the periodontal patient. On the other hand, the periodontist is often challenged to treat the more difficult cases and at the same time driven to incorporate the latest (and sometimes unproven) techniques and products into their practice.

The goal of this issue of the *Dental Clinics of North America* is to bring together various experts in the field of periodontology to write about topics that are pertinent to the practice of periodontics in the general practice setting. All of the authors who have been kind enough to sacrifice their valuable time to write an article are experts in the topic for which they write. First, foundational knowledge on the etiology, pathogenesis, epidemiology, and risk factors of periodontal diseases are presented. This updated knowledge is essential for decision-making regarding the diagnosis and treatment of the periodontal patient. Lately, there has also been considerable interest in the systemic effects of periodontal disease that has burgeoned into the new field of periodontal medicine. Recent findings in this area are thus also presented. A series of articles follow that provide a contemporary view of various aspects of prevention and treatment of periodontal disease in general practice. Finally, an article that speculates on how the practice of periodontics might change over the next 10 years is provided.

Together, it is our hope that these articles will be of use to the general practitioner who wishes to add to his or her knowledge to better treat the periodontal patient.

Frank A. Scannapieco, DMD, PhD
Department of Oral Biology
School of Dental Medicine
University at Buffalo
State University of New York
109 Foster Hall
Buffalo, NY 14214, USA

E-mail address: fas1@buffalo.edu

ELSEVIER
SAUNDERS

THE DENTAL
CLINICS
OF NORTH AMERICA

Dent Clin N Am 49 (2005) 491–516

Etiology and Pathogenesis of Periodontal Diseases

Dimitris N. Tatakis, DDS, PhD*,
Purnima S. Kumar, BDS, MDS

*Section of Periodontology, College of Dentistry,
The Ohio State University, P.O. Box 182357, 305 West 12th Avenue, #193,
Columbus, OH 43218-2357, USA*

According to the most recent classification that resulted from a 1999 international workshop [1], diseases of the periodontium comprise a long list of conditions involving the supporting structures of the tooth. The two most prevalent and most investigated periodontal diseases are dental plaque–induced gingivitis and chronic periodontitis. Aggressive periodontitis, which encompasses several previous clinical entities such as localized juvenile periodontitis (currently termed localized aggressive periodontitis, LAP), generalized juvenile periodontitis and rapidly progressing periodontitis (now collectively classified as generalized aggressive periodontitis), periodontitis associated with systemic diseases, and necrotizing ulcerative periodontal diseases (ie, necrotizing ulcerative gingivitis and periodontitis), round out the list of the most significant and common periodontal diseases. The last 10 to 15 years have seen the emergence of several important new findings and concepts regarding the etiopathogenesis of periodontal diseases. These findings include the recognition of dental bacterial plaque as a biofilm, identification and characterization of genetic defects that predispose individuals to periodontitis, host-defense mechanisms implicated in peri-odontal tissue destruction, and the interaction of risk factors with the host defenses and bacterial plaque. This article reviews current aspects of the etiology and pathogenesis of periodontal diseases.

This work was supported by the Section of Periodontology, College of Dentistry, The Ohio State University.

* Corresponding author.

E-mail address: tatakis.1@osu.edu (D.N. Tatakis).

dental.theclinics.com

Etiology and pathogenesis of periodontal diseases

Gingivitis and periodontitis are inflammatory conditions of infectious nature [2]. The unequivocal role of dental bacterial plaque in the development of these diseases was established almost 40 years ago [3–7]. Gingivitis is a reversible inflammatory reaction of the marginal gingiva to plaque accumulation, whereas periodontitis is a destructive, nonreversible condition resulting in loss of tooth connective-tissue attachment to bone, which ultimately leads to loss of the involved teeth. Existing evidence indicates that gingivitis precedes the onset of periodontitis; however, not all gingivitis cases develop into periodontitis [5,8,9]. The reason for this is that accumulation of plaque bacteria is necessary but not sufficient by itself for the development of periodontitis: a susceptible host is necessary [5,9,10].

The role of dental plaque

The presence of bacteria in the oral cavity has been known since the time of Anton von Leeuwenhoek, who described the presence of "animalcules" in dental plaque. The bacterial etiology of periodontal diseases has been explored for over 100 years, evolving along with technologic advances in identification and characterization. Although early studies indicated that periodontal diseases occurred in response to plaque mass (nonspecific plaque hypothesis), current thinking implicates specific microbial species in disease causation (specific plaque hypothesis) [11,12]. This bacterial etiology of periodontal disease is strongly supported by clinical studies that have reported that mechanical and chemical antibacterial treatment can prevent or treat gingivitis and periodontitis [12,13].

The identification of specific causative species, or periodontopathogens, has been hampered by some of the unique features of periodontal diseases. The foremost of these features is that disease occurs in a site already colonized by a bacterial population. Thus, disease might be caused by overgrowth of one or more species in the resident population or by colonization by exogenous pathogens. For example, it has been shown that *Capnocytophaga* spp are seen in high levels before the onset of gingivitis, whereas *Prevotella* spp are detected in areas with established gingivitis. Thus, it may be interpreted that *Capnocytophaga* spp are more likely to be etiologic agents and *Prevotella* spp may be present as a consequence of the disease process [14]. Colonization by exogenous pathogens is thought to contribute to the episodic nature of disease progression [15]; that is, not all sites with baseline-attachment loss demonstrate the same rate of disease progression or disease activity at the same time points.

Many methods have been used to study the composition of plaque bacteria. Initial studies were based on cultivation and microscopic visualization. Research studies using detection systems based on specific antibodies were useful in determining the presence and levels of species of interest. With the advent of molecular methods, however, the diversity of the oral flora has been extensively explored. Studies by Kroes et al [16], Paster et al [17], and Choi et al [18] have revealed that over half of the plaque accumulated is composed of heretofore uncultivated species. Culture-based studies have not been able to explore the diversity of this polymicrobial infection. Thus, it is possible that as-yet-undetected species are responsible for disease.

One of the most significant recent developments in the understanding of periodontal disease etiology is the recognition of dental plaque as a biofilm. A biofilm is defined as single cells and microcolonies enclosed in a highly hydrated, predominantly anionic exopolymer matrix [19]. These sessile cells behave in profoundly different ways from their free-floating (planktonic) counterparts.

Dental plaque as a biofilm—development

Research on plaque development has shown that oral bacteria colonize nonshedding hard surfaces and shedding soft tissue surfaces. The physical and morphologic characteristics of these surfaces create different ecosystems or niches with distinct bacterial profiles. These niches are the result of a dynamic equilibrium that exists between the adhesion forces of micro-organisms and swallowing and mastication forces, salivary and crevicular flow, and oral hygiene measures.

Bacterial adhesion to oral surfaces is a function of bacterial surface characteristics and the receptivity of the host epithelium. Studies on bacterial colonization of other niches in the body have shown that epithelial cells of individuals susceptible to infection harbor as many as five times more pathogenic bacteria than resistant individuals [20]. Studies using animal models suggest that the same might be true of periodontal disease [21].

Plaque formation follows several distinct phases, beginning with adsorption onto the tooth surface of a conditioning film derived from bacterial and host molecules that forms immediately following tooth eruption or tooth cleaning [22]. This adsorption is followed by passive transport of bacteria mediated by weak, long-range forces of attraction. Covalent and hydrogen bonds create strong, short-range forces that result in irreversible attachment [23]. The primary colonizers form a biofilm by autoaggregation (attraction between same species) and coaggregation (attraction between different species). Coaggregation results in a functional organization of plaque bacteria and formation of different morphologic structures such as corncobs and rosettes. The microenvironment now changes from aerobic/capnophilic to facultative anaerobic. The attached bacteria multiply and secrete an extracellular matrix, which results in a mature mixed-population biofilm [24]. Transmission occurs from other sites, leading to incorporation of new members into the biofilm and the formation of a climax community.

A biofilm environment confers certain properties to bacteria that are not seen in the planktonic state, a fact that explains the importance of recognizing dental plaque as a biofilm and not as bacteria in the planktonic state. In the following sections, some of the properties of a biofilm are reviewed.

Cell–cell communication. An important characteristic seen only in biofilm-associated bacteria is quorum sensing, or cell density–mediated gene expression. This process is mediated by two groups of compounds known as autoinducer 1 and autoinducer 2. Gram-positive and gram-negative cells secrete molecules known as autoinducer-2, which is encoded by the *luxS* gene [25]. In *Streptococcus gordonii*, *luxS* turns on expression of *sspA* and *sspB* genes, which encode for a protein that provides a binding site for the major fimbriae of *Porphyromonas gingivalis* [26–29]. Thus, *Porphyromonas gingivalis*, a secondary colonizer, is capable of preferential binding in the presence of *S gordonii*, an early colonizer.

Gene transfer. Biofilm-associated bacteria communicate with each other by way of horizontal gene transfer. In *S mutans*, quorum sensing is mediated by competence-stimulating peptide. Genes of the competence-stimulating peptide signaling system (*comC*, *comD*, *comE*, and *comX*) are responsible for multiple functions: biofilm formation, competence (ability to accept foreign DNA), and acid tolerance [30,31].

Antimicrobial resistance. The biofilm provides a protected environment against antimicrobial agents. The biofilm acts as a barrier to diffusion due to the presence of neutralizing enzymes (β-lactamase, IgA protease) and a diffusion-resistant matrix [32]. Cells in the biofilm can develop antibiotic resistance from horizontal gene transfer and mutations and by expressing efflux pumps. Penicillin [33] and tetracycline [34] resistance occurs among bacteria by conjugative transfer of mobile genetic elements. Further, cells in a biofilm have a slower rate of cell division and might therefore not be as susceptible to antibiotics as actively dividing planktonic cells. This resistance provided by biofilm living must be taken into account when selecting antibiotics. In vitro antibiotic susceptibility tests are typically conducted on planktonic cells whose behavior is significantly different from that of biofilm-associated cells. Thus, it has been argued that "biofilm inhibitory concentration" is a more realistic estimate of antimicrobial activity than the current measures [35].

Regulation of gene expression. Biofilm living has been shown to regulate gene expression in certain bacteria. For example, exposure of *S gordonii* to saliva results in the induction of genes (*sspA/B*) that mediate host-surface binding and coaggregation with *Porphyromonas gingivalis* and *Actinomyces* spp [36,37]. Similarly, genes encoding glucan (*gtf*) and fructan (*ftf*) synthesis are differentially regulated in biofilm-associated *S mutans* [38].

Bacterial antigens and virulence factors in the biofilm

Recent studies have focused on "virulence factors" associated with putative periodontopathogens. A virulence factor is any microbial component that is necessary for causing disease in the host. These factors may be essential for host colonization or may be "true" antigens capable of causing an immune response by the host. In vitro studies of biofilms have enabled the study of the antigenic potential of biofilms [39].

Virulence factors can be differentially expressed in response to the environment. *Actinobacillus actinomycetemcomitans*, for example, produces leukotoxin, a 116-kd protein antigen capable of immunomodulation [40]. Leukotoxin causes apoptosis (programmed cell death of leukocytes), the first line of defense against bacterial invasion. Because the organism grows optimally at pH 7.0 to 8.0, it is suggested that the more virulent strains of *Actinobacillus actinomycetemcomitans* are present on the surface of subgingival plaque [40]. Similarly, *Porphyromonas gingivalis* strain W50 shows maximal growth and proteolytic activity in conditions of pH 7.0 to 8.0 and hemin excess, suggesting it becomes more virulent in an inflamed gingival crevice [41]. Among the specific virulence factors associated with putative periodontopathogens are the following molecules (Table 1).

Lipopolysaccharide. The outer membranes of most gram-negative bacteria display repeating polysaccharide units attached to the O-side chains of a lipid component (lipopolysaccharide). Lipopolysaccharide is highly antigenic and capable of inducing the release of inflammatory mediators and cytokines such as prostaglandin E_2, interleukin (IL)-1α, IL-1β, tumor necrosis factor-α (TNF-α), and IL-8 through CD14 and Toll-like receptor–mediated activation of several host cells. The structure of lipopolysaccharide also allows classification of bacteria based on its structure. For example, *Actinobacillus actinomycetemcomitans* can be classified into six distinct serotypes of varying virulence based on lipopolysaccharide structure [42]. Unlike other bacteria, lipopolysaccharide of *Porphyromonas gingivalis* activates the cytokine cascade through Toll-like receptors, perhaps because of its unique three-dimensional structure [43].

Heat shock proteins. When eukaryotic and bacterial cells are exposed to environmental stress (eg, temperature, pH, redox potential), they synthesize stress proteins such as heat shock proteins [44]. These proteins act as molecular chaperones in the assembly and folding of proteins and thus protect the cell from the damaging effects of environmental stress. Heat shock protein homologs such as GroEL, GroES, DnaK, and HtpG have been studied in oral bacteria. Heat shock proteins from *Actinobacillus actinomycetemcomitans* stimulate osteoclast activation and epithelial

Table 1
Bacterial virulence factors and their effects on the host

Factor	Produced by	Effects on host cells
Lipopoly-saccharide	Gram negative bacteria including *Actinobacillus actinomycetemcomitans, Treponema denticola, Porphyromonas gingivalis, Tannerella forsythia*	Increases cytokine release from PMNs, macrophages, fibroblasts Induces nitric oxide secretion in macrophages Increases differentiation of osteoclast precursors Activates osteoclasts Supports osteoclast survival Stimulates T-helper cell proliferation
Heat shock proteins	*Actinobacillus actinomycetemcomitans, Tannerella forsythia, Porphyromonas gingivalis, Campylobacter rectus, Fusobacterium nucleatum, Streptococcus mutans, Prevotella* spp, *Capnocytophaga* spp	Induce gingival epithelial cell proliferation in low doses Osteolytic activity PDL epithelial cell proliferation Molecular mimicry between bacterial and host heat shock proteins, leading to autoimmune response
Extracellular proteolytic enzymes	*Tannerella forsythia, Porphyromonas gingivalis, Treponema denticola*	Degrade fibrinogen, fibronectin, albumin, laminin Hydrolyze collagen IV, IgG, IgA
Fimbriae	*Actinobacillus actinomycetemcomitans, Porphyromonas gingivalis*	Important in colonization Role in invasion of host cells
Outer membrane proteins	*Actinobacillus actinomycetemcomitans, Porphyromonas gingivalis*	Enhance innate immune response through cytokines Suppress proliferation of T and B cells Suppress proliferation of fibroblasts, monocytes, osteoblasts
Leukotoxin	*Actinobacillus actinomycetemcomitans*	Promotes apoptosis of T cells, natural killer cells, PMNs (in low concentration) Causes cell death by necrosis (in high concentration)
Flagellum	*Treponema denticola*	Role in adherence, due to fibronectin binding
Capsule	*Porphyromonas gingivalis*	Increases resistance to phagocytosis by PMNs Inhibits fibroblast attachment to root surface

Abbreviations: PDL, periodontal ligament; PMNs, polymorphonuclear leukocytes.

proliferation at low concentrations and are cytotoxic at high doses [45]. Microbial heat shock proteins are highly immunogenic and have been shown to be associated with autoimmune diseases such as rheumatoid arthritis and atherosclerosis. It has been suggested that chronic infections such as periodontitis may result from prolonged exposure to heat shock proteins, thereby promoting autoimmune disease. The evidence, however, is tenuous, as seen with *Porphyromonas gingivalis* GroEL [46,47].

Fimbriae. Fimbriae are found in oral bacteria such as *Actinobacillus actinomycetemcomitans* and *Porphyromonas gingivalis.* They are long protein filaments, present singly or in bundles on the surface of cells. The major component is fimbrillin, a highly antigenic protein encoded by *fimA* in *Porphyromonas gingivalis* and *flp* in *Actinobacillus actinomycetemcomitans*. In both bacteria, fimbriae are thought to be important in colonization because fimbrial-deficient mutants show reduced ability to bind and invade epithelial cells and fibroblasts [48]. Fimbriae-mediated epithelial invasion stimulates expression of host cell adhesion molecules such as intercellular adhesion molecule, vascular cell adhesion molecule, P-selectin, and E-selectin, thus inducing a massive leukocytic response at the site. *Porphyromonas gingivalis* fimbriae also stimulate IL-1α, IL-1β, TNF-α, and granulocyte-macrophage colony–stimulating factor, leading to bone resorption.

Extracellular proteolytic enzymes. Tannerella forsythia, Porphyromonas gingivalis, Treponema denticola, and other oral bacteria produce proteolytic enzymes often displayed on their cell surfaces. Dentilisin (*Treponema denticola*), PrtH (*Tannerella forsythia*), and RgpA, RgpB, and Kgp (*Porphyromonas gingivalis*) are the best-characterized enzymes in this group [49]. The RgpA/B and Kgp proteinases, major virulence factors of *Porphyromonas gingivalis*, degrade fibrinogen, fibronectin, laminin, adhesion molecules, and several types of collagen [50–52]. *Tannerella forsythia* with the *prtH* genotype is found to be more common in chronic periodontitis than in health. Dentilisin has been shown to hydrolyze fibrinogen, albumin, laminin, collagen type IV, IgG, and IgA.

Although there is compelling evidence that bacteria and bacterial products present a challenge to the host defense system, there is no single bacterial product that induces all the changes observed in periodontal disease. Henderson and coworkers [53] proposed that bacterial modulins are responsible for immunomodulation of the host cells. Modulins are bioactive bacterial compounds such as exotoxins, endotoxins, and metabolic end products produced by commensal and pathogenic organisms that can induce host cytokine networks. What is evident from the preceding description of the various virulence factors is that bacteria can cause direct tissue damage; however, by triggering several host cells to release inflammatory cytokines and other mediators (see later discussion), bacteria can also cause indirect tissue damage. It seems that the host response to the bacteria renders most of the damage seen in periodontal disease.

Specific microorganisms associated with periodontal health and disease

Different periodontal diseases have somewhat unique profiles of associated bacteria (Table 2). This characteristic and the fact that disease occurs in sporadic bursts in the mouth strengthens the evidence for the role of specific microorganisms in disease causation and progression.

Table 2
Bacterial species associated with periodontal health and disease

Condition	Associated microorganisms	Strength of evidence	Techniques used
Periodontal health	Gram (+) anaerobe		
	Atopobium rimae	CS	m
	Gram (+) facultative		
	Streptococcus sanguis	CS, LS	C, M, I, c, m
	Streptococcus mitis	CS, LS	C, M, I, c, m
	Gram (−) anaerobe		
	Bacteroides sp oral clone BU063	CS	m
	Veillonella spp	CS, LS	C, M, I, c, m
	Gemella spp	CS, LS	C, M, I, c, m
	Capnocytophaga spp	CS, LS	C, M, I, c, m
Gingivitis	Gram (+) anaerobe		
	Actinomyces viscosus	CS	C, M, I, c
	Peptostreptococcus micros	CS, LS	C, M, I, c
	Gram (+) facultative		
	Streptococcus spp	CS, LS	C, M, I, c
	Gram (−) anaerobe		
	Campylobacter gracilis	CS, LS	C, M, I, c
	Fusobacterium nucleatum	CS, LS	C, M, I, c
	Prevotella intermedia	CS, LS	C, M, I, c
	Veillonella parvula	CS, LS	C, M, I, c
Chronic periodontitis	Gram (+) anaerobe		
	Peptostreptococcus micros	CS	C, M, I, c, m
	Gram (−) anaerobe		
	Porphyromonas gingivalis	CS, LS	C, M, I, c, m
	Tannerella forsythia	CS, LS	C, M, I, c, m
	Prevotella intermedia	CS, LS	C, M, I, c, m
	Campylobacter rectus	CS, LS	C, M, I, c, m
	Eikenella corrodens	CS	C, M, I, c, m
	Fusobacterium nucleatum	CS, LS	C, M, I, c, m
	Actinobacillus actinomycetemcomitans	CS	C, I, c, m
	Treponema spp	CS, LS	C, M, I, c, m
	Filifactor alocis	CS	C, I, c, m
	Megasphaera sp oral clone BB166	CS	m
	Deferribacteres sp oral clone BH017	CS	m
	Desulfobulbus sp oral clone R004	CS	m
	Bacteroides sp oral clone AU126	CS	m
Aggressive periodontitis	Gram (−) anaerobe		
	Actinobacillus actinomycetemcomitans	CS, LS	C, c, m
	Porphyromonas gingivalis	CS, LS	C, I, c, m
	Campylobacter rectus	CS	C
	Eikenella corrodens	CS	C
Acute necrotizing gingivitis	Gram (−) anaerobe		
	Treponema spp	CS	C, M, m
	Prevotella intermedia	CS	m
	Rothia dentocariosa	CS	m
	Fusobacterium spp	CS	m
	Achromobacter spp	CS	m

Table 2 (*continued*)

Condition	Associated microorganisms	Strength of evidence	Techniques used
Periodontal abscess	*Propionibacterium acnes*	CS	m
	Capnocytophaga spp	CS	m
	Gram (+) anaerobe		
	Peptostreptococcus micros	CS	C
	Gram (−) anaerobe		
	Fusobacterium nucleatum	CS	C
	Prevotella intermedia	CS	C
	Tannerella forsythia	CS	C
	Campylobacter rectus	CS	C

Abbreviations: c, checkerboard; C, culture; CS, cross-sectional studies; I, immunodetection; LS, longitudinal studies; m, molecular methods; M, microscopy.

Periodontal health

Bacteria that are associated with periodontal health include primary or early colonizers such as *S sanguis*, *S mitis*, *Gemella* spp, *Atopobium* spp, *Fusobacterium nucleatum*, and *Capnocytophaga* spp [54–56]. Species belonging to the genera *Veillonella*, *Streptococcus*, and *Capnocytophaga* are thought to be beneficial to the host [55]. Recent molecular analysis has shown the presence of certain uncultivated species such as *Bacteroides* oral clone BU063 to be strongly associated with periodontal health [57].

Gingivitis

Gram-positive species (eg, *Streptococcus* spp, *Actinomyces viscosus*, *Peptostreptococcus micros*) and gram-negative species (eg, *Campylobacter gracilis*, *F nucleatum*, *Prevotella intermedia*, *Veillonella*) have been associated with gingivitis [13,58,59]. Pregnancy-associated gingivitis, however, appears to have a microflora with a high proportion of *Prevotella intermedia* [60].

Chronic periodontitis

The bacterial profile of chronic periodontitis has been explored in cross-sectional and longitudinal studies. The effect of various treatment methods in changing the microbial ecology has also been investigated. *Porphyromonas gingivalis*, *Tannerella forsythia*, *Prevotella intermedia*, *Campylobacter rectus*, *Eikenella corrodens*, *F nucleatum*, *Actinobacillus actinomycetemcomitans*, *Peptostreptococcus micros*, and *Treponema* spp have been most commonly found to be associated with chronic periodontitis. *Porphyromonas gingivalis*, *Tannerella forsythia*, *Prevotella intermedia*, *Campylobacter rectus*, and *F nucleatum* have been reported at higher levels in sites with active disease or with progressing disease [61–64]. Clinical resolution of disease following treatment is also associated with a decrease in the levels of these species. More recent molecular approaches have also found previously uncultivated bacterial species such as *Desulfobulbus* sp oral clone R004, *Deferribacteres* sp oral clones BH017 and D084, and *Bacteroides* sp oral clone AU126 to be associated with periodontitis [17,54].

Localized aggressive periodontitis

Studies have implicated *Actinobacillus actinomycetemcomitans* as an important organism in the etiology of LAP [65–67]. This species has been found as the predominant cultivable species in as many as 90% of sites with LAP. It should be noted, however, that not all studies support the association of *Actinobacillus actinomycetemcomitans* in aggressive periodontitis. This organism is not always found in disease sites; further, it has also been found in healthy children, albeit in low numbers, suggesting that it is a member of the healthy microbial flora [68]. Other species such as *Porphyromonas gingivalis*, *E corrodens*, and *Campylobacter rectus* have been found in high levels in certain cases of LAP [69]. Viruses such as Epstein Barr virus and human cytomegalovirus have also been associated with this disease [70].

Generalized aggressive periodontitis

The microbial etiology of generalized aggressive periodontitis is not as well defined as the other forms of periodontal diseases due to changes in disease nomenclature over time. The disease now encompasses entities such as periodontosis, prepubertal periodontitis, and rapidly progressing periodontitis. Nevertheless, available evidence suggests that the bacterial profile of generalized aggressive periodontitis is not significantly different from that of chronic periodontitis [71–73].

Necrotizing ulcerative gingivitis

The bacterial flora of necrotizing ulcerative gingivitis has been demonstrated to be composed, for the most part, of fusobacteria and spirochetes. Recent studies have isolated previously unsuspected spirochetes (eg, *Treponema putidum*, a proteolytic treponeme) from lesions of necrotizing ulcerative gingivitis [74]. Other bacteria reported in these lesions include *Rothia dentocariosa*, *Treponema* spp, *Achromobacter* spp, *Propionibacterium acnes*, *Capnocytophaga* spp, and *Prevotella intermedia* [56].

Periodontal abscess

A periodontal abscess is a localized purulent infection within the tissues adjacent to the periodontal pocket. *F nucleatum*, *Prevotella intermedia*, *Peptostreptococcus micros*, *Tannerella forsythia*, *Campylobacter rectus, and Porphyromonas gingivalis* have been recovered from these lesions [75,76].

The role of host susceptibility

As mentioned earlier, plaque bacteria are necessary but not sufficient for the development of periodontitis: a susceptible host is necessary. This aspect of periodontal pathogenesis is addressed in the following paragraphs.

Gingivitis

Although development of gingivitis after plaque accumulation appears to be a universal finding, the rate or speed of development and the degree of the clinical inflammatory response is variable between individuals, even under similar plaque accumulation conditions [77]. In contrast to the voluminous literature on periodontitis, there are few studies addressing potential host-dependent variations in susceptibility to gingivitis [77,78]. Based on studies using the experimental gingivitis model, one can estimate that approximately 13% of all individuals represent a "resistant" group [77,79,80]. Several factors have been shown to modulate the clinical expression of gingival inflammation in response to plaque accumulation. Some factors result in exacerbated gingival response to plaque, including metabolic factors such as puberty and pregnancy, genetic factors such as Down syndrome, nutritional factors such as vitamin C deficiency, the intake of drugs such as those leading to gingival enlargement, systemic diseases such as leukemia, immune deficiencies, and diabetes mellitus, and other conditions such as stress [77]. Recent evidence also suggests that genetic polymorphisms such as those in the IL-1 gene cluster may contribute to susceptibility to gingivitis [81]. The clinical significance of these factors is that patients who have them (eg, pregnant women or children born with Down syndrome) are more susceptible to gingivitis and are therefore at greater risk for disease. Consequently, these patients require more stringent plaque control practices. Other factors such as smoking and anti-inflammatory drugs lead to a muted response [77], which results in gingiva appearing healthier than expected based on the amount of plaque present. This muted gingival response in smokers could mask severe underlying disease (ie, periodontal attachment loss) unless the clinician performs a complete periodontal examination that includes periodontal probing.

Periodontitis

Ample evidence suggests that susceptibility to periodontitis varies considerably among individuals, with approximately 10% being highly susceptible and 10% being highly resistant [9]. This difference in susceptibility has largely been attributed to genetic factors [82,83]. In a study of adult twins, it was estimated that 50% of the risk for chronic periodontitis is accounted for by heredity [83]. The specific genes that might be implicated in chronic periodontitis have not been determined. A specific genetic marker (IL-1 genotype) has been associated with greater susceptibility to periodontitis in some populations and with poorer long-term prognosis (ie, greater tooth loss) following treatment [84,85]. Similar to the findings for chronic periodontitis, genetically determined susceptibility has also been demonstrated for LAP, although no specific gene mutations have been identified to date [86]. Although there are no reliable means at present to predict susceptibility to periodontitis, evidence suggests that susceptibility to periodontitis may be linked to susceptibility to gingivitis [77].

Genetic diseases associated with periodontitis, such as Down syndrome [87] and Papillon-Lefèvre syndrome [88], highlight the importance of hereditary factors in determining susceptibility to periodontal disease. Furthermore, when the primary genetic defect and the ensuing biochemical and physiologic implications are known, such diseases can provide significant insights regarding pathogenesis. The recent identification of specific gene defects underlying systemic diseases whose phenotype includes periodontitis—cyclic neutropenia [89,90], severe congenital neutropenia [91,92], Chédiak-Higashi syndrome [93–95], Papillon-Lefèvre syndrome [88,96,97], leukocyte adhesion deficiency [98,99], and Cohen syndrome [100,101]—has enhanced the understanding of how molecules and cells can be implicated in periodontal destruction (Table 3). Cyclic neutropenia, severe congenital neutropenia, Cohen syndrome, and Chédiak-Higashi syndrome represent various forms of quantitative neutrophil defects, underscoring the protective function of neutrophils (polymorphonuclear leukocytes; PMNs) against infections (see later discussion). Immunologic abnormalities common to Chédiak-Higashi and Papillon-Lefèvre syndrome include abnormalities in natural killer cells (see later discussion). Leukocyte adhesion deficiency is characterized by PMNs that cannot migrate to the site of injury or infection; this defect results in absence of extravascular PMNs despite increased PMN numbers in the circulation. It should be noted that in addition to those already described, other specific immunologic and genetic defects might be associated with the aforementioned diseases. An individual's genetic background, which cannot be modified, is not the only factor that can influence disease susceptibility. Several acquired or

Table 3
Genetic diseases associated with periodontitis

Genetic disease	Implicated gene	Affected protein	Year identified [reference]
Leukocyte adhesion deficiency	ITGB2	Integrin, beta-2	1986 [99]
Chédiak-Higashi syndrome	LYST	Lysosomal trafficking regulator	1996 [95]
Papillon-Lefèvre syndrome	CTSC	Cathepsin C	1999 [88,97]
Cyclic neutropenia	ELA2	Neutrophil elastase	1999 [90]
Severe congenital neutropenia	ELA2	Neutrophil elastase	2000 [92]
Cohen syndrome	COH1	COH1	2003 [101]

environmental factors, most of them modifiable, have been strongly implicated (see the article by Albandar within this issue for further exploration of this topic). The two most significant risk factors are smoking and diabetes mellitus. Smoking, in a dose-dependent manner [102], greatly increases the risk for chronic periodontitis and generalized aggressive periodontitis [103–106]. Smokers, compared with nonsmokers, have deeper probing depths, more attachment loss, greater bone loss, more rapid disease progression, and more tooth loss; in addition, they respond less well to periodontal therapy and are more prone to lose teeth during maintenance [106]. The various mechanisms through which smoking increases susceptibility to periodontitis include negative effects on PMN functions, on humoral and cellular immune responses, on fibroblast function, and on the vascular bed, among others [106]. The only positive aspect of the strong relation of smoking to periodontitis susceptibility is the fact that smoking is a modifiable factor; smoking cessation has been shown to be of significant benefit in reducing the risk of disease activity [105,106]. There are several treatment modalities available to the clinician to help his or her patients achieve a smoke-free lifestyle [106,107], therefore decreasing their susceptibility to periodontitis.

Diabetes is reaching epidemic proportions in the United States and elsewhere [108,109], and persons with diabetes are twice as likely to have periodontitis as nondiabetics [104,110]. Diabetes increases susceptibility to periodontitis and other infectious diseases through several mechanisms. One essential mechanism appears to be the nonenzymatic glycation of proteins and lipids, resulting in the formation of advanced glycation end products (AGEs) [111,112]. AGEs appear to preferentially alter the functionality of the target cells of diabetes (eg, endothelial cells and monocytes) through specific cell surface receptors such as the receptor for AGEs. When the AGE-induced activation of cell surface receptor for AGEs is experimentally blocked in diabetic animals, periodontitis-associated alveolar bone loss is decreased [111]. The altered functionality of endothelial and monocytic cells results in vascular changes and in exacerbated inflammatory responses; the inflammatory responses include increased levels of inflammatory cytokines such as TNF-α and matrix-degrading enzymes such as collagenase [111,112].

Host cells and molecules implicated in periodontal pathogenesis

The accumulated dental bacterial plaque has the potential to cause periodontal tissue damage directly, through mechanisms such as matrix-degrading enzymes and molecules that impair the functions of host cells as described previously. It appears, however, that plaque elicits most periodontal tissue injury through indirect mechanisms dependent on initiation and propagation of inflammatory host tissue reactions. The classic studies of Page and Schroeder [113] provided the basic understanding of gingivitis and periodontitis histopathology and inflammation. The inflammatory infiltrate of periodontitis is characterized by PMNs, macro-phages, lymphocytes, plasma cells, and substantial loss of collagen. This inflammatory infiltrate has cellular elements associated with acute (PMN) and chronic (lymphocytes, plasma cells) reactions. There are complex interactions between these host defense cells and the periodontal structural elements. The major cellular structural elements of the periodontium are the epithelial cells, the periodontal ligament and gingival fibroblasts, and the cells of the alveolar bone (eg, osteoblasts and osteoclasts). Molecular structural elements are the extracellular matrix components such as the various collagens and the noncollagenous proteins (eg, elastin and connective tissue proteoglycans). The nature of the interactions between these components determines whether a typical response to plaque accumulation results in marginal clinical inflammation (gingivitis) alone or in irreversible destruction of the attachment apparatus (periodontitis). The following paragraphs review the role of specific host cells and molecules, focusing on recent findings.

Neutrophils

The primary purpose of an inflammatory reaction, be it acute or chronic, is to contain or eliminate the injury-causing agent (eg, bacterial lipopoly-saccharide) and to initiate the cascade of events that will result in repair of any tissue damage. In this regard, PMNs are the first line of defense against bacteria, and proper PMN functionality is essential for protecting the integrity of the periodontium [114]. In most patients with LAP and other conditions associated with periodontitis, PMNs have been shown to exhibit defects in chemotaxis or phagocytosis [114]. The strong association of periodontitis with genetic diseases characterized by quantitative (eg, cyclic neutropenia) or qualitative (eg, leukocyte adhesion deficiency syndrome) PMN defects provides convincing evidence of the critical protective role of PMNs. PMNs and other host components essential for defense against microorganisms, however, may also be central participants in the tissue destruction seen in periodontitis and other infectious/inflammatory diseases [115]. For example, activated PMNs have been shown to cause damage to gingival epithelial cells [116] and periodontal ligament fibroblasts [117]. The significance of the PMNs in this aspect of periodontal disease pathogenesis is also supported by other findings. Increased tissue levels of PMNs have been associated with active (destructive) periodontal lesions [118], whereas salivary or gingival crevicular fluid levels of neutrophil proteolytic enzymes such as collagenase and elastase correlate with disease activity or clinical indices of disease [119,120].

Elastase (a neutrophil enzyme that has indirect antibacterial properties) and collagenase can degrade several components of the extracellular matrix (eg, various collagens and elastin), thus destroying the three-dimensional scaffolding necessary for tissue organization. The significance of collagenase in periodontitis tissue damage has been clinically exploited by the introduction of nonantimicrobial-dose doxycycline therapy [121–123]; low-dose doxycycline inhibits host collagenase without having any discernible effect on the microflora present [121,123]. In addition to the aforementioned PMN proteolytic enzymes, the neutrophil may contribute to tissue destruction through the release of reactive (toxic) oxygen metabolites [116,124]. These reactive oxygen-containing molecules can also degrade periodontal matrix molecules directly [125] and indirectly through activation of latent enzymes [126] or inactivation of enzyme inhibitors [127].

Recent evidence from LAP studies suggests that a hyper-responsive or "hyperfunctional" PMN, as opposed to a "hypofunctional" or "deficient" one, may cause enhanced tissue damage in this disease [128]. PMN hyper-responsiveness, which may manifest as increased levels of intracellular signaling molecules [129] and reactive oxygen metabolites [130], appears to be genetic in origin.

Macrophages

Macrophages are mononuclear cells responsible for orchestrating an immune response and that participate in the early, nonspecific, or innate defense against microorganisms and in specific immunity through their antigen-presenting function. Macrophages can modulate these responses through the various cytokines they produce. Studies in the last decade have shown that macrophages present in periodontitis lesions have varied phenotypes or subsets [131], suggesting diverse functionality. Unlike what has been shown for PMNs [118], there is no evidence of significant changes in the number of macrophages when tissues from healthy, gingivitis, and periodontitis sites are compared [132,133]. Furthermore, there is little evidence of macrophage activation in periodontitis lesions [133]. The significance of the various macrophage subsets to the disease process remains to be elucidated.

Natural killer cells

Natural killer cells are a lymphocyte subset involved in the innate immune response. Natural killer cells play a vital role in host defenses against infected and malignant cells by recognizing and killing such cells and by producing cytokines such as TNF-α and interferon-γ that in turn help regulate other immune cells. Natural killer cell levels increase significantly from healthy human gingiva to diseased periodontal tissues [134,135], suggesting their involvement in the immune response to plaque accumulation. Impaired natural killer cell functionality has been recently described in various systemic conditions associated with periodontitis (eg, Papillon-Lefèvre syndrome [136], Chédiak-Higashi syndrome [137], and smoking [138]), suggesting that natural killer cells serve a protective function in the periodontium.

T lymphocytes

T cells, one of two major lymphocyte subsets, are mononuclear cells whose activation is essential for cell-mediated immunity. There are several types of T cells, which are categorized by their surface antigens and functional properties; the two most common are helper and cytotoxic T cells. Helper ($CD4^+$) T cells, the target of HIV infection, function primarily by proliferating and activating ("helping") other lymphocytes such as B cells and other T cells that ultimately are directly involved in the specific immune response against a pathogen or antigen. Cytotoxic ($CD8^+$) T cells, as their name implies, function as destroyers of target cells (typically infected or cancerous cells) that express specific antigens on their surface. $CD4^+$ and $CD8^+$ T cells are present in periodontitis lesions; their ratio and relative numbers are thought to reflect the regulatory status of the local immune response [139,140]. One of the most exciting recent findings about T cells and their contribution to periodontal pathogenesis involves the under-standing of their direct involvement in periodontal bone resorption [141,142]. This understanding stems from the discovery of osteoprotegerin ligand, a molecule that is critical for osteoclast formation and lymphocyte and lymph node development and regulation. T cells activated by periodontopathogens produce osteoprotegerin ligand, which directly stimulates the formation of osteoclasts through its binding to receptor activator of nuclear factor kappa B (RANK). RANK is a cell surface receptor molecule that is highly expressed on osteoclast precursors and osteoclasts and is critical for osteoclast differentiation and activation. In addition to osteoprotegerin ligand and RANK, a third related molecule is involved in bone homeostasis: osteoprotegerin. Osteoprotegerin, produced by osteoblasts and other cells, is a decoy receptor that circulates and binds osteoprotegerin ligand and thus prevents osteoprotegerin ligand from activating RANK [143]. Osteoprotegerin ligand and osteoprotegerin are produced by periodontal cells, and their ratio is altered, favoring osteoprotegerin ligand, in diseased periodontal tissues [144–146]. Exogenous osteoprotegerin administration can inhibit bacteria-induced alveolar bone resorption [141] and represents a promising future treatment modality to prevent periodontal and peri-implant bone loss.

B cells

B cells, the second major lymphocyte subset, are essential for humoral immunity. A B cell, preprogrammed to recognize a specific antigen, gives rise to plasma cells that produce specific antibodies when triggered by the antigen and other regulatory cells. The numbers of B cells increase from health to gingivitis to periodontitis [113,147], as does the ratio of B cells to T cells [132]. The presence of significantly higher B-cell levels in active periodontitis lesions suggests that B-cell activation contributes to disease progression [148].

Proinflammatory cytokines and lipid mediators

The vast array of signaling molecules participating in the complex cellular interactions taking place in the tissue can be categorized as proinflammatory and anti-inflammatory (Table 4). In many instances, it is the balance between these two types of signals that determines the tissue response and the initiation or progression of disease. The following proinflammatory mediators are some of the best studied in relation to periodontal disease pathogenesis.

Interleukin-1. The contributions of IL-1α and IL-1β (two distinct but related molecules, collectively referred to as IL-1 here) to alveolar bone loss and periodontal disease have received considerable attention [149]. IL-1, produced by monocytic, epithelial, osteoblastic, and other cells, is a potent stimulator of bone resorption and inhibitor of bone formation. Several periodontopathogens can stimulate IL-1 production by host cells (see the Lipopolysaccharide section above), and IL-1 levels are elevated in diseased periodontal tissues. In humans, local levels of IL-1 increase in gingivitis [150] and in periodontitis [151], whereas periodontal therapy significantly decreases such levels [151]. In recent nonhuman primate experiments, use of a specific IL-1 inhibitor resulted in significant reduction of periodontopathogen-induced attachment loss, bone resorption, and inflammation [152]. These results suggest that IL-1 inhibitors might be useful in the management of periodontitis.

Tumor necrosis factor-α. TNF-α is a molecularly distinct cytokine that shares many biologic activities with IL-1. TNF-α has been implicated in the periodontal disease process because of its ability to stimulate bone resorption and other catabolic processes. The use of TNF inhibitors (in combination with IL-1 inhibitors) results in decreased inflammation and tissue destruction in nonhuman primates [153,154]. Recent clinical studies and complementary evidence from animal experiments suggest that TNF-α may be of particular significance in the exacerbated periodontal tissue destruction associated with diabetes [111,155,156].

Prostaglandins and thromboxanes. Prostaglandin E_2 and thromboxane B_2 are lipid molecules produced by many host cells through the cyclooxygenase pathway, one of the two major paths of arachidonic acid metabolism. Among other studies, the use of flurbiprofen (a nonsteroidal anti-inflammatory drug that inhibits prostaglandin E_2 and thromboxane B_2

Table 4
Host molecules regulating the inflammatory response

Molecules	Proinflammatory	Anti-inflammatory
Cytokines	IL-1α, IL-1β, TNF-α	IL-10
Lipid molecules	Prostaglandin E_2, thromboxane B_2	Lipoxin A_4

production) helped demonstrate that these mediators contribute to the redness and bleeding of gingivitis [157] and the alveolar bone loss of periodontitis [158].

Anti-inflammatory cytokines and lipid mediators

The discovery of host-derived anti-inflammatory molecules is a much more recent development compared with the isolation of their proinflammatory counterparts.

Interleukin-10. IL-10 is a cytokine with potent anti-inflammatory properties that regulates humoral and cellular immune responses and the production of several proinflammatory cytokines such as IL-1 and TNF. Recent animal studies demonstrate that lack of IL-10 leads to significantly greater alveolar bone loss [159,160], whereas recent clinical evidence indicates that gingival tissue IL-10 levels are significantly greater in healthy compared with periodontitis sites [161,162]. These and other results suggest that IL-10 might be of use as biologic therapy in periodontitis.

Lipoxins. Lipoxins are produced through the lipoxygenase pathway, the second major path of arachidonic acid metabolism. Recent evidence suggests that lipoxin A_4, in addition to other molecules in this class, can modulate the host response to promote resolution of inflammation, in general, and in response to periodontopathogens, in particular [163,164]. This evidence raises the possibility of active anti-inflammatory therapy with lipoxins (or analogs thereof) as means to control the inflammation-induced tissue damage in periodontitis.

Summary

The last decade or so has brought significant advances to the understanding of periodontal disease pathogenesis. These advances include the discovery of new, uncultivated, disease-associated bacterial species; the recognition of dental plaque as a biofilm; the identification and characterization of genetic defects that predispose to periodontitis; the role of risk factors in disease susceptibility; and the discovery of new host-derived cellular and molecular mechanisms implicated in periodontal tissue destruction. Many of these discoveries hold promise for the future as foundation for the engineering of new prevention and treatment modalities.

References

[1] Armitage GC. Development of a classification system for periodontal diseases and conditions. Ann Periodontol 1999;4:1–6.

[2] Williams RC. Periodontal disease. N Engl J Med 1990;322:373–82.

[3] Löe H, Holm-Pedersen P. Absence and presence of fluid from normal and inflamed gingivae. Periodontics 1965;3:171–7.

[4] Theilade E, Wright WH, Jensen SB, et al. Experimental gingivitis in man. II. A longitudinal clinical and bacteriological investigation. J Periodontal Res 1966;1:1–13.

[5] Lindhe J, Hamp S, Löe H. Experimental periodontitis in the beagle dog. J Periodontal Res 1973;8:1–10.

[6] Slots J, Hausmann E. Longitudinal study of experimentally induced periodontal disease in *Macaca arctoides*: relationship between microflora and alveolar bone loss. Infect Immun 1979;23:260–9.

[7] Holt SC, Ebersole J, Felton J, et al. Implantation of *Bacteroides gingivalis* in nonhuman primates initiates progression of periodontitis. Science 1988;239:55–7.

[8] Listgarten MA, Schifter CC, Laster L. 3-year longitudinal study of the periodontal status of an adult population with gingivitis. J Clin Periodontol 1985;12:225–38.

[9] Löe H, Anerud A, Boysen H, et al. Natural history of periodontal disease in man. Rapid, moderate and no loss of attachment in Sri Lankan laborers 14 to 46 years of age. J Clin Periodontol 1986;13:431–45.

[10] Page RC. Milestones in periodontal research and the remaining critical issues. J Periodontal Res 1999;34:331–9.

[11] Loesche WJ, Grossman NS. Periodontal disease as a specific, albeit chronic, infection: diagnosis and treatment [table of contents]. Clin Microbiol Rev 2001;14:727–52.

[12] Loesche WJ. Chemotherapy of dental plaque infections. Oral Sci Rev 1976;9:65–107.

[13] Theilade E, Wright WH, Jensen SB, et al. Experimental gingivitis in man. II. A longitudinal clinical and bacteriological investigation. J Periodontal Res 1966;1:1–13.

[14] Mombelli A, Lang NP, Burgin WB, et al. Microbial changes associated with the development of puberty gingivitis. J Periodontal Res 1990;25:331–8.

[15] Goodson JM, Tanner AC, Haffajee AD, et al. Patterns of progression and regression of advanced destructive periodontal disease. J Clin Periodontol 1982;9:472–81.

[16] Kroes I, Lepp PW, Relman DA. Bacterial diversity within the human subgingival crevice. Proc Natl Acad Sci USA 1999;96:14547–52.

[17] Paster BJ, Boches SK, Galvin JL, et al. Bacterial diversity in human subgingival plaque. J Bacteriol 2001;183:3770–83.

[18] Choi BK, Paster BJ, Dewhirst FE, et al. Diversity of cultivable and uncultivable oral spirochetes from a patient with severe destructive periodontitis. Infect Immun 1994;62: 1889–95.

[19] Costerton JW. Overview of microbial biofilms. J Ind Microbiol 1995;15:137–40.

[20] Danino J, Joachims HZ, Barak M. Predictive value of an adherence test for acute otitis media. Otolaryngol Head Neck Surg 1998;118:400–3.

[21] Isogai E, Isogai H, Sawada H, et al. Bacterial adherence to gingival epithelial cells of rats with naturally occurring gingivitis. J Periodontol 1986;57:225–30.

[22] Al-Hashimi I, Levine MJ. Characterization of in vivo salivary-derived enamel pellicle. Arch Oral Biol 1989;34:289–95.

[23] Jenkinson HF, Lamont RJ. Streptococcal adhesion and colonization. Crit Rev Oral Biol Med 1997;8:175–200.

[24] Kolenbrander PE. Oral microbial communities: biofilms, interactions, and genetic systems. Annu Rev Microbiol 2000;54:413–37.

[25] Kolenbrander PE, Andersen RN, Blehert DS, et al. Communication among oral bacteria [table of contents]. Microbiol Mol Biol Rev 2002;66:486–505.

[26] Chung WO, Park Y, Lamont RJ, et al. Signaling system in *Porphyromonas gingivalis* based on a LuxS protein. J Bacteriol 2001;183:3903–9.

[27] Fong KP, Chung WO, Lamont RJ, et al. Intra- and interspecies regulation of gene expression by *Actinobacillus actinomycetemcomitans* LuxS. Infect Immun 2001;69: 7625–34.

[28] Lamont RJ, El-Sabaeny A, Park Y, et al. Role of the *Streptococcus gordonii* SspB protein in the development of *Porphyromonas gingivalis* biofilms on streptococcal substrates. Microbiol 2002;148:1627–36.

[29] McNab R, Ford SK, El-Sabaeny A, et al. LuxS-based signaling in *Streptococcus gordonii*: autoinducer 2 controls carbohydrate metabolism and biofilm formation with *Porphyromonas gingivalis*. J Bacteriol 2003;185:274–84.

[30] Li YH, Lau PC, Tang N, et al. Novel two-component regulatory system involved in biofilm formation and acid resistance in *Streptococcus mutans*. J Bacteriol 2002;184: 6333–42.

[31] Li YH, Tang N, Aspiras MB, et al. A quorum-sensing signaling system essential for genetic competence in *Streptococcus mutans* is involved in biofilm formation. J Bacteriol 2002;184: 2699–708.

[32] Stewart PS. Diffusion in biofilms. J Bacteriol 2003;185:1485–91.

[33] Dowson CG, Hutchison A, Woodford N, et al. Penicillin-resistant viridans streptococci have obtained altered penicillin-binding protein genes from penicillin-resistant strains of *Streptococcus pneumoniae*. Proc Natl Acad Sci USA 1990;87:5858–62.

[34] Roberts AP, Cheah G, Ready D, et al. Transfer of TN916-like elements in microcosm dental plaques. Antimicrob Agents Chemother 2001;45:2943–6.

[35] Anwar H, Dasgupta MK, Costerton JW. Testing the susceptibility of bacteria in biofilms to antibacterial agents. Antimicrob Agents Chemother 1990;34:2043–6.

[36] Kolenbrander PE, Phucas CS. Effect of saliva on coaggregation of oral *Actinomyces* and *Streptococcus* species. Infect Immun 1984;44:228–33.

[37] Du LD, Kolenbrander PE. Identification of saliva-regulated genes of *Streptococcus gordonii* DL1 by differential display using random arbitrarily primed PCR. Infect Immun 2000;68:4834–7.

[38] Li Y, Burne RA. Regulation of the gtfBC and ftf genes of *Streptococcus mutans* in biofilms in response to pH and carbohydrate. Microbiol 2001;147:2841–8.

[39] Bradshaw DJ, Marsh PD. Use of continuous flow techniques in modeling dental plaque biofilms. Methods Enzymol 1999;310:279–96.

[40] Ohta H, Miyagi A, Kato K, et al. The relationships between leukotoxin production, growth rate and the bicarbonate concentration in a toxin-production-variable strain of *Actinobacillus actinomycetemcomitans*. Microbiol 1996;142(Pt 4):963–70.

[41] Marsh PD, McDermid AS, McKee AS, et al. The effect of growth rate and haemin on the virulence and proteolytic activity of *Porphyromonas gingivalis* W50. Microbiol 1994; 140(Pt 4):861–5.

[42] Zambon JJ, Slots J, Genco RJ. Serology of oral *Actinobacillus actinomycetemcomitans* and serotype distribution in human periodontal disease. Infect Immun 1983;41:19–27.

[43] Netea MG, van Deuren M, Kullberg BJ, et al. Does the shape of lipid A determine the interaction of LPS with Toll-like receptors? Trends Immunol 2002;23:135–9.

[44] Goulhen F, Grenier D, Mayrand D. Oral microbial heat-shock proteins and their potential contributions to infections. Crit Rev Oral Biol Med 2003;14:399–412.

[45] Paju S, Goulhen F, Asikainen S, et al. Localization of heat shock proteins in clinical *Actinobacillus actinomycetemcomitans* strains and their effects on epithelial cell proliferation. FEMS Microbiol Lett 2000;182:231–5.

[46] Yamazaki K, Ohsawa Y, Tabeta K, et al. Accumulation of human heat shock protein 60-reactive T cells in the gingival tissues of periodontitis patients. Infect Immun 2002;70: 2492–501.

[47] Ueki K, Tabeta K, Yoshie H, et al. Self-heat shock protein 60 induces tumour necrosis factor-alpha in monocyte-derived macrophage: possible role in chronic inflammatory periodontal disease. Clin Exp Immunol 2002;127:72–7.

[48] Njoroge T, Genco RJ, Sojar HT, et al. A role for fimbriae in *Porphyromonas gingivalis* invasion of oral epithelial cells. Infect Immun 1997;65:1980–4.

[49] Curtis MA, Kuramitsu HK, Lantz M, et al. Molecular genetics and nomenclature of proteases of *Porphyromonas gingivalis*. J Periodontal Res 1999;34:464–72.

[50] Kesavalu L, Ebersole JL, Machen RL, et al. *Porphyromonas gingivalis* virulence in mice: induction of immunity to bacterial components. Infect Immun 1992;60:1455–64.

[51] Kesavalu L, Holt SC, Ebersole JL. *Porphyromonas gingivalis* virulence in a murine lesion model: effects of immune alterations. Microb Pathog 1997;23:317–26.

[52] Chen Z, Casiano CA, Fletcher HM. Protease-active extracellular protein preparations from *Porphyromonas gingivalis* W83 induce N-cadherin proteolysis, loss of cell adhesion, and apoptosis in human epithelial cells. J Periodontol 2001;72:641–50.

[53] Henderson B, Poole S, Wilson M. Bacterial modulins: a novel class of virulence factors which cause host tissue pathology by inducing cytokine synthesis. Microbiol Rev 1996;60: 316–41.

[54] Kumar PS, Griffen AL, Barton JA, et al. New bacterial species associated with chronic periodontitis. J Dent Res 2003;82:338–44.

[55] Socransky SS, Haffajee AD. The bacterial etiology of destructive periodontal disease: current concepts. J Periodontol 1992;63:322–31.

[56] Paster BJ, Falkler WA Jr, Enwonwu CO, et al. Prevalent bacterial species and novel phylotypes in advanced noma lesions. J Clin Microbiol 2002;40:2187–91.

[57] Leys EJ, Lyons SR, Moeschberger ML, et al. Association of *Bacteroides forsythus* and a novel *Bacteroides* phylotype with periodontitis. J Clin Microbiol 2002;40:821–5.

[58] Macuch PJ, Tanner AC. *Campylobacter* species in health, gingivitis, and periodontitis. J Dent Res 2000;79:785–92.

[59] Kremer BH, Loos BG, van der Velden U, et al. *Peptostreptococcus micros* smooth and rough genotypes in periodontitis and gingivitis. J Periodontol 2000;71:209–18.

[60] Kornman KS, Loesche WJ. The subgingival microbial flora during pregnancy. J Periodontal Res 1980;15:111–22.

[61] Dzink JL, Socransky SS, Haffajee AD. The predominant cultivable microbiota of active and inactive lesions of destructive periodontal diseases. J Clin Periodontol 1988;15:316–23.

[62] Haffajee AD, Socransky SS, Dzink JL, et al. Clinical, microbiological and immunological features of subjects with destructive periodontal diseases. J Clin Periodontol 1988;15:240–6.

[63] Dzink JL, Tanner AC, Haffajee AD, et al. Gram negative species associated with active destructive periodontal lesions. J Clin Periodontol 1985;12:648–59.

[64] Dzink JL, Gibbons RJ, Childs WC III, et al. The predominant cultivable microbiota of crevicular epithelial cells. Oral Microbiol Immunol 1989;4:1–5.

[65] Zambon JJ. *Actinobacillus actinomycetemcomitans* in adult periodontitis. J Periodontol 1994;65:892–3.

[66] Zambon JJ. *Actinobacillus actinomycetemcomitans* in human periodontal disease. J Clin Periodontol 1985;12:1–20.

[67] Haraszthy VI, Hariharan G, Tinoco EM, et al. Evidence for the role of highly leukotoxic *Actinobacillus actinomycetemcomitans* in the pathogenesis of localized juvenile and other forms of early-onset periodontitis. J Periodontol 2000;71:912–22.

[68] Gafan GP, Lucas VS, Roberts GJ, et al. Prevalence of periodontal pathogens in dental plaque of children. J Clin Microbiol 2004;42:4141–6.

[69] Kornman KS, Robertson PB. Clinical and microbiological evaluation of therapy for juvenile periodontitis. J Periodontol 1985;56:443–6.

[70] Michalowicz BS, Ronderos M, Camara-Silva R, et al. Human herpesviruses and *Porphyromonas gingivalis* are associated with juvenile periodontitis. J Periodontol 2000; 71:981–8.

[71] Kamma JJ, Nakou M, Gmur R, et al. Microbiological profile of early onset/aggressive periodontitis patients. Oral Microbiol Immunol 2004;19:314–21.

[72] Takeuchi Y, Umeda M, Ishizuka M, et al. Prevalence of periodontopathic bacteria in aggressive periodontitis patients in a Japanese population. J Periodontol 2003;74:1460–9.

[73] Lee JW, Choi BK, Yoo YJ, et al. Distribution of periodontal pathogens in Korean aggressive periodontitis. J Periodontol 2003;74:1329–35.

[74] Wyss C, Moter A, Choi BK, et al. *Treponema putidum* sp. nov., a medium-sized proteolytic spirochaete isolated from lesions of human periodontitis and acute necrotizing ulcerative gingivitis. Int J Syst Evol Microbiol 2004;54:1117–22.

[75] Newman MG, Sims TN. The predominant cultivable microbiota of the periodontal abscess. J Periodontol 1979;50:350–4.

[76] Herrera D, Roldan S, Gonzalez I, et al. The periodontal abscess (I). Clinical and microbiological findings. J Clin Periodontol 2000;27:387–94.

[77] Tatakis DN, Trombelli L. Modulation of clinical expression of plaque-induced gingivitis. I. Background review and rationale. J Clin Periodontol 2004;31:229–38.

[78] Trombelli L, Tatakis DN, Scapoli C, et al. Modulation of clinical expression of plaque-induced gingivitis. II. Identification of "high-responder" and "low-responder" subjects. J Clin Periodontol 2004;31:239–52.

[79] Wiedemann W, Lahrsow J, Naujoks R. Über den Einfluss der Parodontalen Resistenze auf die Experimentelle Gingivitis. [The effect of periodontal resistance on experimental gingivitis.] Dtsch Zahnarztl Z 1979;34:6–9 [in German].

[80] van der Weijden GA, Timmerman MF, Danser MM, et al. Effect of pre-experimental maintenance care duration on the development of gingivitis in a partial mouth experimental gingivitis model. J Periodontal Res 1994;29:168–73.

[81] Scapoli C, Tatakis DN, Mamolini E, et al. Modulation of clinical expression of plaque-induced gingivitis: interleukin-1 gene cluster polymorphisms. J Periodontol 2005;76:49–56.

[82] Hart TC, Kornman KS. Genetic factors in the pathogenesis of periodontitis. Periodontol 2000 1997;14:202–15.

[83] Michalowicz BS, Diehl SR, Gunsolley JC, et al. Evidence of a substantial genetic basis for risk of adult periodontitis. J Periodontol 2000;71:1699–707.

[84] McGuire MK, Nunn ME. Prognosis versus actual outcome. IV. The effectiveness of clinical parameters and IL-1 genotype in accurately predicting prognoses and tooth survival. J Periodontol 1999;70:49–56.

[85] Greenstein G, Hart TC. A critical assessment of interleukin-1 (IL-1) genotyping when used in a genetic susceptibility test for severe chronic periodontitis. J Periodontol 2002;73: 231–47.

[86] Li Y, Xu L, Hasturk H, et al. Localized aggressive periodontitis is linked to human chromosome 1q25. Hum Genet 2004;114:291–7.

[87] Amano A, Kishima T, Akiyama S, et al. Relationship of periodontopathic bacteria with early-onset periodontitis in Down's syndrome. J Periodontol 2001;72:368–73.

[88] Hart TC, Hart PS, Bowden DW, et al. Mutations of the cathepsin C gene are responsible for Papillon-Lefevre syndrome. J Med Genet 1999;36:881–7.

[89] Rylander H, Ericsson I. Manifestations and treatment of periodontal disease in a patient suffering from cyclic neutropenia. J Clin Periodontol 1981;8:77–87.

[90] Horwitz M, Benson KF, Person RE, et al. Mutations in ELA2, encoding neutrophil elastase, define a 21-day biological clock in cyclic haematopoiesis. Nat Genet 1999;23: 433–6.

[91] Saglam F, Atamer T, Onan U, et al. Infantile genetic agranulocytosis (Kostmann type). A case report. J Periodontol 1995;66:808–10.

[92] Dale DC, Person RE, Bolyard AA, et al. Mutations in the gene encoding neutrophil elastase in congenital and cyclic neutropenia. Blood 2000;96:2317–22.

[93] Gillig JL, Caldwell CH. The Chediak-Higashi syndrome: case report. ASDC J Dent Child 1970;37:527–9.

[94] Blume RS, Wolff SM. The Chédiak-Higashi syndrome: studies in four patients and a review of the literature. Medicine (Baltimore) 1972;51:247–80.

[95] Nagle DL, Karim MA, Woolf EA, et al. Identification and mutation analysis of the complete gene for Chédiak-Higashi syndrome. Nat Genet 1996;14:307–11.

[96] Haneke E. The Papillon-Lefèvre syndrome: keratosis palmoplantaris with periodontopathy. Report of a case and review of the cases in the literature. Hum Genet 1979;51:1–35.

[97] Toomes C, James J, Wood AJ, et al. Loss-of-function mutations in the cathepsin C gene result in periodontal disease and palmoplantar keratosis. Nat Genet 1999;23:421–4.

[98] Waldrop TC, Anderson DC, Hallmon WW, et al. Periodontal manifestations of the heritable Mac-1, LFA-1, deficiency syndrome. Clinical, histopathologic and molecular characteristics. J Periodontol 1987;58:400–16.

[99] Marlin SD, Morton CC, Anderson DC, et al. LFA-1 immunodeficiency disease. Definition of the genetic defect and chromosomal mapping of alpha and beta subunits of the lymphocyte function-associated antigen 1 (LFA-1) by complementation in hybrid cells. J Exp Med 1986;164:855–67.

[100] Alaluusua S, Kivitie-Kallio S, Wolf J, et al. Periodontal findings in Cohen syndrome with chronic neutropenia. J Periodontol 1997;68:473–8.

[101] Kolehmainen J, Black GC, Saarinen A, et al. Cohen syndrome is caused by mutations in a novel gene, COH1, encoding a transmembrane protein with a presumed role in vesicle-mediated sorting and intracellular protein transport. Am J Hum Genet 2003;72: 1359–69.

[102] Gonzalez YM, De Nardin A, Grossi SG, et al. Serum cotinine levels, smoking, and periodontal attachment loss. J Dent Res 1996;75:796–802.

[103] Schenkein HA, Gunsolley JC, Koertge TE, et al. Smoking and its effects on early-onset periodontitis. J Am Dent Assoc 1995;126:1107–13.

[104] Grossi SG, Zambon JJ, Ho AW, et al. Assessment of risk for periodontal disease. I. Risk indicators for attachment loss. J Periodontol 1994;65:260–7.

[105] Grossi SG, Zambon J, Machtei EE, et al. Effects of smoking and smoking cessation on healing after mechanical periodontal therapy. J Am Dent Assoc 1997;128:599–607.

[106] Johnson GK, Hill M. Cigarette smoking and the periodontal patient. J Periodontol 2004; 75:196–209.

[107] Tomar SL. Dentistry's role in tobacco control. J Am Dent Assoc 2001;132(Suppl):30S–5S.

[108] Engelgau MM, Geiss LS, Saaddine JB, et al. The evolving diabetes burden in the United States. Ann Intern Med 2004;140:945–50.

[109] Alberti G, Zimmet P, Shaw J, et al. Type 2 diabetes in the young: the evolving epidemic: the international diabetes federation consensus workshop. Diabetes Care 2004;27: 1798–811.

[110] Soskolne WA, Klinger A. The relationship between periodontal diseases and diabetes: an overview. Ann Periodontol 2001;6:91–8.

[111] Lalla E, Lamster IB, Feit M, et al. Blockade of RAGE suppresses periodontitis-associated bone loss in diabetic mice. J Clin Invest 2000;105:1117–24.

[112] Lalla E, Lamster IB, Stern DM, et al. Receptor for advanced glycation end products, inflammation, and accelerated periodontal disease in diabetes: mechanisms and insights into therapeutic modalities. Ann Periodontol 2001;6:113–8.

[113] Page RC, Schroeder HE. Pathogenesis of inflammatory periodontal disease. A summary of current work. Lab Invest 1976;34:235–49.

[114] Van Dyke TE, Levine MJ, Genco RJ. Neutrophil function and oral disease. J Oral Pathol 1985;14:95–120.

[115] Weiss SJ. Tissue destruction by neutrophils. N Engl J Med 1989;320:365–76.

[116] Altman LC, Baker C, Fleckman P, et al. Neutrophil-mediated damage to human gingival epithelial cells. J Periodontal Res 1992;27:70–9.

[117] Deguchi S, Hori T, Creamer H, et al. Neutrophil-mediated damage to human periodontal ligament-derived fibroblasts: role of lipopolysaccharide. J Periodontal Res 1990;25:293–9.

[118] Schroeder HE, Lindhe J. Conversion of stable established gingivitis in the dog into destructive periodontitis. Arch Oral Biol 1975;20:775–82.

[119] Gangbar S, Overall CM, McCulloch CA, et al. Identification of polymorphonuclear leukocyte collagenase and gelatinase activities in mouthrinse samples: correlation with periodontal disease activity in adult and juvenile periodontitis. J Periodontal Res 1990;25: 257–67.

[120] Zafiropoulos GG, Flores-de-Jacoby L, Todt G, et al. Gingival crevicular fluid elastase-inhibitor complex: correlation with clinical indices and subgingival flora. J Periodontal Res 1991;26:24–32.

[121] Caton JG, Ciancio SG, Blieden TM, et al. Treatment with subantimicrobial dose doxycycline improves the efficacy of scaling and root planing in patients with adult periodontitis. J Periodontol 2000;71:521–32.

[122] Reddy MS, Geurs NC, Gunsolley JC. Periodontal host modulation with antiproteinase, anti-inflammatory, and bone-sparing agents. A systematic review. Ann Periodontol 2003;8: 12–37.

[123] Gapski R, Barr JL, Sarment DP, et al. Effect of systemic matrix metalloproteinase inhibition on periodontal wound repair: a proof of concept trial. J Periodontol 2004;75: 441–52.

[124] Waddington RJ, Moseley R, Embery G. Reactive oxygen species: a potential role in the pathogenesis of periodontal diseases. Oral Dis 2000;6:138–51.

[125] Bartold PM, Wiebkin OW, Thonard JC. The effect of oxygen-derived free radicals on gingival proteoglycans and hyaluronic acid. J Periodontal Res 1984;19:390–400.

[126] Saari H, Suomalainen K, Lindy O, et al. Activation of latent human neutrophil collagenase by reactive oxygen species and serine proteases. Biochem Biophys Res Commun 1990;171: 979–87.

[127] Weiss SJ, Curnutte JT, Regiani S. Neutrophil-mediated solubilization of the subendothelial matrix: oxidative and nonoxidative mechanisms of proteolysis used by normal and chronic granulomatous disease phagocytes. J Immunol 1986;136:636–41.

[128] Kantarci A, Oyaizu K, Van Dyke TE. Neutrophil-mediated tissue injury in periodontal disease pathogenesis: findings from localized aggressive periodontitis. J Periodontol 2003; 74:66–75.

[129] Tyagi SR, Uhlinger DJ, Lambeth JD, et al. Altered diacylglycerol level and metabolism in neutrophils from patients with localized juvenile periodontitis. Infect Immun 1992;60: 2481–7.

[130] Shapira L, Borinski R, Sela MN, et al. Superoxide formation and chemiluminescence of peripheral polymorphonuclear leukocytes in rapidly progressive periodontitis patients. J Clin Periodontol 1991;18:44–8.

[131] Schlegel Gomez R, Langer P, Pelka M, et al. Variational expression of functionally different macrophage markers (27E10, 25F9, RM3/1) in normal gingiva and inflammatory periodontal disease. J Clin Periodontol 1995;22:341–6.

[132] Lappin DF, Koulouri O, Radvar M, et al. Relative proportions of mononuclear cell types in periodontal lesions analyzed by immunohistochemistry. J Clin Periodontol 1999; 26:183–9.

[133] Chapple CC, Srivastava M, Hunter N. Failure of macrophage activation in destructive periodontal disease. J Pathol 1998;186:281–6.

[134] Wynne SE, Walsh LJ, Seymour GJ, et al. In situ demonstration of natural killer (NK) cells in human gingival tissue. J Periodontol 1986;57:699–702.

[135] Cobb CM, Singla O, Feil PH, et al. Comparison of NK-cell (Leu-7+ and Leu-11b+) populations in clinically healthy gingiva, chronic gingivitis and chronic adult periodontitis. J Periodontal Res 1989;24:1–7.

[136] Lundgren T, Parhar RS, Renvert S, et al. Impaired cytotoxicity in Papillon-Lefèvre syndrome. J Dent Res 2005;84:414–7.

[137] Orange JS. Human natural killer cell deficiencies and susceptibility to infection. Microbes Infect 2002;4:1545–58.

[138] Zeidel A, Beilin B, Yardeni I, et al. Immune response in asymptomatic smokers. Acta Anaesthesiol Scand 2002;46:959–64.

[139] Stoufi ED, Taubman MA, Ebersole JL, et al. Phenotypic analyses of mononuclear cells recovered from healthy and diseased human periodontal tissues. J Clin Immunol 1987;7: 235–45.

[140] Cole KL, Seymour GJ, Powell RN. Phenotypic and functional analysis of T cells extracted from chronically inflamed human periodontal tissues. J Periodontol 1987;58:569–73.

[141] Teng YT, Nguyen H, Gao X, et al. Functional human T-cell immunity and osteoprotegerin ligand control alveolar bone destruction in periodontal infection. J Clin Invest 2000;106: R59–67.

[142] Taubman MA, Kawai T. Involvement of T-lymphocytes in periodontal disease and in direct and indirect induction of bone resorption. Crit Rev Oral Biol Med 2001;12:125–35.

[143] Kostenuik PJ, Shalhoub V. Osteoprotegerin: a physiological and pharmacological inhibitor of bone resorption. Curr Pharm Des 2001;7:613–35.

[144] Mogi M, Otogoto J, Ota N, et al. Differential expression of RANKL and osteoprotegerin in gingival crevicular fluid of patients with periodontitis. J Dent Res 2004;83:166–9.

[145] Kanzaki H, Chiba M, Shimizu Y, et al. Periodontal ligament cells under mechanical stress induce osteoclastogenesis by receptor activator of nuclear factor kappaB ligand up-regulation via prostaglandin E2 synthesis. J Bone Miner Res 2002;17:210–20.

[146] Wada N, Maeda H, Tanabe K, et al. Periodontal ligament cells secrete the factor that inhibits osteoclastic differentiation and function: the factor is osteoprotegerin/osteoclasto-genesis inhibitory factor. J Periodontal Res 2001;36:56–63.

[147] Seymour GJ, Powell RN, Davies WI. Conversion of a stable T-cell lesion to a progressive B-cell lesion in the pathogenesis of chronic inflammatory periodontal disease: an hypothesis. J Clin Periodontol 1979;6:267–77.

[148] Reinhardt RA, Bolton RW, McDonald TL, et al. In situ lymphocyte subpopulations from active versus stable periodontal sites. J Periodontol 1988;59:656–70.

[149] Tatakis DN. Interleukin-1 and bone metabolism: a review. J Periodontol 1993;64:416–31.

[150] Giannopoulou C, Cappuyns I, Mombelli A. Effect of smoking on gingival crevicular fluid cytokine profile during experimental gingivitis. J Clin Periodontol 2003;30:996–1002.

[151] Holmlund A, Hanstrom L, Lerner UH. Bone resorbing activity and cytokine levels in gingival crevicular fluid before and after treatment of periodontal disease. J Clin Periodontol 2004;31:475–82.

[152] Delima AJ, Karatzas S, Amar S, et al. Inflammation and tissue loss caused by periodontal pathogens is reduced by interleukin-1 antagonists. J Infect Dis 2002;186:511–6.

[153] Assuma R, Oates T, Cochran D, et al. IL-1 and TNF antagonists inhibit the inflammatory response and bone loss in experimental periodontitis. J Immunol 1998;160:403–9.

[154] Graves DT, Delima AJ, Assuma R, et al. Interleukin-1 and tumor necrosis factor antagonists inhibit the progression of inflammatory cell infiltration toward alveolar bone in experimental periodontitis. J Periodontol 1998;69:1419–25.

[155] Salvi GE, Collins JG, Yalda B, et al. Monocytic TNF alpha secretion patterns in IDDM patients with periodontal diseases. J Clin Periodontol 1997;24:8–16.

[156] Nishimura F, Iwamoto Y, Mineshiba J, et al. Periodontal disease and diabetes mellitus: the role of tumor necrosis factor-alpha in a 2-way relationship. J Periodontol 2003;74: 97–102.

[157] Heasman PA, Offenbacher S, Collins JG, et al. Flurbiprofen in the prevention and treatment of experimental gingivitis. J Clin Periodontol 1993;20:732–8.

[158] Williams RC, Jeffcoat MK, Howell TH, et al. Altering the progression of human alveolar bone loss with the non-steroidal anti-inflammatory drug flurbiprofen. J Periodontol 1989; 60:485–90.

[159] Al-Rasheed A, Scheerens H, Rennick DM, et al. Accelerated alveolar bone loss in mice lacking interleukin-10. J Dent Res 2003;82:632–5.

[160] Sasaki H, Okamatsu Y, Kawai T, et al. The interleukin-10 knockout mouse is highly susceptible to *Porphyromonas gingivalis*-induced alveolar bone loss. J Periodontal Res 2004;39:432–41.

[161] Suarez LJ, Ocampo AM, Duenas RE, et al. Relative proportions of T-cell subpopulations and cytokines that mediate and regulate the adaptive immune response in patients with aggressive periodontitis. J Periodontol 2004;75:1209–15.

[162] Goutoudi P, Diza E, Arvanitidou M. Effect of periodontal therapy on crevicular fluid interleukin-1beta and interleukin-10 levels in chronic periodontitis. J Dent 2004;32:511–20.

[163] Serhan CN, Jain A, Marleau S, et al. Reduced inflammation and tissue damage in transgenic rabbits overexpressing 15-lipoxygenase and endogenous anti-inflammatory lipid mediators. J Immunol 2003;171:6856–65.

[164] Van Dyke TE, Serhan CN. Resolution of inflammation: a new paradigm for the pathogenesis of periodontal diseases. J Dent Res 2003;82:82–90.

THE DENTAL
CLINICS
OF NORTH AMERICA

Dent Clin N Am 49 (2005) 517–532

Epidemiology and Risk Factors of Periodontal Diseases

Jasim M. Albandar, DDS, DMD, PhD[a,b,c,*]

[a]Department of Periodontology, Temple University School of Dentistry,
3223 North Broad Street, Philadelphia, PA 19140, USA
[b]Periodontal Diagnostics Research Laboratory, Temple University School of Dentistry,
3223 North Broad Street, Philadelphia, PA 19140, USA
[c]Temple University Graduate School, Room 3A07, 3223 North Broad Street,
Philadelphia, PA 19140, USA

Periodontal diseases and dental caries are the main chronic infectious diseases of the oral cavity and the principal causes of tooth loss in humans. Periodontal diseases include a group of chronic inflammatory diseases that affect the periodontal supporting tissues of teeth and encompass destructive and nondestructive diseases [1]. Gingivitis is inflammation of the soft tissue without apical migration of the junctional epithelium. It is a reversible, nondestructive disease that does not involve loss of periodontal tissues [2]. Periodontitis is inflammation of the periodontium that is accompanied by apical migration of the junctional epithelium, leading to destruction of the connective tissue attachment and alveolar bone loss [3,4].

Chronic periodontitis is the most common form of destructive periodontal diseases [3,5] and shows a slow disease progression characterized by bursts of disease activity separated by quiescent periods of varying durations [6–8]. Aggressive periodontitis encompasses aggressive, rapidly progressive forms of periodontitis [9], which often commence during adolescence and early adulthood, and hence classified as early-onset periodontitis [10–12]. Two other groups of destructive periodontal diseases exist, including periodontitis as a manifestation of systemic diseases [13] and necrotizing periodontal diseases [14].

Periodontal diseases share common etiologic factors and have several predisposing factors [15–17]. Most periodontal diseases are infectious in

---

* Department of Periodontology, Temple University School of Dentistry, 3223 North Broad Street, Philadelphia, PA 19140.
  E-mail address: jasim.albandar@temple.edu

0011-8532/05/$ - see front matter
doi:10.1016/j.cden.2005.03.003

nature, initiated as a consequence of dental plaque biofilm formation [18–20]. Another common feature of these diseases is that host factors play an important role in their development [21] and therefore show some similarities in their histopathogenesis. Nevertheless, various types of periodontal diseases also show distinctive differences in etiology and risk predisposition. As a result, host factors may play different roles in the development of various periodontal diseases. In addition, the occurrence, clinical features, and progression pattern of these diseases differ significantly.

Goals of epidemiologic studies of periodontal diseases

Epidemiology is the study of health and disease in populations and the effect of various biologic, demographic, environmental, and lifestyles on these states. Epidemiologic studies are conducted to describe the health status of populations, elucidate the etiology of diseases, identify risk factors, forecast disease occurrence, and assist in disease prevention and control. Epidemiologic research often involves the measurement of parameters of disease and health, the estimation of their occurrence in populations, and the use of population estimates to carry out statistical testing of hypotheses related to disease-associated variables. Population-based measurements may include the estimation of the percentage of the population that currently exhibit the disease (prevalence), the percentage of the population that may acquire the disease during a given time interval (incidence), and the probability of occurrence of the disease in the population during a given time interval in the future (risk).

Population studies of the distribution and risk factors of periodontal diseases offer a unique investigational model that provides power and generalization to observations made among more limited populations. By contributing to a better understanding of the causal relationships between risk factors and occurrence of disease, epidemiologic studies form the basis of the disciplines of "risk assessment" and "disease control." Information about the distribution of periodontal diseases in the population, current knowledge about the pathogenesis and methods of control of these diseases, and the population's perception of the disease constitute the foundation for determining periodontal treatment needs and making resource allocation decisions for disease control.

Diagnostic criteria and measurement methods

Gingivitis is identified clinically as inflammation of the gingiva causing one or more soft tissue changes including redness, edema, increase in thickness, ulceration, or bleeding. Several indices have been described for the measurement of gingivitis [2]. More recently, however, diagnostic criteria and indices that assess the presence, extent, or severity of gingival bleeding [22,23] have been used because they provide more objective methods of assessing the degree of gingival inflammation.

Studies have assessed periodontal health and the severity of periodontitis in populations using a wide range of approaches and methodologies. One common approach has been the assessment of periodontal soft or hard tissue loss, with or without assessment of the degree of inflammation. Probing pocket depth has often been used as a measure of local periodontal tissue inflammation and tissue loss, even though assessments of the status of epithelial attachment have often been overlooked, and the validity of periodontal disease estimates based on this measure may therefore be questioned. Hence, differences in disease parameters measured in different studies may partly explain the differences in study findings.

Indices are measurement instruments used in some studies to assess the periodontal health of populations. Simplifying the assessment method and the potential reduction in measurement errors are important advantages of using periodontal indices. Hence, indices may allow a more straightforward approach to gathering and interpreting data. Russell's Periodontal Index [24] and Ramfjord's Periodontal Disease Index [25] were commonly used in periodontal surveys from the 1950s to 1970s but have seldom been used thereafter because of major validity limitations [26,27]. The Community Periodontal Index of Treatment Needs [28] and its newer incarnation, the Community Periodontal Index [29], are widely used today; however, both indices have been criticized for their limited validity for the assessment of periodontal diseases [27,30].

More recently, the Periodontitis Index [26,31] was described to assess the prevalence and severity of periodontitis in the population. This index can use full-mouth data or partial measurements typically used in large national surveys. The Periodontitis Index classifies subjects as having mild, moderate, or advanced periodontitis or not having periodontitis. Because this index does not combine parameters of different diseases, it does not endure some of the validity limitations found in the other indices mentioned earlier. The index uses measurements of attachment loss and probing depth in the evaluation of the severity of disease. The probing depth is measured to indicate only the depth of the true pocket (ie, the probing depth apical to the cementoenamel junction). In the absence of periodontal inflammation and pocketing, the Periodontitis Index does not regard presence of attachment loss alone as a measure of periodontitis.

Because of lack of resources or the desire to simplify the examination process, many epidemiologic studies of periodontal diseases have used partial recording methods to assess the occurrence and severity of disease. Partial recording protocols, however, systematically underestimate periodontal disease prevalence, and the degree of underestimation is influenced by the type of protocol used [22,32].

Epidemiology of periodontal diseases

Gingivitis

Epidemiologic studies show that gingivitis is ubiquitous in populations of children and adults globally. It has been estimated that more than 82% of adolescents in the United States have overt gingivitis and signs of gingival bleeding [33]. Similar or higher prevalence of gingivitis has been reported in children and adolescents in other parts of the world [34–38]. A high prevalence of gingivitis is found also in adults. For instance, it has been estimated that more than half of United States adults have gingival bleeding [26,39,40]. Adjusting for the measurement bias due to the use of partial recording protocols in the United States national surveys (as described by Kingman and Albandar [22]), more than 75% of American adults have gingival bleeding and a high percentage have dental calculus, suggesting poor oral hygiene. Other populations show similar or even higher levels of gingival inflammation [38].

Gingivitis is a reversible condition, which except for indicating the level of oral hygiene in the population, has unclear significance as a predictor of future periodontal tissue loss [41,42]. Nonetheless, a high prevalence and extent of gingival bleeding in the population may be detrimental, which is supported by data showing that young subjects who have overt gingival inflammation may show a higher frequency of future periodontal attachment loss than subjects without inflammation [43].

Chronic periodontitis

Nonaggressive forms of periodontitis (chronic periodontitis) are common worldwide. They may occur in most age groups but are most prevalent among adults and seniors [44]. The estimates of chronic periodontitis in various populations vary significantly, in part because populations differ in their demographics and levels of exposure to various etiologic and risk factors of periodontitis. In addition, studies often have used inconsistent study design and many lack standardization of disease definition and measurement methods. Hence, it may be difficult to draw valid conclusions about the prevalence and severity of disease in different populations based on published reports.

Chronic periodontitis in children and adolescents shows a wide frequency range in various geographic regions and racial/ethnic groups [35,44–46]. Low disease frequencies among young Caucasians in Western Europe and North America and relatively high frequencies in Africa and Latin America have been reported. In the age group 11 to 25 years, it is estimated that the disease affects 1% to 3% in Western Europe, 2% to 5% in North America, 4% to 8% in South America, 5% to 8% in Asia, and 10% to 20% in Africa [35]. The estimates by racial/ethnic groups are 1% to 3% of Caucasians, 5% to 8% of Asians, 5% to 10% of Hispanics and Latin Americans, and 8% to 20% of Africans and African Americans.

Two recent surveys, the National Survey of Employed Adults and Seniors (EAS survey, 1985–1986) and the Third National Health and Nutrition Examination Survey (NHANES III, 1988–1994), have provided invaluable information about the epidemiology of periodontal and other oral diseases in the United States population. The EAS survey used a multistage sampling design using United States business establishments (adults, 18–64 years old) and senior centers (65 years and older) as sampling frames. This survey found that approximately 24% and 14% of employed adults and 68% and 52% of seniors had one or more teeth with ≥4 mm and ≥5 mm attachment loss, respectively; 14% and 4% of adults and 22% and 8% of seniors had teeth with ≥4 mm and ≥5 mm probing depth, respectively; and 84% and 89% of adults and seniors had dental calculus, respectively [26].

The NHANES III also used a multistage sampling design but was household based, targeting the civilian noninstitutionalized United States population. Among 30- to 90-year-olds, 33% and 20% had ≥4 mm and ≥5 mm attachment loss, respectively, and 23% and 9% had ≥4 mm and ≥5 mm probing depth, respectively [31]. In the age group 65 years and older, more than 80% and 40% had attachment loss of ≥3 mm and ≥5 mm, respectively, and about 60% and 10% had probing depth of ≥3 mm and ≥5 mm, respectively [26].

It is important to note that the EAS survey and the NHANES III used partial-mouth examinations whereby only the midbuccal and mesiobuccal tooth surfaces of one maxillary and one mandibular quadrants were examined. Kingman and Albandar [22] showed that this method significantly underestimates the prevalence of attachment loss and suggested a method to adjust for the bias in these estimates. Using this approach to adjust the disease estimates in the EAS survey and the NHANES III, it may be concluded that about 41% and 22% of employed adults aged 18 to 64 years and 100% and 83% of seniors aged 65 years and older had one or more teeth with ≥4 mm and ≥5 mm attachment loss, respectively (Table 1). Similarly, in the NHANES III, 56% and 32% of subjects 30 to 90 years old had corresponding attachment loss. The estimates in subjects aged 65 years and older were 100% and 60% had ≥3 mm and ≥5 mm attachment loss, respectively, 90% and 15% had ≥3 mm and ≥5 mm probing depth, respectively, and 75% and 22% had ≥3 mm and ≥5 mm gingival recession, respectively. Population studies in American seniors [47–49] have typically used partial recording protocols similar to the one used in recent United States national surveys. Adjusting for the measurement bias due to this design shows that United States seniors have a very high level of chronic periodontitis and tissue loss comparable to the rates reported in the EAS survey and the NHANES III.

Albandar et al [31] assessed the prevalence and severity of chronic periodontitis in the United States adult population. Estimates based on partial recordings showed that from 1988 to 1994, about 35% of United States dentate adults aged 30 years and older had periodontitis. These adults included 22%, 10%, and 3% with mild, moderate, and advanced

Table 1

Percentage of subjects by degree of attachment loss and probing depth assessed in two recent United States national surveys using a partial recording system (random half-mouth and two sites per tooth) and the estimated true prevalence rates using an inflation factor to adjust for measurement bias

Parameter	Partial recording system			Inflation factor	Full-mouth estimates		
	EAS 18–64 y	EAS 65+ y	NHANES 30–90 y		EAS 18–64 y	EAS 65+ y	NHANES 30–90 y
Attachment loss ≥4 mm	24.1	68.2	32.7	1.7	41.0	100.0	55.6
Attachment loss ≥5 mm	13.6	51.7	19.9	1.6	21.8	82.7	31.8
Probing depth ≥4 mm	14.3	22.2	23.1	1.4	20.0	31.1	32.3
Probing depth ≥5 mm	4.3	7.6	8.9	1.6	6.9	12.2	14.2
Mild periodontitis	—	—	21.8	1.4	—	—	30.5
Moderate periodontitis	—	—	9.5	1.4	—	—	13.3
Severe periodontitis	—	—	3.1	1.4	—	—	4.3

Data from Albandar JM. Periodontal diseases in North America. Periodontol 2000 2002; 29:31–69; and Albandar JM, Brunelle JA, Kingman A. Destructive periodontal disease in adults 30 years of age and older in the United States, 1988–1994. J Periodontol 1999;70(1):13–29.

periodontitis, respectively (see Table 1). Adjusting for the measurement error due to the partial recordings suggests that approximately 48% of United States adults had chronic periodontitis, including 31%, 13%, and 4% with mild, moderate, and advanced periodontitis, respectively.

In Europe, a high percentage of adults have moderate probing depth and mild to moderate periodontal attachment loss. It is estimated that between 13% and 54% of 35- to 44-year-olds have 3.5- to 5.5-mm probing depths [50]. These estimates, however, may be conservative because they were derived from poorly documented surveys. A large survey in the United Kingdom found that 42% of 35- to 44-year-olds and 70% of 55- to 64-year-olds had attachment loss >3.5 mm [51]. Generally, a higher prevalence of periodontal disease is reported in Western European compared with Eastern European populations.

Credible data from other regions of the world are scarce. Most studies in Central and South America used convenience samples, and the criteria and measures of periodontal disease were not clearly defined. It has been common to use the Community Periodontal Index of Treatment Needs for evaluating periodontal status, and measurement of periodontal attachment loss is seldom reported. Given these inaccuracies, the estimates of disease in this region are uncertain. It has been estimated that approximately 38% to 67% of the population in Central and South America have moderate or advanced chronic periodontitis, including 28% to 52% with moderate disease and 4% to 19% with severe disease [37]. A recent survey used a representative sample of the adult urban population in southern Brazil and showed that 79% and 52% of subjects aged 30 years and older had attachment loss of ≥5 and ≥7 mm, respectively, and poor oral hygiene and dental calculus were prevalent [52]. Periodontitis is widespread among the older age groups, with approximately 70% to 100% of adults aged 50 years and older having moderate or advanced chronic periodontitis [37,53].

Studies also show that African populations have poor oral hygiene, abundant calculus, and a high prevalence of moderate probing depth and attachment loss. Disease estimates in this continent, however, may not be accurate due to the scarcity of reliable studies. Among adults aged 30 years and older, the prevalence range of ≥4 mm attachment loss is 44% to 84% in Uganda, 79% to 98% in Tanzania, and 91% to 99% in Kenya [27].

The continent of Asia includes more than half of the world's population, with groups of diverse ethnicity and marked differences in wealth and other socioeconomic characteristics. Generally, studies report a very high prevalence of gingival bleeding and dental calculus and a low prevalence of healthy periodontal status irrespective of age cohort or the country's level of development [54]. Periodontal diseases are more prevalent in high-income countries compared with low-income countries, particularly in the younger age groups, whereas these differences are less pronounced in seniors.

Early-onset aggressive periodontitis

Aggressive periodontitis is a disease characterized by severe and rapid loss of periodontal attachment that affects the permanent dentition and may commence at or after the circumpubertal age [1,11]. This nomenclature has been recommended to replace earlier classifications, including early-onset, juvenile, and rapidly progressive periodontitis [10]. For the most part, epidemiologic studies of aggressive periodontitis have many of the same inherent weaknesses of disease definition and study design as studies of chronic periodontitis. Thus, issues such as disease misclassification and inconsistent exclusion criteria of cases make inferences exigent.

Aggressive periodontitis shows a wide range of occurrence frequencies in various geographic regions and demographic groups, and the variance seems particularly large between different racial/ethnic groups. Prevalence estimates in the age group 11 to 25 years are 0.1% to 0.5% in Western Europe, 0.4% to 0.8% in North America, 0.3% to 1.0% in South America, 0.4% to 1.0% in Asia, and 0.5% to 5.0% in Africa [35]. Estimates of disease occurrence by racial/ethnic groups are 0.1% to 0.2% of Caucasians, 0.4% to 1.0% of Asians, 0.5% to 1.0% of Hispanics and Latin Americans, and 1.0% to 3.0% of Africans and African Americans.

Gingival recession

Periodontitis is often followed by recession of the periodontal soft tissues, which results in exposure of the root surfaces of teeth. Gingival recession also may be related to factors other than inflammatory periodontal disease. These include physical trauma, anatomical factors, and other etiological factors. This clinical condition has several negative outcomes, including increased sensitivity of teeth, esthetic grievance, and susceptibility to root caries. It is important to delineate the prevalence, severity, and risk factors of this condition; however, only a few studies have investigated this.

Studies in United States adults show that 23% of 30- to 90-year-olds and 50% of 65- to 90-year-olds had ≥3 mm gingival recession and that 15% of 65- to 90-year-olds had ≥5 mm recession [39]. After adjusting for the bias due to partial recording, these rates correspond to approximately 35%, 75%, and 23%, respectively. High frequencies of gingival recession have also been reported in other populations [27,53]. In an urban South American population aged 14 years and older, 52% and 22% of the subjects had ≥3 mm and ≥5 mm recession, respectively, and about half of those 40 years and older had ≥5 mm recession [53]. These findings suggest that gingival recession is common in various populations.

Etiologic and risk factors of periodontal diseases

Chronic and aggressive periodontitis are multifactorial diseases [15,16,55]. Microorganisms and microbial products in dental plaque are the main etiologic factors responsible for the initiation of the inflammatory reaction leading to periodontal tissue loss [19,20]. Several other local and systemic factors, however, have been shown to play important modifying roles in enhancing the inflammatory or destructive effects of microorganisms.

The significance of different risk factors for the pathogenesis of disease and for the development of tissue loss may vary in different forms of periodontal diseases. Profound progress in risk assessment has been made in recent years, and studies suggest that certain factors possess true risk-modifying effects, whereas others are merely risk indicators or surrogates of other effects. Certain local factors can enhance dental plaque accumulation or influence the composition of the dental plaque biofilm and may thereby potentiate the harmful effects of plaque microorganisms [17,55–58]. In addition, the gingival inflammatory response to plaque accumulation seems to differ substantially among individuals [59].

Age, gender, and socioeconomic status

Epidemiologic studies show that the prevalence and severity of attachment loss increase with age [26,60–63]. It is unclear, however, whether this increase is attributed to an increased risk of destructive periodontitis in older individuals or due to the cumulative effect of time [26,60,64,65]. Several studies also show an association between gender and attachment loss in adults, with men having higher prevalence and severity of periodontal destruction than women [26,31,51,63,66]. Recent data suggest that this finding may be related to gender-dependent genetic predisposing factors [67] or other sociobehavioral factors. Socioeconomic status is an important risk indicator of periodontal disease, in that individuals with low socioeconomic status have a higher occurrence of attachment loss and probing depth than those with high socioeconomic status [68–72].

Race/ethnicity

The level of attachment loss is also influenced by race/ethnicity, although the exact role of this factor is not fully understood. Certain racial/ethnic groups, particularly subjects of African and Latin American background, have a higher risk of developing periodontal tissue loss than other groups. In the United States population, subjects of African or Mexican heritage have greater attachment loss than Caucasians [31]. The association of periodontal disease with race/ethnicity is significantly attenuated when certain effects such as cigarette smoking and income are accounted for [73]. This effect modification suggests that certain racial/ethnic characteristics are indicators of or confounded by certain other effects. For instance, African Americans generally have lower socioeconomic status than Caucasians. Hence, the increased risk of periodontitis in certain racial/ethnic groups may be partly attributed to socioeconomic, behavioral, and other disparities [74]. On the other hand, there is evidence that increased risk may also be partly related to biologic/genetic predisposition [75–78].

Specific microorganisms

Although there is sufficient evidence that accumulation and maturation of a plaque biofilm is necessary for the initiation and progression of periodontal diseases, studies show that bacterial species colonizing the gingival pocket play variable roles in the pathogenesis of these diseases and may therefore possess different levels of risk of periodontal tissue loss [79]. For instance, the microorganism *Actinobacillus actinomycetemcomitans* has often been identified in the subgingival sites in persons with severe attachment loss or rapid disease progression [80–82]. This bacterium was detected in about 50% of sites with new incidence of radiographic bone loss in young subjects followed over 8 years [83]. Furthermore, specific genetic variants of *A actinomycetemcomitans* possessing significantly enhanced leukotoxin production have been shown to significantly correlate with a higher prevalence of aggressive periodontitis mainly in individuals of African descent [76,78].

There is also evidence that *Porphyromonas gingivalis* is strongly associated with chronic periodontitis [80]. This bacterium is consistently detected in high levels in persons with severe attachment loss, deep probing depth, or with rapidly progressive disease [84,85]. Cross-sectional studies showed that presence of *P gingivalis* and *Tannerella forsythensis* (*Bacteroides forsythus*) in the subgingival flora was associated with significant increased risks for periodontal tissue loss. In one study, the odds ratios of the presence of the two respective species with clinical attachment loss and severe bone loss were 1.7 and 2.5 [86,87], whereas the reported risks were significantly higher in another study (odds ratios: 12.3 and 10.4, respectively) [88].

Active infections with human cytomegalovirus and other herpesviruses have been proposed as possible risk factors for destructive periodontal diseases, including chronic periodontitis, aggressive periodontitis, and necrotizing periodontal diseases [89]. One study found that presence of herpesviruses in subgingival sites was associated with subgingival colonization of these sites with periodontopathic bacteria and with a threefold to fivefold increased risk of severe chronic periodontitis [90].

Oral hygiene

Oral hygiene has been consistently associated with higher occurrence of periodontal diseases in various populations [26,64,73]. A study of the natural history of periodontal diseases showed that attachment loss in a Sri Lankan population was significantly associated with dental calculus [91]. In addition, there is evidence that sites with gingival inflammation show a higher progression of attachment loss than sites without gingival inflammation [43,92]. Comprehensive oral hygiene programs are effective in preventing or reducing the level of gingival inflammation in children and adults [93,94]. These programs, however, may not be viable in preventing aggressive periodontitis [95], and it may be difficult to achieve a satisfactory level of oral hygiene in the general population to prevent chronic periodontitis and periodontal tissue loss effectively [51,96].

Smoking

Smoking behaviors have consistently been associated with attachment loss in most studies [55,97]. Smokers have a significantly higher risk of developing chronic periodontal disease [70,73,86,98] and show a higher rate of periodontal destruction over time than nonsmokers [71,99]. There is a dose-effect relationship between cigarette smoking and the severity of periodontal disease such that heavy smokers and those with a longer history of smoking show more severe tissue loss than light smokers [98,100]. Generally, studies show that cigarette smoking is associated with a twofold to sevenfold increased risk of having attachment loss compared with nonsmokers, with a more pronounced risk in young smokers [86,87, 97,99,101,102]. The population risk due to cigarette smoking has been studied in large surveys and it is estimated that in the United States population, approximately 42% and 11% of periodontitis cases may be attributed to current and former cigarette smoking, respectively [98]. A recent survey in Brazilian adults estimated that 12% of periodontitis cases may be attributable to cigarette smoking [103]. Cigar and pipe smoking have been shown to have detrimental effects on periodontal health similar to those attributed to cigarette smoking [104,105].

Systemic diseases

Certain systemic diseases have been associated with an increased risk of attachment loss. The association between diabetes mellitus and periodontal diseases has been studied extensively, and the evidence suggests that diabetics have considerably higher risk of attachment loss than nondiabetics [55,106–108]. There is incomplete information about the relationship of periodontal tissue loss with other systemic diseases and conditions such as osteopenia and osteoporosis [109,110] and arthritis [56,111]. Certain systemic diseases such as AIDS [112] and Down syndrome [113] are significant risk factors for periodontal disease, and a high percentage of cases show moderate to advanced periodontitis.

Gene polymorphisms

Several gene polymorphisms have been investigated, some of which have been shown to be associated with an increased risk of periodontitis [114–117]. Various genetic risk factors, however, may explain only a part of the variance in the occurrence of periodontitis [118]. In addition, significant interactions seem to exist between genetic, environmental, and demographic factors [15,55]. For example, there are data suggesting a modifying effect of smoking and variability in the occurrence of certain genotypes in different racial/ethnic groups. Hence, more studies are needed to better understand the role of these and other factors in the increased susceptibility to destructive periodontal diseases.

Summary

Periodontal surveys enable the determination of the prevalence, extent, and severity of periodontal diseases in populations and can generally be conducted in a reasonable time frame at a relatively moderate cost. The main disadvantage of surveys is that they provide only a "snapshot in time" of the occurrence in the population of the disease and of various exposures (potential risk factors) associated with the disease. Therefore, surveys do not provide convincing proof of causal relationships. All inferences derived from these surveys must take into account the potential confounding effects from correlated, noncausal study variables, which can lead to spurious inferences. In addition, the lack of standardization of study design, definition of disease, and methods of disease detection and measurement may significantly limit the use of results of population studies of periodontal diseases. The significance of using clear definitions of diseases and properly described measurement parameters in epidemiologic studies cannot be overemphasized because this practice helps facilitate reproduction and validation of study findings by other independent investigators.

References

[1] Armitage GC. Development of a classification system for periodontal diseases and conditions. Ann Periodontol 1999;4(1):1–6.

[2] Ciancio SG. Current status of indices of gingivitis. J Clin Periodontol 1986;13(5):375–82.

[3] Flemmig TF. Periodontitis. Ann Periodontol 1999;4(1):32–8.

[4] Suzuki JB. Diagnosis and classification of the periodontal diseases. Dent Clin N Am 1988; 32(2):195–216.

[5] Lindhe J, Ranney R, Lamster I, et al. Consensus report: chronic periodontitis. Ann Periodontol 1999;4(1):38.

[6] Albandar JM. A 6-year study on the pattern of periodontal disease progression. J Clin Periodontol 1990;17(7 Pt 1):467–71.

[7] Albandar JM, Rise J, Gjermo P, et al. Radiographic quantification of alveolar bone level changes. A 2-year longitudinal study in man. J Clin Periodontol 1986;13(3):195–200.

[8] Socransky SS, Haffajee AD, Goodson JM, et al. New concepts of destructive periodontal disease. J Clin Periodontol 1984;11(1):21–32.

[9] Lang N, Bartold M, Cullinan M, et al. Consensus report: aggressive periodontitis. Ann Periodontol 1999;4(1):53.

[10] Albandar JM, Brown LJ, Löe H. Clinical features of early-onset periodontitis. J Am Dent Assoc 1997;128(10):1393–9.

[11] Albandar JM, Brown LJ, Genco RJ, et al. Clinical classification of periodontitis in adolescents and young adults. J Periodontol 1997;68(6):545–55.

[12] Tonetti MS, Mombelli A. Early-onset periodontitis. Ann Periodontol 1999;4(1):39–53.

[13] Lindhe J, Ranney R, Lamster I, et al. Consensus report: periodontitis as a manifestation of systemic diseases. Ann Periodontol 1999;4:64.

[14] Lang N, Soskolne WA, Greenstein G, et al. Consensus report: necrotizing periodontal diseases. Ann Periodontol 1999;4:78.

[15] Albandar JM, Rams TE. Risk factors for periodontitis in children and young persons. Periodontol 2000 2002;29:207–22.

[16] Nunn ME. Understanding the etiology of periodontitis: an overview of periodontal risk factors. Periodontol 2000 2003;32:11–23.

[17] Ezzo PJ, Cutler CW. Microorganisms as risk indicators for periodontal disease. Periodontol 2000 2003;32:24–35.

[18] Socransky SS, Haffajee AD. Dental biofilms: difficult therapeutic targets. Periodontol 2000 2002;28:12–55.

[19] Lindhe J, Hamp SE, Löe H. Plaque-induced periodontal disease in beagle dogs. J Periodontal Res 1975;10:243–55.

[20] Löe H, Theilade E, Jensen SB. Experimental gingivitis in man. J Periodontol 1965;36: 177–87.

[21] Kinane DF, Lappin DF. Clinical, pathological and immunological aspects of periodontal disease. Acta Odontol Scand 2001;59(3):154–60.

[22] Kingman A, Albandar JM. Methodological aspects of epidemiological studies of periodontal diseases. Periodontol 2000 2002;29:11–30.

[23] Newbrun E. Indices to measure gingival bleeding. J Periodontol 1996;67(6):555–61.

[24] Russell AL. A system of classification and scoring for prevalence surveys of periodontal disease. J Dent Res 1956;35:350–9.

[25] Ramfjord SP. Indices for prevalence and incidence of periodontal disease. J Periodontol 1959;30:51–9.

[26] Albandar JM. Periodontal diseases in North America. Periodontol 2000 2002;29:31–69.

[27] Baelum V, Scheutz F. Periodontal diseases in Africa. Periodontol 2000 2002;29:79–103.

[28] Ainamo J, Barmes D, Beagrie G, et al. Development of the World Health Organization (WHO) Community Periodontal Index of Treatment Needs (CPITN). Int Dent J 1982;32: 281–91.

[29] World Health Organization. Oral health surveys. Basic methods. Geneva (Switzerland): World Health Organization; 1997.

[30] Baelum V, Papapanou PN. CPITN and the epidemiology of periodontal disease. Community Dent Oral Epidemiol 1996;24(6):367–8.

[31] Albandar JM, Brunelle JA, Kingman A. Destructive periodontal disease in adults 30 years of age and older in the United States, 1988–1994. J Periodontol 1999;70(1):13–29.

[32] Susin C, Kingman A, Albandar JM. Effect of partial recording protocols on estimates of prevalence of periodontal disease. J Periodontol 2005;76:262–7.

[33] Albandar JM, Brown LJ, Brunelle JA, et al. Gingival state and dental calculus in early-onset periodontitis. J Periodontol 1996;67(10):953–9.

[34] Cunha ACP, Chambrone LA. Prevalência de gengivite em criancas. Revista Periodontia 1998;7:1–5.

[35] Albandar JM, Tinoco EM. Global epidemiology of periodontal diseases in children and young persons. Periodontol 2000 2002;29:153–76.

[36] Cunha ACP, Chambrone LA. [Prevalência de gengivite em criancas de um nivel social baixo.] Revista Periodontia 1998;7:6–10 [in Portugese].

[37] Gjermo P, Rosing CK, Susin C, et al. Periodontal diseases in Central and South America. Periodontol 2000 2002;29:70–8.

[38] Petersen PE, Kaka M. Oral health status of children and adults in the Republic of Niger, Africa. Int Dent J 1999;49(3):159–64.

[39] Albandar JM, Kingman A. Gingival recession, gingival bleeding, and dental calculus in adults 30 years of age and older in the United States, 1988–1994. J Periodontol 1999;70(1): 30–43.

[40] Oliver RC, Brown LJ, Löe H. Periodontal diseases in the United States population. J Periodontol 1998;69(2):269–78.

[41] Lang NP, Adler R, Joss A, et al. Absence of bleeding on probing. An indicator of periodontal stability. J Clin Periodontol 1990;17(10):714–21.

[42] Haffajee AD, Socransky SS, Goodson JM. Clinical parameters as predictors of destructive periodontal disease activity. J Clin Periodontol 1983;10(3):257–65.

[43] Albandar JM, Kingman A, Brown LJ, et al. Gingival inflammation and subgingival calculus as determinants of disease progression in early-onset periodontitis. J Clin Periodontol 1998;25(3):231–7.

[44] Albandar JM, Rams TE. Global epidemiology of periodontal diseases: an overview. Periodontol 2000 2002;29:7–10.

[45] Albandar JM. Prevalence of incipient radiographic periodontal lesions in relation to ethnic background and dental care provisions in young adults. J Clin Periodontol 1989;16(10): 625–9.

[46] Löe H, Brown LJ. Early onset periodontitis in the United States of America. J Periodontol 1991;62(10):608–16.

[47] Beck JD, Koch GG, Rozier RG, et al. Prevalence and risk indicators for periodontal attachment loss in a population of older community-dwelling blacks and whites. J Periodontol 1990;61(8):521–8.

[48] Douglass CW, Jette AM, Fox CH, et al. Oral health status of the elderly in New England. J Gerontol 1993;48(2):M39–46.

[49] Fox CH, Jette AM, McGuire SM, et al. Periodontal disease among New England elders. J Periodontol 1994;65(7):676–84.

[50] Sheiham A, Netuveli GS. Periodontal diseases in Europe. Periodontol 2000 2002;29: 104–21.

[51] Morris AJ, Steele J, White DA. The oral cleanliness and periodontal health of UK adults in 1998. Br Dent J 2001;191(4):186–92.

[52] Susin C, Dalla Vecchia CF, Oppermann RV, et al. Periodontal attachment loss in an urban population of Brazilian adults, and the effect of demographic, behavioral and environmental risk indicators. J Periodontol 2004;75(7):1033–41.

[53] Susin C, Haas AN, Oppermann RV, et al. Gingival recession: epidemiology and risk indicators in a representative urban Brazilian population. J Periodontol 2004;75(10): 1377–86.

[54] Corbet EF, Zee KY, Lo EC. Periodontal diseases in Asia and Oceania. Periodontol 2000 2002;29:122–52.

[55] Albandar JM. Global risk factors and risk indicators for periodontal diseases. Periodontol 2000 2002;29:177–206.

[56] Albandar JM. Some predictors of radiographic alveolar bone height reduction over 6 years. J Periodontal Res 1990;25(3):186–92.

[57] Albandar JM, Buischi YA, Axelsson P. Caries lesions and dental restorations as predisposing factors in the progression of periodontal diseases in adolescents. A 3-year longitudinal study. J Periodontol 1995;66(4):249–54.

[58] Kinane DF. Causation and pathogenesis of periodontal disease. Periodontol 2000 2001;25: 8–20.

[59] Tatakis DN, Trombelli L. Modulation of clinical expression of plaque-induced gingivitis. I. Background review and rationale. J Clin Periodontol 2004;31(4):229–38.

[60] Papapanou PN, Lindhe J, Sterrett JD, et al. Considerations on the contribution of ageing to loss of periodontal tissue support. J Clin Periodontol 1991;18(8):611–5.

[61] Yoneyama T, Okamoto H, Lindhe J, et al. Probing depth, attachment loss and gingival recession. Findings from a clinical examination in Ushiku, Japan. J Clin Periodontol 1988; 15(9):581–91.

[62] Burt BA. Periodontitis and aging: reviewing recent evidence. J Am Dent Assoc 1994;125(3): 273–9.

[63] Corbet EF, Wong MC, Lin HC. Periodontal conditions in adult Southern Chinese. J Dent Res 2001;80(5):1480–5.

[64] Abdellatif HM, Burt BA. An epidemiological investigation into the relative importance of age and oral hygiene status as determinants of periodontitis. J Dent Res 1987;66(1): 13–8.

[65] Ship JA, Beck JD. Ten-year longitudinal study of periodontal attachment loss in healthy adults. Oral Surg Oral Med Oral Pathol Oral Radiol Endod 1996;81(3):281–90.

[66] Grossi SG. Effect of estrogen supplementation on periodontal disease. Compend Contin Educ Dent Suppl 1998;22:S30–6.

[67] Reichert S, Stein J, Gautsch A, et al. Gender differences in HLA phenotype frequencies found in German patients with generalized aggressive periodontitis and chronic periodontitis. Oral Microbiol Immunol 2002;17(6):360–8.

[68] Borrell LN, Burt BA, Gillespie BW, et al. Periodontitis in the United States: beyond black and white. J Public Health Dent 2002;62(2):92–101.

[69] Drury TF, Garcia I, Adesanya M. Socioeconomic disparities in adult oral health in the United States. Ann N Y Acad Sci 1999;896:322–4.

[70] Dolan TA, Gilbert GH, Ringelberg ML, et al. Behavioral risk indicators of attachment loss in adult Floridians. J Clin Periodontol 1997;24(4):223–32.

[71] Elter JR, Beck JD, Slade GD, et al. Etiologic models for incident periodontal attachment loss in older adults. J Clin Periodontol 1999;26(2):113–23.

[72] Gamonal JA, Lopez NJ, Aranda W. Periodontal conditions and treatment needs, by CPITN, in the 35–44 and 65–74 year-old population in Santiago, Chile. Int Dent J 1998; 48(2):96–103.

[73] Hyman JJ, Reid BC. Epidemiologic risk factors for periodontal attachment loss among adults in the United States. J Clin Periodontol 2003;30(3):230–7.

[74] Poulton R, Caspi A, Milne BJ, et al. Association between children's experience of socioeconomic disadvantage and adult health: a life-course study. Lancet 2002;360(9346): 1640–5.

[75] Schenkein HA, Best AM, Gunsolley JC. Influence of race and periodontal clinical status on neutrophil chemotactic responses. J Periodontal Res 1991;26(3 Pt 2):272–5.

[76] Haubek D, Ennibi OK, Abdellaoui L, et al. Attachment loss in Moroccan early onset periodontitis patients and infection with the JP2-type of *Actinobacillus actinomycetemcomitans*. J Clin Periodontol 2002;29(7):657–60.

[77] Albandar JM, DeNardin AM, Adesanya MR, et al. Associations of serum concentrations of IgG, IgA, IgM and interleukin-1beta with early-onset periodontitis classification and race. J Clin Periodontol 2002;29(5):421–6.

[78] DiRienzo JM, Slots J, Sixou M, et al. Specific genetic variants of *Actinobacillus actinomycetemcomitans* correlate with disease and health in a regional population of families with localized juvenile periodontitis. Infect Immun 1994;62(8):3058–65.

[79] Wolff L, Dahlen G, Aeppli D. Bacteria as risk markers for periodontitis. J Periodontol 1994;65(Suppl 5):498–510.

[80] Slots J, Ting M. *Actinobacillus actinomycetemcomitans* and *Porphyromonas gingivalis* in human periodontal disease: occurrence and treatment. Periodontol 2000 1999;20: 82–121.

[81] Slots J. The predominant cultivable organisms in juvenile periodontitis. Scand J Dent Res 1976;84:1–10.

[82] Slots J. Bacterial specificity in adult periodontitis. A summary of recent work. J Clin Periodontol 1986;13(10):912–7.

[83] Aass AM, Rossow I, Preus HR, et al. Incidence of early periodontitis in a group of young individuals during 8 years: associations with selected potential predictors. J Periodontol 1994;65(9):814–9.

[84] Albandar JM, Olsen I, Gjermo P. Associations between six DNA probe-detected periodontal bacteria and alveolar bone loss and other clinical signs of periodontitis. Acta Odontol Scand 1990;48(6):415–23.

[85] Albandar JM, Brown LJ, Löe H. Putative periodontal pathogens in subgingival plaque of young adults with and without early-onset periodontitis. J Periodontol 1997;68(10): 973–81.

[86] Grossi SG, Zambon JJ, Ho AW, et al. Assessment of risk for periodontal disease. I. Risk indicators for attachment loss. J Periodontol 1994;65(3):260–7.

[87] Grossi SG, Genco RJ, Machtei EE, et al. Assessment of risk for periodontal disease. II. Risk indicators for alveolar bone loss. J Periodontol 1995;66(1):23–9.

[88] van Winkelhoff AJ. Loos BG, van der Reijden WA, et al. *Porphyromonas gingivalis*, *Bacteroides forsythus* and other putative periodontal pathogens in subjects with and without periodontal destruction. J Clin Periodontol 2002;29(11):1023–8.

[89] Kamma JJ, Slots J. Herpesviral-bacterial interactions in aggressive periodontitis. J Clin Periodontol 2003;30(5):420–6.

[90] Contreras A, Umeda M, Chen C, et al. Relationship between herpesviruses and adult periodontitis and periodontopathic bacteria. J Periodontol 1999;70(5):478–84.

[91] Neely AL, Holford TR, Loe H, et al. The natural history of periodontal disease in man. Risk factors for progression of attachment loss in individuals receiving no oral health care. J Periodontol 2001;72(8):1006–15.

[92] Schatzle M, Loe H, Burgin W, et al. Clinical course of chronic periodontitis. I. Role of gingivitis. J Clin Periodontol 2003;30(10):887–901.

[93] Albandar JM, Buischi YA, Mayer MP, et al. Long-term effect of two preventive programs on the incidence of plaque and gingivitis in adolescents. J Periodontol 1994; 65(6):605–10.

[94] Axelsson P, Lindhe J, Nystrom B. On the prevention of caries and periodontal disease. Results of a 15-year longitudinal study in adults. J Clin Periodontol 1991;18(3):182–9.

[95] Albandar JM, Buischi YA, Oliveira LB, et al. Lack of effect of oral hygiene training on periodontal disease progression over 3 years in adolescents. J Periodontol 1995;66(4): 255–60.

[96] Löe H. Oral hygiene in the prevention of caries and periodontal disease. Int Dent J 2000; 50(3):129–39.

[97] Gelskey SC. Cigarette smoking and periodontitis: methodology to assess the strength of evidence in support of a causal association. Community Dent Oral Epidemiol 1999;27(1): 16–24.

[98] Tomar SL, Asma S. Smoking-attributable periodontitis in the United States: findings from NHANES III. National Health and Nutrition Examination Survey. J Periodontol 2000; 71(5):743–51.

[99] Bergstrom J, Eliasson S, Dock J. A 10-year prospective study of tobacco smoking and periodontal health. J Periodontol 2000;71(8):1338–47.

[100] Jette AM, Feldman HA, Tennstedt SL. Tobacco use: a modifiable risk factor for dental disease among the elderly. Am J Public Health 1993;83(9):1271–6.

[101] Bergstrom J. Tobacco smoking and risk for periodontal disease. J Clin Periodontol 2003; 30(2):107–13.

[102] Linden GJ, Mullally BH. Cigarette smoking and periodontal destruction in young adults. J Periodontol 1994;65(7):718–23.

[103] Susin C, Oppermann RV, Haugejorden O, et al. Periodontal attachment loss attributable to cigarette smoking in an urban Brazilian population. J Clin Periodontol 2004;31:951–9.

[104] Krall EA, Garvey AJ, Garcia RI. Alveolar bone loss and tooth loss in male cigar and pipe smokers. J Am Dent Assoc 1999;130(1):57–64.

[105] Albandar JM, Streckfus CF, Adesanya MR, et al. Cigar, pipe, and cigarette smoking as risk factors for periodontal disease and tooth loss. J Periodontol 2000;71(12):1874–81.

[106] Lalla E, Lamster IB, Feit M, et al. Blockade of RAGE suppresses periodontitis-associated bone loss in diabetic mice. J Clin Invest 2000;105(8):1117–24.

[107] Taylor GW. Periodontal treatment and its effects on glycemic control: a review of the evidence. Oral Surg Oral Med Oral Pathol Oral Radiol Endod 1999;87(3):311–6.

[108] Thomson WM, Slade GD, Beck JD, et al. Incidence of periodontal attachment loss over 5 years among older South Australians. J Clin Periodontol 2004;31(2):119–25.

[109] Payne JB, Reinhardt RA, Nummikoski PV, et al. Longitudinal alveolar bone loss in postmenopausal osteoporotic/osteopenic women. Osteoporos Int 1999;10(1):34–40.

[110] Reinhardt RA, Payne JB, Maze CA, et al. Influence of estrogen and osteopenia/ osteoporosis on clinical periodontitis in postmenopausal women. J Periodontol 1999;70(8): 823–8.

[111] Miranda LA, Fischer RG, Sztajnbok FR, et al. Periodontal conditions in patients with juvenile idiopathic arthritis. J Clin Periodontol 2003;30(11):969–74.

[112] Alpagot T, Duzgunes N, Wolff LF, et al. Risk factors for periodontitis in HIV patients. J Periodontal Res 2004;39(3):149–57.

[113] Agholme MB, Dahllof G, Modeer T. Changes of periodontal status in patients with Down syndrome during a 7-year period. Eur J Oral Sci 1999;107(2):82–8.

[114] Cullinan MP, Westerman B, Hamlet SM, et al. A longitudinal study of interleukin-1 gene polymorphisms and periodontal disease in a general adult population. J Clin Periodontol 2001;28(12):1137–44.

[115] Michalowicz BS, Diehl SR, Gunsolley JC, et al. Evidence of a substantial genetic basis for risk of adult periodontitis. J Periodontol 2000;71(11):1699–707.

[116] Li Y, Xu L, Hasturk H, et al. Localized aggressive periodontitis is linked to human chromosome 1q25. Hum Genet 2004;114(3):291–7.

[117] Noack B, Gorgens H, Hoffmann T, et al. Novel mutations in the cathepsin C gene in patients with pre-pubertal aggressive periodontitis and Papillon-Lefevre syndrome. J Dent Res 2004;83(5):368–70.

[118] Diehl SR, Wang Y, Brooks CN, et al. Linkage disequilibrium of interleukin-1 genetic polymorphisms with early-onset periodontitis. J Periodontol 1999;70(4):418–30.

ELSEVIER
SAUNDERS

THE DENTAL
CLINICS
OF NORTH AMERICA

Dent Clin N Am 49 (2005) 533–550

Systemic Effects of Periodontal Diseases

Frank A. Scannapieco, DMD, PhD

*Department of Oral Biology, School of Dental Medicine, University at Buffalo,
State University of New York, 109 Foster Hall, Buffalo, NY 14214, USA*

The possibility that a localized oral condition such as periodontal disease (PD) may have systemic effects seems to be of interest to the average person. The notion that a condition that is often ignored (or dealt with only when causing pain) may have long-term systemic consequences gets people's attention. To some constituencies of the dental profession, this attention is a good thing; perhaps some of those who have ignored their oral health will now pay attention to their mouth and seek regular dental care. This notion has considerable public health significance because if it is true, then treatment of periodontal inflammation would contribute to reduction in the risk of many prevalent, often fatal chronic diseases.

To what extent are the putative associations between PD and systemic conditions such as atherosclerosis, myocardial infarction, stroke, pneumonia, diabetes mellitus, and adverse pregnancy outcomes based on proven fact? To what extent can these potential associations be explained by a plausible pathogenic mechanism? Will provision of periodontal therapy reduce the risk of these systemic diseases? The goal of this article is to briefly review the history of this concept, describe the biologically plausible circumstances that may underlie these potential associations, and provide a summary of the published literature that supports or refutes them.

History of the focal infection hypothesis

The concept that oral infection may contribute to various systemic diseases is not new. Indeed, the possibility that a localized, or focal, infection such as PD could have systemic effects was a popular idea at the turn of the twentieth century [1,2]. A focal infection is a chronic, localized infection that can disseminate microorganisms or toxic microbial products to contiguous or

---

E-mail address: fas1@buffalo.edu

distant tissues. In addition to the teeth and jaws, other common sites of focal infection were considered to be tonsils, sinuses, fingers and toes, bronchi, the gastrointestinal tract including appendicitis and ulcers, the urinary tract, and lymph nodes. It was thought that many focal infections led to indolent systemic diseases such as arthritis, nephritis, conjunctivitis and iritis, otitis media, endocarditis, and anemia. As a result of this theory, many physicians of the era often recommended preventive full-mouth extractions in subjects suspected of having a focal infection causing systemic diseases.

Over time, a variety of arguments developed against the focal infection theory. In many patients, extraction of the teeth did not reverse the course of the systemic disease. Most of these early ideas were based on anecdotal evidence, not on evidence obtained from carefully designed epidemiologic studies or controlled trials (to be fair, such studies were rarely if ever performed in those days). Thus, by the 1950s, the focal infection hypothesis fell from favor.

In recent years, evidence has come forth supporting the notion that localized infectious diseases such as PD may indeed influence a number of systemic diseases (Fig. 1). This view holds that bacteria from dental plaque enter the blood stream through discontinuities of the oral tissues (ulcerated sulcular epithelium; infected root canals) and travel through the blood to cause infection at a distant site. It may also be possible that PD bacteria

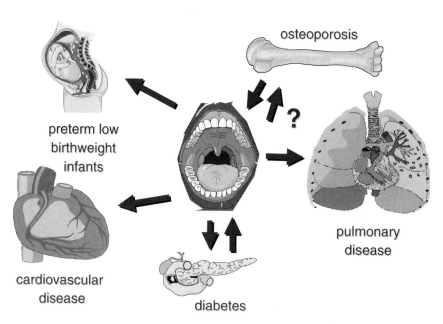

Fig. 1. Recent evidence suggests the possibility that poor oral health, particularly PD, may influence the initiation or the progression of several important and prevalent systemic diseases and conditions.

stimulate the release of pro-inflammatory cytokines or acute-phase proteins at a distant site (eg, liver, pancreas, skeleton, arteries). These products may initiate or intensify a disease process (eg, atherosclerosis, diabetes). Bacteria may also travel from oral sites to other mucosal surfaces (lung, gut) to cause inflammation and infection (pneumonia, gastric ulcers). This article reviews recent studies that address the association of oral infection with systemic conditions such as atherosclerosis, pulmonary disease, and pregnancy complications.

Association of periodontal disease with atherosclerosis, cardiovascular disease, and stroke

Most cases of coronary heart disease and cerebrovascular disease (stroke) result from atherosclerosis, an aberrant biologic process that causes narrowing of arteries due to deposition of cholesterol and cholesterol esters on the surface of blood vessel walls. The cholesterol-rich plaques also contain cells, including fibroblasts and immune cells [3]. Not all individuals suffer atherosclerosis equally; some individuals have higher risk for this disease process than others. Well-recognized risk factors for atherosclerosis include chronically elevated blood levels of cholesterol and triglyceride, hypertension, diabetes mellitus, and cigarette smoking.

Cholesterol, a lipid necessary for normal cell function, is synthesized in the liver and absorbed through the gut from dietary sources and transported in the blood bound to low-density lipoproteins. These low-density lipoproteins bind to specific transmembrane receptor proteins for transport into the cell through receptor-mediated endocytosis. Cholesterol uptake is reduced in some people and excess cholesterol accumulates in the blood to eventually form atherosclerotic plaques. If these plaques occlude blood flow in brain arteries, the result can be stroke; if they occur in coronary arteries, it can lead to myocardial infarction.

A recent and growing literature implicates chronic inflammation, infection, and possibly autoimmunity in the pathogenesis of atherosclerosis [4]. Arterial inflammation may be locally increased by lipid imbalances, hemodynamic stress, and immune reactions directed against the vascular wall, eventually leading to the formation of complicated atherosclerotic lesions [5]. This inflammation-mediated damage may initiate or contribute to the progression of the atherosclerotic plaque. A number of infectious agents appear to be associated with atherosclerosis, and alterations in the immune response may compromise clearance of such agents from these plaques. One of the best studied of these association's involves *Chlamydia pneumoniae,* an intracellular bacterium that commonly causes pneumonia and milder respiratory tract infections. *C pneumoniae* DNA and proteins have been detected in arteries of patients with giant cell arteritis [6] and in endarterectomy samples [7]. Elevated levels of antibody against *C pneumoniae* are found in patients with coronary heart disease compared with controls [8].

Other chronic infections such as PD have also been implicated as inciting agents for cardiovascular inflammation and disease. The first article of the recent era to report a relationship between PD and cardiovascular disease was a case-control study published by Simonka et al [9] in 1988. These researchers age matched 211 men with previous heart attack to 336 patients without heart attack. They found significantly more evidence of PD and need for periodontal surgery in patients over 50 years old with heart attack compared with those without heart attack. Since then, several additional case-control studies on this subject have been published [10–13]. Of these, all except one [12] reported a positive association between indicators of poor dental health and outcomes of atherosclerosis (cerebrovascular disease). The one study reporting the absence of a positive association was of very elderly subjects. It is possible that the cumulative effects of various disease processes that contribute to atherosclerosis in the elderly could have obscured the effect of oral disease on these processes. Another recent study determined whether a combination of clinical variables in a functional risk diagram enhanced the ability to differentiate between subjects with or without an immediate history of acute myocardial infarction [14]. Eighty-eight subjects with recent acute myocardial infarction and 80 matched control subjects with no history of acute myocardial infarction were compared. It was found that alveolar bone loss ≥ 4.0 mm was significantly greater in subjects with acute myocardial infarction. Taken together, these studies support a positive association between PD and the prevalence of cardiovascular events.

Stimulated by the early case-control studies, a number of cross-sectional studies provided further evidence in support of the association between PD with cerebrovascular disease, after controlling for other cardiovascular risk factors, particularly smoking [15–23]. As an example, Table 1 demonstrates the moderate risk for a history of heart attack in subjects with periodontal attachment loss [20]. In addition, several other studies have shown a positive association between PD and stroke [18,24–26], and one study associated PD with peripheral vascular disease, another sequela of atherosclerosis [27].

It has been suggested that the association observed between atherosclerosis-induced disease and PD may be the result of etiologic factors common

Table 1
Risk of heart attack in subjects with various levels of periodontal attachment loss

Sites with periodontal attachment loss ≥ 3 mm (%)	Odds ratio (95% confidence interval) for yes versus no: "Has your doctor ever told you that you had a heart attack?"
0	1.00 (reference)
>0–33	1.38 (0.75–2.254)
>33–67	2.28 (1.18–4.39)
>67–100	3.77 (1.46–9.74)

Data from Arbes SJ Jr, Slade GD, Beck JD. Association between extent of periodontal attachment loss and self-reported history of heart attack: an analysis of NHANES III data. J Dent Res 1999;78(12):1779.

to both disease processes, such as lifestyle practices like cigarette smoking, and therefore coincidental [28–31]. Determining the role of lifestyle factors independent from the effect of PD on atherosclerosis requires the conduct of large prospective longitudinal epidemiologic studies of never smokers in addition to large randomized controlled clinical trials to determine whether periodontal intervention prevents the initiation or progression of athero-sclerosis-induced diseases.

Because of the great heterogeneity in methodologies used between studies in assessment of oral disease, it is difficult to directly compare the results of one study to others. Nevertheless, the available data suggest that PD is modestly associated with atherosclerosis-induced diseases such as cardio-vascular disease, stroke, and peripheral vascular disease.

Association of periodontal disease with pneumonia

Pneumonia is defined as an inflammation of the lungs caused by fungal, viral, parasitic, or bacterial infection. Bacterial pneumonia, the most common and treatable form of the disease, is initiated following colonization of the oral cavity and pharyngeal mucosa by potential respiratory pathogens, aspiration of the colonized pathogens into the lower airway, and failure of defense mechanisms to eliminate the bacteria from the airway mucosa [32]. Aspiration of oral secretions, a somewhat frequent event even in normal, healthy in-dividuals who may aspirate small quantities of secretions during sleep, is more frequent in patients with altered consciousness [33]. Other conditions predisposing to aberrant aspiration include stroke, Parkinson's disease, alcohol abuse, and sedative use [34]. Multiple defense mechanisms operate within the healthy respiratory tract to eliminate aspirated material from the lower airway, but their effectiveness can be impaired by a variety of conditions such as malnutrition, smoking, chronic obstructive pulmonary disease (COPD), diabetes, corticosteroid use, and endotracheal or nasogastric intubation.

Bacterial pneumonia can be classified as either community-acquired pneumonia or hospital-acquired (nosocomial) pneumonia. Up to 5.6 million cases of community-acquired pneumonia occur annually in the United States [35] and the overall mortality rate is <5%. Among the community-acquired pneumonia cases that require hospitalization, the mortality rate can be as high as 40% in those admitted to ICUs. Community-acquired pneumonia is typically caused by aspiration of bacteria that normally reside in the oropharynx, such as *Streptococcus pneumoniae, Haemophilus influenzae*, and *Mycoplasma pneumoniae*.

Nosocomial pneumonia occurs in institutionalized subjects such as hospitalized patients admitted to ICUs and nursing home patients. Nosocomial pneumonia accounts for 10% to 15% of all hospital-acquired infections, with a mortality rate as high as 25%. In contrast to community-acquired pneumonia, a different set of bacteria causes nosocomial pneumonia, including species such as *Staphylococcus aureus* and gram-negative bacteria such as *Pseudomonas aeruginosa* and the enteric species *Klebsiella pneumoniae, Escherichia coli,* and *Enterobacter* spp.

Several studies have demonstrated that the oral cavity may serve as a reservoir for respiratory pathogen colonization and infection. One of the first studies to document this finding [36] compared oral hygiene and the rate of dental plaque or buccal mucosal colonization by potential respiratory pathogens in ICU subjects with age- and gender-matched outpatients at their initial visit to a dental school clinic. The ICU patients demonstrated significantly more plaque than the control subjects. Colonization of dental plaque or oral mucosa by potential respiratory pathogens was found in 65% of the ICU patients but in only 16% of the preventive dentistry clinic patients. The potential respiratory pathogens identified in the ICU patients included *Staphylococcus aureus, Pseudomonas aeruginosa,* and a number of different enteric gram-negative bacteria. Several patients had oropharyngeal colonization by two or more potential pathogens. Oral colonization by respiratory pathogens was associated with antibiotic usage.

This observation was also noted in a subsequent study [37] in which an association was noted between poor oral health status (including dental caries, dental plaque, and colonization of dental plaque by respiratory pathogens) and onset on pneumonia in 57 ICU patients. The relative risk for pneumonia was increased 9.6-fold when the dental plaque was colonized by a pathogen between days 0 and 5 following ICU admission. Furthermore, the pathogen causing pneumonia was noted to first colonize the dental plaque.

Recent studies have also assessed the relationship between oral health, respiratory pathogen oral colonization, and pneumonia in nursing home populations. For example, 134 geriatric patients (34 inpatients, 53 long-term care patients, and 47 outpatients) were assessed for oral conditions such as xerostomia, caries, PD, and salivary IgA levels [38]. These subjects were also assessed for a diagnosis of aspiration pneumonia based on body temperature $>2\,^\circ$C above baseline, clinical deterioration, elevated white blood cell count, and infiltrates on chest radiograph. They noted that 27% of dentate inpatients and 19% of dentate long-term care patients developed aspiration pneumonia, whereas only 5% edentulous patients developed pneumonia, suggesting that teeth may serve as a reservoir of respiratory pathogen colonization in these subjects. A study of the relationship of oral health status and lung infection in 302 nursing home residents was reported by Mojon et al [39] who found an increased risk of respiratory tract infection in subjects with teeth in comparison to edentulous subjects. Another study [40] of 189 elderly male outpatients, hospital inpatients, and nursing-home patients over 60 years of age found significant associations between pneumonia and the number of decayed teeth, the frequency of brushing teeth, and being dependent for oral care. A subsequent study found the dental plaque of 12 of 28 (43%) elderly patients recently admitted to a hospital were colonized by gram-negative bacillary pathogens, suggesting the possibility that dental plaque may serve as a reservoir for lung infections [41]. When 28 chronic-care nursing home residents were compared with 30 dental clinic outpatients over 65 years of age, matched for gender and race, it was found that the dental plaque scores were significantly higher in the nursing home residents than in the outpatient controls (Fig. 2). In addition, 14.3% of chronic-care subjects showed dental plaque colonization with respiratory pathogens compared with 0% of the control dental outpatients [42].

Finally, 358 veterans aged 55 years and older were found to have an elevated risk of aspiration pneumonia if they had teeth and (1) if their teeth were carious, (2) when the periodontopathogen *Porphyromonas gingivalis* was detected in dental plaque, and (3) when the respiratory pathogen *Staphylococcus aureus* was detected in saliva [43].

Oral intervention trials to prevent pneumonia

The findings reviewed in the previous section suggest that the oral cavity may serve as a reservoir for lower airway infection, especially in in-stitutionalized subjects. This observation further suggests that improved oral hygiene could reduce or eliminate respiratory pathogens from the mouth

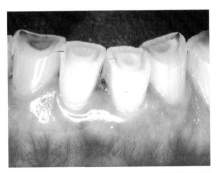

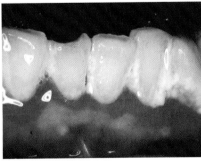

Fig. 2. (*Upper panel*) Example of oral hygiene status of elderly subject presenting for the first time to a dental school clinic. (*Lower panel*) Example of oral hygiene status of elderly nursing home resident. Subjects enrolled in the study are described in Russell et al [42]. (Courtesy of S. Russell, DDS, MPH, New York, NY.)

and thus prevent the onset of serious respiratory infection in vulnerable subjects. Although oral hygiene measures are a component of nursing care, implementation of such measures is difficult in some patients such as those who are orally intubated. Several intervention studies show, however, that improved oral hygiene measures can reduce the incidence of ventilator-associated pneumonia (VAP).

Several approaches have been taken to reduce the numbers of bacterial pathogens in the oral cavity of subjects with high risk of pneumonia. One approach uses topical nonabsorbable antibiotics (eg, 150 mg polymyxin B sulfate, 1 g neomycin sulfate, 1 g vancomycin hydrochloride in 60 mL of 5% dextrose) [44]. The 25 ICU test patients had the antibiotic mixture applied to the retropharynx every 24 hours and then swallowed. These patients were compared with 27 in a placebo group who received topical 5% dextrose. Application of the antibiotic paste reduced tracheobronchial colonization by gram-negative respiratory pathogens and *Staphylococcus aureus* and reduced the rate of pneumonia fivefold compared with the control treatment.

The effectiveness of oral topical chlorhexidine gluconate to reduce pneumonia was examined in mechanically ventilated patients following cardiac surgery [45]. Patients were randomly assigned to two groups: one group received 0.12% chlorhexidine gluconate (treatment) applied twice daily to buccal, pharyngeal, gingival, tongue, and tooth surfaces. The second group received the vehicle alone (placebo) applied in a similar fashion. Patients in both groups also received standard oral care according to the ICU's protocol. The topical chlorhexidine gluconate treatment reduced the incidence of total respiratory tract infections by 69% ($P < 0.05$) compared with placebo (Table 2). This intervention also significantly reduced total mortality (1.16% versus 5.56%) and the need for systemic antibiotics.

In another study, a test group of 30 patients received 0.2% chlorhexidine gel three times a day [46], whereas a similar-sized control group received an oral rinse with bicarbonate isotonic serum and oropharyngeal aspiration four times a day. The results showed that oral antiseptic decontamination

Table 2
Reduction of nosocomial respiratory infection by the use of oral 0.12% chlorhexidine gluconate

	Experimental group	Placebo control group
No. of patients	173	180
No. of respiratory infections	5	17*
No. of cases in which gram-negative bacteria was cause of pneumonia	8	20

*$P < 0.05$.

Data from DeRiso AJ II, Ladowski JS, Dillon TA, et al. Chlorhexidine gluconate 0.12% oral rinse reduces the incidence of total nosocomial respiratory infection and nonprophylactic systemic antibiotic use in patients undergoing heart surgery. Chest 1996;109(6):1558.

with 0.2% chlorhexidine gel significantly reduced the incidence of nos-ocomial pneumonia.

A subsequent prospective study [47] provides additional evidence that oral topical antimicrobial agents reduce the risk of pneumonia. Three groups of patients admitted to three ICUs over a 2-year period were enrolled in this study. The test group of 87 patients received a 2% gentamycin/colostin/vancomycin paste every 6 hours. A placebo group of 78 patients received Orabase without antibiotics. A control group of 61 patients received no treatment. The topical antibiotic treatment prevented acquired oropharyngeal colonization (10% versus 59% in the placebo group and 63% in the control group, $P < 0.0001$ and $P < 0.00001$, respectively) and the incidence of VAP (10% versus 31% in the placebo group and 23% in the control group, $P = 0.001$ and $P = 0.04$, respectively).

There have also been several preliminary trials testing oral hygiene interventions to reduce the incidence of pneumonia in nursing home subjects [48,49]. For example, 366 elderly residents from 11 nursing homes were studied; a test group of 184 subjects received supervised toothbrushing after each meal, and topical povidone iodine 1% once a day; the control group of 182 subjects received no intervention. A 2-year follow-up found that the relative risk of pneumonia in the group with no active oral care was 67% greater compared with the oral care group ($P = 0.04$).

Association of periodontal disease with chronic obstructive pulmonary disease

Poor oral hygiene and PD also may be associated with other respiratory diseases such as COPD, a very prevalent chronic disease [35]. COPD is defined as a spectrum of conditions characterized by chronic obstruction to airflow due to emphysema and/or chronic bronchitis. Although no study has established that PD influences the pathophysiology of COPD, several studies have demonstrated a statistical association between the two con-ditions. For example, an analysis of 23,808 community-dwelling individuals enrolled in the First National Health and Nutrition Examination Survey data [50] found 365 individuals reporting a respiratory condition confirmed by a study physician. These subjects were categorized as having a confirmed chronic respiratory disease (chronic bronchitis or emphysema), acute respiratory disease (influenza, pneumonia, acute bronchitis), or not having a respiratory disease. Logistic regression analysis revealed that poor oral hygiene and smoking status were statistically associated with chronic respiratory disease. Additional data in support of this concept found that PD (measured as alveolar bone loss assessed from periapical radiographs) was an independent risk factor for COPD in adult men enrolled in the VA Normative Aging study [51].

To verify these results, a cross-sectional, retrospective analysis of data from the Third National Health and Nutrition Examination Survey

(NHANES III) was performed. The NHANES III documented the general health and nutritional status of randomly selected United States subjects from 1988 to 1994 [52]. Of 13,792 subjects ≥20 years of age having at least six natural teeth, those with a history of bronchitis or emphysema were considered together as having COPD. Subjects with COPD had, on average, more periodontal attachment loss (mean clinical attachment level [CAL] 1.48 ± 1.35) than those without COPD (mean CAL 1.17 ± 1.09). Taking into account a variety of risk factors common to COPD and PD (eg, gender, age, race, education, income, dental treatment history, alcohol consumption, diabetes status, smoking status), logistic regression analysis found risk of COPD to be significantly elevated when the mean attachment loss was ≥2.0 mm compared with periodontally healthy individuals (mean attachment loss <2.0 mm; odds ratio 1.35; 95% confidence interval [CI]: 1.07–1.71). In addition, the trend was noted that lung function appeared to diminish as the amount of attachment loss increased. No such trend was apparent when gingival bleeding was considered.

A more recent study evaluated the role of smoking in a possible relationship between PD and COPD [53]. The authors re-evaluated 7625 NHANES III participants ≥30 years of age who received a spirometric examination. After adjustment for potential confounders, no statistically significant association between PD and COPD was found among former smokers or nonsmokers. Current smokers with ≥4 mm mean loss of attachment, however, had an odds ratio of 3.71 (95% CI: 1.74, 7.89) for COPD. The investigators concluded that cigarette smoking is a cofactor in the relationship between PD and COPD. Because smoking is important in the etiology of PD and COPD, it is difficult to separate the contribution of PD and smoking to the etiology of COPD. It is likely that smoking is the major initiator and contributor to COPD and may contribute to disease progression by way of several pathways [32].

In summary, oral colonization by respiratory pathogens appears to be a risk factor for lung infection in high-risk subjects. Oral interventions that improve oral hygiene and possibly reduce oral inflammation may prove to be a simple, inexpensive, and effective means to lower risk of pneumonia in institutionalized populations. Further studies are required to verify the apparent association between PD and COPD.

Adverse pregnancy outcomes and periodontal disease

Preterm low birth weight (PTLBW) continues to be a significant cause of infant morbidity and mortality. PTLBW is associated with elevated risk for mortality in the first year of life, for developmental problems in childhood, and for several diseases in adulthood. Most perinatal deaths occur in infants born prematurely, especially in infants delivered before 32 weeks' gestation [54]. The prevalence of preterm birth varies from 6% to 15% of all deliveries depending on the population studied in developed countries, and the prevalence has risen in recent years. Risk factors that appear to contribute to adverse pregnancy outcomes include low socioeconomic status, race, multiple births, the mother's age, history of a preterm birth or delivery of a low birth weight infant, parity, past reproductive history, drug and alcohol abuse, and systemic maternal infection. Bacterial vaginosis is a clinical condition caused by overgrowth of the vaginal mucosa by certain aerobic and anaerobic bacteria. Several studies have shown that the onset of bacterial vaginosis during pregnancy is associated with spontaneous abortion, preterm labor, premature birth, premature rupture of the membranes, amniotic fluid infection, postpartum endometriosis, and postcesarean wound infections.

It is also possible that infectious processes occurring elsewhere in the body may contribute to neonatal morbidity and mortality. It has been suggested that PD may be one such infection. The first report of a possible association between PTLBW and PD examined 93 mothers who gave birth to preterm or low birth weight children [55]. These mothers were matched with 31 control mothers who gave birth to children of normal term and birth weight. PTLBW was defined as birth weight less than 2500 g, spontaneous abortion before 12 weeks gestation, preterm labor requiring medical intervention, or premature rupture of the membranes before 36 weeks of gestational age of birth, with gestational age less than 36 weeks. It was found that the risk of PTLBW was 7.5-fold greater if the mother had evidence of PD (diagnosed as having clinical attachment loss) compared with mothers without evidence of PD. Several additional studies have since been published that provide evidence supporting the contention that women with PD have a greater risk of having preterm or low birth weight children [56–60].

In contrast, a case-control study of 236 mothers with PTLBW and 507 normal-birth controls [61] found no association between maternal PD and increased risk of PTLBW. In fact, these investigators found that increasing mean pocket depth at the time of delivery was associated with a reduction in the risk of PTLBW. Other studies since published have not supported this association [62–64].

These conflicting results demonstrate the need for large-scale, multicenter randomized trials of PD treatment to establish causal relationships between periodontal status and PTLBW. Recently, several studies have been published that have tested the effect of periodontal intervention to reduce adverse pregnancy outcomes [65,66]. One study examined 200 pregnant women who received periodontal treatment before 28 weeks of gestation. These women were compared with 200 mothers who received periodontal treatment after delivery (Table 3). Although this trial was randomized, it was not double blinded. Oral intervention included plaque control instruction, scaling, and root planing, with oral rinsing once a day. It was found that periodontal therapy before 28 weeks' gestation significantly reduced the rate of PTLBW in women with PD. Another study [67] compared 74 subjects who

Table 3
Incidence of preterm births, low birth weight, and preterm/low birth weight in treatment and control groups

	Treatment group (N = 163)		Control group (N = 188)		
	n	%	n	%	P
Preterm birth	2	1.10	12	6.38	0.017
Low birth weight	1	0.55	7	3.72	0.083
Preterm/low birth weight	3	1.63	19	10.11	0.001

Treatment consisted of plaque control instructions, rinse once a day with 0.12% chlorhexidine, scaling, and root planing performed under local anesthesia. The control group subjects received no intervention.

Modified from Lopez NJ, Smith PC, Gutierrez J. Periodontal therapy may reduce the risk of preterm low birth weight in women with periodontal disease: a randomized controlled trial. J Periodontol 2002;73(8):916.

received mechanical dental plaque control instructions and scaling and root planing of all teeth compared with 90 control subjects who did not receive periodontal intervention. Significant reduction in the incidence of PTLBW was found in women who received periodontal therapy during pregnancy. These preliminary intervention studies provide provocative evidence that periodontal therapy before 28 weeks of gestation may significantly reduce the incidence of PTLBW children.

Diabetes mellitus

Diabetes mellitus (diabetes) is a metabolic derangement characterized by impairment in glucose use. Diabetes occurs in two major forms: type 1 diabetes is the result of a reduction in or the elimination of insulin production by beta cells in the pancreas. Insulin functions through interaction with muscle and liver cells to regulate glucose metabolism. Reduced insulin production is most often the result of destruction of the beta cells, probably due to autoimmune or viral disease. Individuals with type 1 diabetes require daily insulin supplementation to properly regulate glucose use. Insulin delivery is usually by injection, although progress has been made with the use of insulin pumps and pancreatic transplantation that provides an endogenous source of insulin.

Type 2 diabetes is characterized by a deficient response to insulin by target cells, although insulin production is typically normal or even enhanced in these individuals. This impairment may be due to changes in the structure or number of the cell receptors for insulin. This form of diabetes is by far the most common (estimated to be 85%–90% of all diabetes). Taken together, type 1 and 2 diabetes now appear to occur in epidemic proportions, with 5% to 10% of all Americans having some form of the disease. Recent studies suggest that the number of cases of diabetes is increasing each year, probably related to the concomitant increase in obesity in the population.

Diabetes is a serious medical condition, with numerous acute and chronic complications. The complications of diabetes are related to chronic elevation of blood glucose levels in peripheral blood (hyperglycemia). One effect of hyperglycemia is the formation of advanced glycation end products (AGEs), the products of nonenzymatic glycation/oxidation of proteins/lipids that accumulate in the blood vessel wall [68]. These AGEs are monitored as the concentration of glycated hemoglobin (HbA1c) in the blood. These molecules bind to the receptor for AGE (RAGE). This interaction leads to recruitment of inflammatory cells and their activation to stimulate inflammatory pathways that exacerbate atherosclerosis and other untoward effects.

Over time, several serious side effects can occur as the result of AGE–RAGE interactions, including so-called "macrovascular" complications such as coronary artery disease, cerebrovascular disease (stroke), and peripheral vascular disease. Microvascular complications include retinopathy, nephropathy, and neuropathy. Detailed descriptions of the clinical signs and symptoms, complications, and treatment are beyond the scope of the present discussion.

Diabetes also seems to impact fibroblast and collagen metabolism. Hyperglycemia has been associated with reduced cellular proliferation and reduced collagen synthesis [69,70]. Hyperglycemia could have untoward effects on wound healing, which is essential in the response to periodontal therapy.

It has been known for several decades that persons with diabetes tend to have more serious PD than nondiabetics. Numerous studies have documented that diabetics show more severe pocket depths, alveolar bone loss, frequent abscess formation, and poor healing following therapy than nondiabetics [71]. Studies of Pima Native Americans, who have a very high rate of diabetes [72], show a higher prevalence and incidence of periodontal attachment loss and alveolar bone loss than control populations [73].

A recent study found a relationship between periodontitis and glucose tolerance status [74]. Patients with deep periodontal pockets (defined as having a mean pocket depth >2.0 mm) were significantly associated with having impaired glucose tolerance and diabetes compared with subjects with shallow pockets (<1.3 mm). Subjects with normal glucose tolerance at baseline and who subsequently developed impaired glucose tolerance were significantly more likely to have deep pockets.

The mechanisms responsible for more aggressive periodontitis in diabetics may involve the same mechanisms involved in chronic complications of diabetes. For example, diabetic mice infected with the human periodontal pathogen *Porphyromonas gingivalis* were treated with soluble RAGE [75]. Soluble RAGE binds ligand and blocks interaction with and activation of cell-surface RAGE. Blockade of RAGE diminished alveolar bone loss, with decreased generation of tumor necrosis factor α and interleukin 6 in gingival tissue and decreased levels of matrix metalloproteinases.

In addition to the finding that individuals with diabetes have a greater risk of PD, recent studies have also suggested that subjects with PD are more likely to have poor glycemic control than diabetics without PD. Infections such as periodontitis may stimulate proinflammatory cytokine synthesis to amplify the production of AGEs in diabetics [76]. Thus, control of chronic periodontal infection may contribute to long-term glycemic control. For example, in one study, 113 Native Americans (81 female and 32 male subjects) with PD and type 2 diabetes were randomized into five treatment groups [77]. Periodontal treatment included ultrasonic scaling and curettage combined with one of the following antimicrobial regimens: (1) topical water and systemic doxycycline, 100 mg, for 2 weeks; (2) topical 0.12% chlorhexidine and systemic doxycycline, 100 mg, for 2 weeks; (3) topical povidone-iodine and systemic doxycycline, 100 mg, for 2 weeks; (4) topical 0.12% chlorhexidine and placebo; and (5) topical water and placebo (control group). The doxycycline-treated groups showed the greatest reduction in probing depth and subgingival *Porphyromonas gingivalis* compared with the control group. In addition, all three groups receiving systemic doxycycline showed significant reductions ($P \leq 0.04$) in mean HbA1c at 3 months, reaching nearly 10% from the pretreatment value. It was unclear from this study what role scaling alone would play in reducing HbA1c in diabetics. In a more recent study, subjects with type 2 diabetes with periodontitis were randomly divided into two groups [78]. Group 1 (15 subjects) received full-mouth scaling and root planing plus amoxicillin/ clavulanic acid, 875 mg. The second group (15 patients) received only full-mouth scaling and root planing. Following therapy, both groups showed reduction in probing depths and reduced levels of HbA1c values after the 3 months; however, the reduction in HbA1c values was statistically significant only for group 2.

Summary

A number of studies suggest that PD is associated with diseases resulting from atherosclerosis, lung diseases such as pneumonia and COPD, and adverse pregnancy outcomes. Presently, the data must be regarded as preliminary. Additional large-scale longitudinal epidemiologic and interventional studies are necessary to validate these associations and to determine whether the associations are causal.

References

[1] Pallasch TJ, Wahl MJ. The focal infection theory: appraisal and reappraisal. J Calif Dent Assoc 2000;28(3):194–200.
[2] Newman HN. Focal infection. J Dent Res 1996;75(12):1912–9.
[3] Ross R. Cell biology of atherosclerosis. Annu Rev Physiol 1995;57:791–804.

[4] Ross R. Atherosclerosis—an inflammatory disease. N Engl J Med 1999;340:115–26.

[5] Ludewig B, Zinkernagel RM, Hengartner H. Arterial inflammation and atherosclerosis. Trends Cardiovasc Med 2002;12(4):154–9.

[6] Wagner AD, Gerard HC, Fresemann T, et al. Detection of *Chlamydia pneumoniae* in giant cell vasculitis and correlation with the topographic arrangement of tissue-infiltrating dendritic cells. Arthritis Rheum 2000;43(7):1543–51.

[7] Chiu B. Multiple infections in carotid atherosclerotic plaques. Am Heart J 1999;138(5 Pt 2): S534–6.

[8] Saikku P, Leinonen M, Tenkanen L, et al. Chronic *Chlamydia pneumoniae* infection as a risk factor for coronary heart disease in the Helsinki Heart Study. Ann Intern Med 1992;116(4): 273–8.

[9] Simonka M, Skaleric U, Hojs D. [Condition of teeth and periodontal tissue in patients who had suffered a heart attack]. Zobozdrav Vestn 1988;43(3–5):81–3 [in Croatian].

[10] Mattila KJ, Nieminen MS, Valtonen VV, et al. Association between dental health and acute myocardial infarction. BMJ 1989;298(6676):779–81.

[11] Mattila KJ, Valle MS, Nieminen MS, et al. Dental infections and coronary atherosclerosis. Atherosclerosis 1993;103:205–11.

[12] Mattila KJ, Asikainen S, Wolf J, et al. Age, dental infections, and coronary heart disease. J Dent Res 2000;79(2):756–60.

[13] Emingil G, Buduneli E, Aliyev A, et al. Association between periodontal disease and acute myocardial infarction. J Periodontol 2000;71(12):1882–6.

[14] Renvert S, Ohlsson O, Persson S, et al. Analysis of periodontal risk profiles in adults with or without a history of myocardial infarction. J Clin Periodontol 2004;31(1):19–24.

[15] DeStefano F, Anda RF, Kahn HS, et al. Dental disease and risk of coronary heart disease and mortality. BMJ 1993;306(6879):688–91.

[16] Paunio K, Impivaara O, Tiekso J, et al. Missing teeth and ischaemic heart disease in men aged 45–64 years. Eur Heart J 1993;14(Suppl K):54–6.

[17] Joshipura KJ, Rimm EB, Douglass CW, et al. Poor oral health and coronary heart disease. J Dent Res 1996;75(9):1631–6.

[18] Beck J, Garcia R, Heiss G, et al. Periodontal disease and cardiovascular disease. J Periodontol 1996;67(Suppl 10):1123–37.

[19] Loesche WJ, Schork A, Terpenning MS, et al. Assessing the relationship between dental disease and coronary heart disease in elderly US veterans. J Am Dent Assoc 1998;129(3): 301–11.

[20] Arbes SJ Jr, Slade GD, Beck JD. Association between extent of periodontal attachment loss and self-reported history of heart attack: an analysis of NHANES III data. J Dent Res 1999; 78(12):1777–82.

[21] Morrison HI, Ellison LF, Taylor GW. Periodontal disease and risk of fatal coronary heart and cerebrovascular diseases. J Cardiovasc Risk 1999;6(1):7–11.

[22] Jansson L, Lavstedt S, Frithiof L, et al. Relationship between oral health and mortality in cardiovascular diseases. J Clin Periodontol 2001;28(8):762–8.

[23] Takata Y, Ansai T, Matsumura K, et al. Relationship between tooth loss and electro-cardiographic abnormalities in octogenarians. J Dent Res 2001;80(7):1648–52.

[24] Syrjanen J, Peltola J, Valtonen V, et al. Dental infections in association with cerebral infarction in young and middle-aged men. J Intern Med 1989;225(3):179–84.

[25] Loesche WJ, Schork A, Terpenning MS, et al. The relationship between dental disease and cerebral vascular accident in elderly United States veterans. Ann Periodontol 1998;3(1): 161–74.

[26] Wu T, Trevisan M, Genco RJ, et al. Periodontal disease and risk of cerebrovascular disease: the First National Health and Nutrition Examination Survey and its follow-up study. Arch Intern Med 2000;160(18):2749–55.

[27] Mendez MV, Scott T, LaMorte W, et al. An association between periodontal disease and peripheral vascular disease. Am J Surg 1998;176(2):153–7.

[28] Hujoel PP, Drangsholt M, Spiekerman C, et al. Periodontal disease and coronary heart disease risk. JAMA 2000;284(11):1406–10.

[29] Hujoel PP, Drangsholt M, Spiekerman C, et al. Examining the link between coronary heart disease and the elimination of chronic dental infections. J Am Dent Assoc 2001;132(7): 883–9.

[30] Howell TH, Ridker PM, Ajani UA, et al. Periodontal disease and risk of subsequent cardiovascular disease in US male physicians. J Am Coll Cardiol 2001;37(2):445–50.

[31] Hujoel PP, Drangsholt M, Spiekerman C, et al. Pre-existing cardiovascular disease and periodontitis: a follow-up study. J Dent Res 2002;81(3):186–91.

[32] Scannapieco FA. Role of oral bacteria in respiratory infection. J Periodontol 1999;70: 793–802.

[33] Huxley EJ, Viroslav J, Gray WR, et al. Pharyngeal aspiration in normal adults and patients with depressed consciousness. Am J Med 1978;64(4):564–8.

[34] Lee-Chiong TL Jr. Pulmonary aspiration. Compr Ther 1997;23(6):371–7.

[35] Niederman MS, Mandell LA, Anzueto A, et al. Guidelines for the management of adults with community-acquired pneumonia. Diagnosis, assessment of severity, antimicrobial therapy, and prevention. Am J Respir Crit Care Med 2001;163(7):1730–54.

[36] Scannapieco FA, Stewart EM, Mylotte JM. Colonization of dental plaque by respiratory pathogens in medical intensive care patients. Crit Care Med 1992;20:740–5.

[37] Fourrier F, Duvivier B, Boutigny H, et al. Colonization of dental plaque: a source of nosocomial infections in intensive care unit patients. Crit Care Med 1998;26:301–8.

[38] Terpenning M, Bretz W, Lopatin D, et al. Bacterial colonization of saliva and plaque in the elderly. Clin Infect Dis 1993;16(Suppl):314–6.

[39] Mojon P, Budtz-Jørgensen E, Michel JP, et al. Oral health and history of respiratory tract infection in frail institutionalised elders. Gerodontol 1997;14(1):9–16.

[40] Langmore SE, Terpenning MS, Schork A, et al. Predictors of aspiration pneumonia: how important is dysphagia? Dysphagia 1998;13:69–81.

[41] Preston AJ, Gosney MA, Noon S, et al. Oral flora of elderly patients following acute medical admission. Gerontology 1999;45(1):49–52.

[42] Russell SL, Boylan RJ, Kaslick RS, et al. Respiratory pathogen colonization of the dental plaque of institutionalized elders. Spec Care Dent 1999;19:1–7.

[43] Terpenning MS, Taylor GW, Lopatin DE, et al. Aspiration pneumonia: dental and oral risk factors in an older veteran population. J Am Geriatr Soc 2001;49:557–63.

[44] Pugin J, Auckenthaler R, Lew DP, et al. Oropharyngeal decontamination decreases incidence of ventilator-associated pneumonia. A randomized, placebo-controlled, double-blind clinical trial. JAMA 1991;265:2704–10.

[45] DeRiso AJ II, Ladowski JS, Dillon TA, et al. Chlorhexidine gluconate 0.12% oral rinse reduces the incidence of total nosocomial respiratory infection and nonprophylactic systemic antibiotic use in patients undergoing heart surgery. Chest 1996;109(6):1556–61.

[46] Fourrier F, Cau-Pottier E, Boutigny H, et al. Effects of dental plaque antiseptic decontamination on bacterial colonization and nosocomial infections in critically ill patients. Intensive Care Med 2000;26:1239–47.

[47] Bergmans DC, Bonten MJ, Gaillard CA, et al. Prevention of ventilator-associated pneumonia by oral decontamination. A prospective, randomized, double-blind, placebo-controlled study. Am J Respir Crit Care Med 2001;164:382–8.

[48] Yoneyama T, Yoshida M, Matsui T, et al. Group at OCW. Oral care and pneumonia [letter]. Lancet 1999;354:515.

[49] Yoneyama T, Yoshida M, Ohrui T, et al. Oral care reduces pneumonia in older patients in nursing homes. J Am Geriatr Soc 2002;50(3):430–3.

[50] Scannapieco FA, Papandonatos GD, Dunford RG. Associations between oral conditions and respiratory disease in a national sample survey population. Ann Periodontol 1998;3:251–6.

[51] Hayes C, Sparrow D, Cohen M, et al. The association between alveolar bone loss and pulmonary function: the VA Dental Longitudinal Study. Ann Periodontol 1998;3(1):257–61.

[52] Scannapieco FA, Ho AW. Potential associations between chronic respiratory disease and periodontal disease: analysis of National Health and Nutrition Examination Survey III. J Periodontol 2001;72:50–6.

[53] Hyman JJ, Reid BC. Cigarette smoking, periodontal disease, and chronic obstructive pulmonary disease. J Periodontol 2004;75(1):9–15.

[54] Slattery MM, Morrison JJ. Preterm delivery. Lancet 2002;360(9344):1489–97.

[55] Offenbacher S, Katz V, Fertik G, et al. Periodontal infection as a possible risk factor for preterm low birth weight. J Periodontol 1996;67(Suppl 10):1103–13.

[56] Dasanayake AP. Poor periodontal health of the pregnant woman as a risk factor for low birth weight. Ann Periodontol 1998;3(1):206–12.

[57] Offenbacher S, Lieff S, Boggess KA, et al. Maternal periodontitis and prematurity. Part I: obstetric outcome of prematurity and growth restriction. Ann Periodontol 2001;6(1):164–74.

[58] Madianos PN, Lieff S, Murtha AP, et al. Maternal periodontitis and prematurity. Part II: maternal infection and fetal exposure. Ann Periodontol 2001;6(1):175–82.

[59] Jeffcoat MK, Geurs NC, Reddy MS, et al. Periodontal infection and preterm birth: results of a prospective study. J Am Dent Assoc 2001;132(7):875–80.

[60] Radnai M, Gorzo I, Nagy E, et al. A possible association between preterm birth and early periodontitis. A pilot study. J Clin Periodontol 2004;31(9):736–41.

[61] Davenport ES, Williams CE, Sterne JA, et al. The East London Study of Maternal Chronic Periodontal Disease and Preterm Low Birth Weight Infants: study design and prevalence data. Ann Periodontol 1998;3(1):213–21.

[62] Moore S, Ide M, Coward PY, et al. A prospective study to investigate the relationship between periodontal disease and adverse pregnancy outcome. Br Dent J 2004;197(5):251–8 [discussion: 247].

[63] Moore S, Ide M, Randhawa M, et al. An investigation into the association among preterm birth, cytokine gene polymorphisms and periodontal disease. Br J Obstet Gynaecol 2004; 111(2):125–32.

[64] Holbrook WP, Oskarsdottir A, Fridjonsson T, et al. No link between low-grade periodontal disease and preterm birth: a pilot study in a healthy Caucasian population. Acta Odontol Scand 2004;62(3):177–9.

[65] Lopez NJ, Smith PC, Gutierrez J. Periodontal therapy may reduce the risk of preterm low birth weight in women with periodontal disease: a randomized controlled trial. J Periodontol 2002;73(8):911–24.

[66] Lopez NJ, Smith PC, Gutierrez J. Higher risk of preterm birth and low birth weight in women with periodontal disease. J Dent Res 2002;81(1):58–63.

[67] Mitchell-Lewis D, Engebretson SP, Chen J, et al. Periodontal infections and pre-term birth: early findings from a cohort of young minority women in New York. Eur J Oral Sci 2001; 109(1):34–9.

[68] Yan SF, Ramasamy R, Naka Y, et al. Glycation, inflammation, and RAGE: a scaffold for the macrovascular complications of diabetes and beyond. Circ Res 2003;93(12):1159–69.

[69] Hasslacher C, Burklin E, Kopischke HG. Inhibition of increased synthesis of glomerular basement membrane collagen in diabetic rats in vivo. Ren Physiol 1981;4(2–3):108–11.

[70] Lien YH, Stern R, Fu JC, et al. Inhibition of collagen fibril formation in vitro and subsequent cross-linking by glucose. Science 1984;225(4669):1489–91.

[71] Soskolne WA. Epidemiological and clinical aspects of periodontal diseases in diabetics. Ann Periodontol 1998;3(1):3–12.

[72] Knowler WC, Pettitt DJ, Saad MF, et al. Diabetes mellitus in the Pima Indians: incidence, risk factors and pathogenesis. Diabetes 1990;6(1):1–27.

[73] Nelson RG, Shlossman M, Budding LM, et al. Periodontal disease and NIDDM in Pima Indians. Diabetes Care 1990;13(8):836–40.

[74] Saito T, Shimazaki Y, Kiyohara Y, et al. The severity of periodontal disease is associated with the development of glucose intolerance in non-diabetics: the Hisayama study. J Dent Res 2004;83(6):485–90.

[75] Lalla E, Lamster IB, Feit M, et al. Blockade of RAGE suppresses periodontitis-associated bone loss in diabetic mice. J Clin Invest 2000;105(8):1117–24.

[76] Grossi SG, Genco RJ. Periodontal disease and diabetes mellitus: a two-way relationship. Ann Periodontol 1998;3(1):51–61.

[77] Grossi SG, Skrepcinski FB, DeCaro T, et al. Treatment of periodontal disease in diabetics reduces glycated hemoglobin. J Periodontol 1997;68(8):713–9.

[78] Rodrigues DC, Taba MJ, Novaes AB, et al. Effect of non-surgical periodontal therapy on glycemic control in patients with type 2 diabetes mellitus. J Periodontol 2003;74(9):1361–7.

ELSEVIER
SAUNDERS

THE DENTAL
CLINICS
OF NORTH AMERICA

Dent Clin N Am 49 (2005) 551–571

Diagnostic Biomarkers for Oral and Periodontal Diseases

Mario Taba, Jr, DDS, PhD[a], Janet Kinney, RDH[a],
Amy S. Kim, DDS[b],
William V. Giannobile, DDS, DMSc[a,b,c,*]

[a]*Department of Periodontics/Prevention/Geriatrics, School of Dentistry,
University of Michigan, 1011 North University Avenue, Ann Arbor, MI 48109-1078, USA*
[b]*Michigan Center for Oral Health Research, University of Michigan,
24 Frank Lloyd Wright Drive, Lobby M, Box 422, Ann Arbor, MI 48106, USA*
[c]*Department of Biomedical Engineering, College of Engineering,
University of Michigan, Ann Arbor, MI, USA*

Periodontitis is a group of inflammatory diseases that affect the connective tissue attachment and supporting bone around the teeth. It is widely accepted that the initiation and the progression of periodontitis are dependent on the presence of virulent microorganisms capable of causing disease. Although the bacteria are initiating agents in periodontitis, the host response to the pathogenic infection is critical to disease progression [1–3]. After its initiation, the disease progresses with the loss of collagen fibers and attachment to the cemental surface, apical migration of the junctional epithelium, formation of deepened periodontal pockets, and resorption of alveolar bone [4]. If left untreated, the disease continues with progressive bone destruction, leading to tooth mobility and subsequent tooth loss. Periodontal disease afflicts over 50% of the adult population in the United States, with approximately 10% displaying severe disease concomitant with early tooth loss [5].

A goal of periodontal diagnostic procedures is to provide useful information to the clinician regarding the present periodontal disease type, location, and severity. These findings serve as a basis for treatment planning

This work was supported by NIDCR grants U01-DE14961 and R43-DE14810 to W.V. Giannobile.

* Corresponding author. Department of Periodontics/Prevention/Geriatrics, School of Dentistry, University of Michigan, 1011 North University Avenue, Ann Arbor, MI 48109-1078.

E-mail address: william.giannobile@umich.edu (W.V. Giannobile).

and provide essential data during periodontal maintenance and disease-monitoring phases of treatment.

Traditional periodontal diagnostic parameters used clinically include probing depths, bleeding on probing, clinical attachment levels, plaque index, and radiographs assessing alveolar bone level [6]. The strengths of these traditional tools are their ease of use, their cost-effectiveness, and that they are relatively noninvasive. Traditional diagnostic procedures are inherently limited, in that only disease history, not current disease status, can be assessed. Clinical attachment loss readings by the periodontal probe and radiographic evaluations of alveolar bone loss measure damage from past episodes of destruction and require a 2- to 3-mm threshold change before a site can be identified as having experienced a significant anatomic event [7]. Advances in oral and periodontal disease diagnostic research are moving toward methods whereby periodontal risk can be identified and quantified by objective measures such as biomarkers (Table 1).

There are several key questions regarding current clinical decision making: How can clinicians assess risk for periodontal disease? What are the useful laboratory and clinical methods for periodontal risk assessment? and What can be achieved by controlling periodontal disease using a risk profile? [8–11]. Risk factors are considered modifiers of disease activity. In association with host susceptibility and a variety of local and systemic conditions, they influence the initiation and progression of periodontitis and successive changes on biomarkers [12–14]. Biomarkers of disease in succession play an important role in life sciences and have begun to assume a greater role in diagnosis, monitoring of therapy outcomes, and drug discovery. The challenge for biomarkers is to allow earlier detection of disease evolution and more robust therapy efficacy measurements. For biomarkers to assume their rightful role in routine practice, it is essential that their relation to the mechanism of disease progression and therapeutic intervention be more fully understood (Table 2) [13].

Table 1
Diagnostic tools to measure periodontal disease at the molecular, cellular, tissue, and clinical levels

Level	Example of process	Example of diagnostic tools
Molecular	Activation of receptors for endotoxin: CD-14; Toll-like receptors	Polymerase chain reaction; DNA-DNA hybridization; laser-capture microdissection
Cellular	Inflammatory cell activation such as neutrophils; osteoclast activation	ELISA; immunohistochemistry
Tissue	Downgrowth of junctional epithelium; bone and connective tissue loss	Histomorphometry; immunohistochemistry
Clinical	Attachment loss Bone loss	Periodontal probing Radiographs

Table 2
Predictors for periodontal diseases

Term	Definition
Risk marker	An attribute or event that is associated with increased probability of disease but is not necessarily a causal factor
Risk indicator	An event that is associated with an outcome only in cross-sectional studies
Risk factor	An action or event that is related statistically in some way to an outcome and is truly causal
Risk determinant	An attribute or event that increases the probability of occurrence of disease
Biomarker	A substance that is measured objectively and evaluated as an indicator of normal biologic processes, pathogenic processes, or pharmacologic responses to a therapeutic intervention

Adapted from Refs. [128,154,155].

There is a need for the development of new diagnostic tests that can detect the presence of active disease, predict future disease progression, and evaluate the response to periodontal therapy, thereby improving the clinical management of periodontal patients. The diagnosis of active phases of periodontal disease and the identification of patients at risk for active disease represent challenges for clinical investigators and practitioners [15]. This article highlights recent advances in the use of biomarker-based disease diagnostics that focus on the identification of active periodontal disease from plaque biofilms [16], gingival crevicular fluid (GCF) [17], and saliva [18]. Mediators that are released into GCF and saliva as biomarkers of disease are shown in Fig. 1. The authors also present an overview of well-studied mediators associated with microbial identification, host response factors, and bone resorptive mediators.

Microbial factors for the diagnosis of periodontal diseases

Of the more than 600 bacterial species that have been identified from subgingival plaque, only a small number have been suggested to play a causal role in the pathogenesis of destructive periodontal diseases in the susceptible host [16]. Furthermore, technologic advances in methodologies such as analysis of 16S ribosomal RNA bacterial genes indicate that as many as several hundred additional species of not-yet-identified bacteria may exist [19]. The presence of bacteria adjacent to the gingival crevice and the intimate contact of bacterial lipopolysaccharide with the host cells trigger monocytes, polymorphonuclear leukocytes (neutrophils), macrophages, and other cells to release inflammatory mediators such as interleukin (IL)-1, tumor necrosis factor (TNF)-α, and prostaglandin E_2 [3]. The role of host response factors derived from GCF and saliva is discussed later.

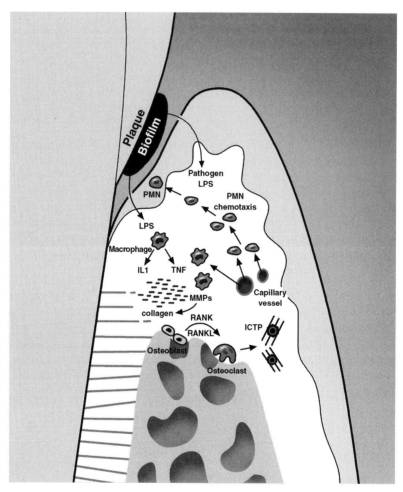

Fig. 1. Schematic representation of the initial events triggered by lipopolysaccharide (LPS) from plaque biofilms on periodontal tissues. Pathogens present in plaque biofilm activate chemotaxis of polymorphonuclear leucocytes (PMN) as a first line of defense against infection. Monocytes and activated macrophages respond to endotoxin by releasing cytokines (tumor necrosis factor [TNF] and interleukin 1 [IL1]) that are mediators for bone resorption. Matrix metalloproteinases (MMPs) released by fibroblast and PMNs are potent collagen destruction enzymes. TNF, IL-1, and receptor activator of NF-κB ligand (RANKL) are elevated in disease sites and play an important role in osteoclastogenesis and bone resorption. Tissue degradation molecules such as pyridinoline cross-linked carboxyterminal telopeptide of type I collagen (ICTP) that are specific to bone resorption are released into the GCF and can be used as biomarkers for periodontal disease and the previously mentioned cytokines and enzymes. RANK, receptor activator of NF-κB.

A number of specific periodontal pathogens have been implicated in periodontal diseases, including *Tanerella forsythensis*, *Porphyromonas gingivalis*, and *Treponema denticola*. These three organisms are members of the "red complex" of bacteria (and exhibit benzoyl-DL-arginine-naphthyla- mide, or BANA, activity) [20,21] that are highly implicated in the progression of periodontal diseases [22]. *Actinobacillus actinomycetemcomi- tans* has been linked with early-onset forms of periodontal disease and aggressive periodontitis, whereas red complex bacteria are associated with chronic periodontitis [23]. The rationale for the use of microbial analysis for periodontitis monitoring is to target pathogens implicated in disease to (1) identify specific periodontal diseases, (2) identify antibiotic susceptibility of infecting organisms colonizing diseased sites, and (3) predict disease activity. Thus, the goal of microbiologic monitoring is twofold (disease monitoring and disease treatment guidance); however, microbial tests (eg, BANA test, DNA probe analysis, or culturing) have failed to predict future disease progression [24]. These findings can be explained by the fact that the presence of specific periodontal pathogens is necessary to initiate periodontal disease but not sufficient to cause disease in the nonsusceptible host [25].

A recent systematic review of the topic asked the focused question, "In patients with periodontal diseases, does microbial identification influence patient management compared with treatment prescribed without this information?" [24]. The answer to this question is central for the clinical utility of microbial-based diagnostic tests for oral and periodontal diseases. If tests do not influence clinical decision making, then in essence, there is no clinical value for the test. Of the 24 studies (a total of 835 subjects) noted in the review, 13 reported microbial identification as an aid in treatment planning [26–38]. The investigators concluded that the literature lacks studies with a high evidence rating; the most-pertinent studies were case reports or case series without controls [24]. Furthermore, although some practitioners consider microbial identification a valuable adjunct to the management of patients with periodontal diseases, there is a lack of strong evidence to support this practice. It is also possible that as-yet-unidentified, uncultivable microbial species are essential to disease initiation and progression. If so, microbial-based tests for these species are obviously unavailable. Future studies are needed in this area to justify the use of microbial testing to predict progression of periodontal diseases [24]. New strategies that combine microbial identification with host response or tissue breakdown factors using discriminant analysis may better improve the ability of microbial analysis to predict future periodontal disease around teeth and dental implants [39,40].

Host response and inflammatory mediators as potential biomarkers

Periodontal inflammation occurs in the gingival tissue in response to plaque bacteria biofilms [3,41]. Gingivitis is characterized by an initial increase in blood flow, enhanced vascular permeability, and the influx of cells (neutrophils and monocyte-macrophages) from the peripheral blood to the gingival crevice [42]. Subsequently, T cells and B cells appear at the infection site. After they appear at the lesion, these cells produce a myriad of cytokines such as IL-1β, IL-6, TNF-α, and immunoglubulins as an antigen-specific response [4]. Initially, tissue degradation is limited to epithelial cells and collagen fibers from the connective tissue. Later on, the inflammatory process may reach periodontal supportive tissue, leading to bone resorption (see Fig. 1) [43].

GCF has been extensively investigated for the release of host response factors. It includes a mixture of molecules from blood, host tissue, and plaque biofilms, such as electrolytes, small molecules, proteins, cytokines, antibodies, bacterial antigens, and enzymes [44–60]. Host cell–derived enzymes such as matrix metalloproteinases (MMPs) are an important group of neutral proteinases implicated in the destructive process of periodontal disease that can be measured in GCF [44,61–67]. The neutrophils are the major cells responsible for MMP release at the infected site, specifically MMP-8 (collagenase-2) and MMP-9 (gelatinase-B) [65]. Although MMP-8 is able to potently degrade interstitial collagens, MMP-9 degrades several extracellular matrix proteins [68–71]. Kinane et al [64] and Mantyla et al [65] presented the use of a rapid chairside test based on the immunologic detection of elevated MMP-8 in GCF to diagnose and monitor the course and treatment of periodontitis. With a threshold of 1 mg/L MMP-8 activity, the test provided a sensitivity of 0.83 and specificity of 0.96, demonstrating value as a potential tool to differentiate periodontitis from gingivitis and healthy sites and to monitor treatment of periodontitis.

Macrophages and polymorphonuclear leukocytes, in response to the chemoattractant effect of bacterial lipopolysaccharide [72], are activated to produce important inflammatory mediators—notably, TNF-α, IL-1, IL-6, and other cytokines [73] related to the host response and tissue destruction [72]. Holmlund et al [74] investigated bone resorption activity, IL-1α, IL-1β, and IL-1 receptor antagonist levels in GCF in sites having no signs of periodontal disease and in sites having horizontal or angular periodontal bone loss. The amounts of IL-1α, IL-1β, and IL-1 receptor antagonist from GCF were quantified by ELISA. It was observed that levels of bone resorption activity, IL-1α, IL-1β, and IL-1 receptor antagonist were significantly higher in GCF from diseased sites compared with healthy sites but did not relate to defect morphology [74].

The severity of periodontitis is associated with local (GCF or tissue) increases in IL-1β, TNF-α, prostaglandins such as prostaglandin E_2 [4], and MMPs [61,67,71], whereas inhibition of these substances produces substantial reductions in periodontal disease. Specifically for IL-1 and TNF, local protein blockade in a monkey model of periodontitis produced significant reductions in bone loss [75,76], highlighting the important role of these mediators in periodontal disease.

Advanced stages of periodontal lesions are populated by a large proportion of B lymphocytes and plasma cells [77–79] and increased levels of immunoglobulins in GCF [54,80–82]. Plombas et al [83] investigated GCF and whole saliva from periodontitis patients and periodontally healthy adults for the presence of IgA and IgG antibodies to *Actinobacillus actinomycetemcomitans, Porphyromonas gingivalis, Prevotella intermedia,* and *Fusobacterium nucleatum.* Compared with healthy patients, the GCF of periodontitis patients contained significantly higher levels of IgA and IgG antibodies to the four microorganisms tested.

Porphyromonas gingivalis and *Actinobacillus actinomycetemcomitans* are examples of well-studied gram-negative pathogens implicated in the immune and inflammatory host response in periodontal disease [84]. *Porphyromonas gingivalis* produces by far the greatest proteolytic activity through peptidases, elastases, trypsinlike proteases, and collagenases [85] that can be monitored by GCF analysis [86,87]. Figueredo et al [62] compared elastase and collagenase activities in GCF before and after nonsurgical periodontal treatment. Improvement in clinical parameters after therapy was accompanied by a significant reduction in the values of total elastase activity, free elastase, MMP-8, and collagenolytic activity in gingivitis and periodontitis sites.

Aspartate aminotransferase, a tissue destruction biomarker released from necrotic cells in GCF, is associated with periodontitis severity [88,89]. Aspartate aminotransferase–positive sites are positively correlated with higher prevalence of *Porphyromonas gingivalis, Streptococcus intermedius, Peptostreptococcus micros, Campylobacter concisus, Bacteroides forsythus, Camplobacter gracilis, Campylobacter rectus,* and *Selenomonas sputigena* [90]. Moreover, to evaluate the relationship between aspartate aminotransferase and periodontal disease, periodontitis subjects were monitored for 12 months using a chairside assay. After nonsurgical therapy, the percentage of sites exhibiting higher levels of aspartate aminotransferase and bleeding on probing was significantly lower at 6 and 12 months compared with baseline. Elevated levels of aspartate aminotransferase, however, were present at sites that did not subsequently exhibit disease progression [89]. Therefore, the biomarker does not discriminate between progressive sites and sites that are stable but inflamed.

In summary, GCF carries multiple molecular factors derived from the host response and is considered a significant protective mechanism in periodontal infection (Table 3) [91]. These host response factors represent important mediators that can aid in the development of periodontal diagnostics.

Bone-specific markers of tissue destruction for periodontal diagnosis

Of the 50 or more different components in GCF and saliva evaluated to date for periodontal diagnosis, most lack specificity to alveolar bone

Table 3
Examples of biomarkers of periodontal disease identified from plaque biofilm, gingival crevicular fluid, or saliva

Category mediator	Examples
Microbial factors	DNA probes or culturing of putative periodontal pathogens (eg, *Porphyromonas gingivalis, Tanerella forsythensis, Treponema denticola*)
Host response factors	IL-1β; TNF-α; aspartate aminotransferase; elastase
Connective tissue breakdown products	Collagen telopeptides; osteocalcin; proteoglycans; fibronection fragments

destruction and essentially constitute soft tissue inflammatory events [92]. When examining the destruction of alveolar bone that is preceded by a microbial infection and inflammatory response, the measurement of connective tissue–derived molecules may lead to a more accurate assessment of tissue breakdown due to the tremendous variability of the host response among individuals [92].

Advances in bone cell biology over the past decade have resulted in several new biochemical markers for the measurement of bone homeostasis. With mounting evidence for a relationship between osteoporosis and oral bone loss, investigators have sought to develop better biologic markers to determine and predict oral bone loss [93]. Two of the more well studied mediators (bone collagen fragments and osteocalcin) are presented in the following text.

Pyridinoline cross-linked carboxyterminal telopeptide of type I collagen

Type I collagen composes 90% of the organic matrix of bone and is the most abundant collagen in osseous tissue [94]. Collagen degradation products have emerged as valuable markers of bone turnover in a multitude of bone resorptive and metabolic diseases [95]. Pyridinoline cross-links represent a class of collagen degradative molecules that include pyridinoline, deoxypyridinoline, N-telopeptides, and C-telopeptides [96]. Pyridinoline and deoxypyridinoline are mature intermolecular cross-links of collagen. Subsequent to osteoclastic bone resorption and collagen matrix degradation, pyridinoline, deoxypyridinoline, and amino- and carboxyterminal cross-linked telopeptides of type I collagen are released into the circulation. Because the cross-linked telopeptides result from post-translational modification of collagen molecules, they cannot be reused during collagen synthesis and are therefore considered specific biomarkers for bone resorption [97]. In addition, the value of pyridinoline cross-links as potential markers of bone turnover relates to their specificity for bone. In skin and other soft tissues, histidine cross-links are the predominant form and no pyridinoline-like structures exist. Recently, a degradation fragment originating from the helical part of type I collagen and consisting of the 620–633 sequence of the α1 chain has been identified to correlate highly with amino- and carboxyterminal telopeptides associated with bone resorption [98].

The pyridinoline cross-linked carboxyterminal telopeptide of type I collagen (ICTP) is a 12- to 20-kd fragment of bone type I collagen released by digestion with trypsin or bacterial collagenase [99]. Elevated serum ICTP and other pyridinoline cross-linked components have been shown to be correlated with the bone resorptive rate in several bone metabolic diseases including osteoporosis [100], rheumatoid arthritis [101], and Paget's disease [102]. Furthermore, pyridinoline cross-links demonstrated significant decreases in postmenopausal osteoporotic subjects after bisphosphonate [103] or estrogen [104] therapy.

Given their specificity for bone resorption, pyridinoline cross-links represent a potentially valuable diagnostic aid in periodontics because biochemical markers specific for bone degradation may be useful in differentiating between the presence of gingival inflammation and active periodontal or peri-implant bone destruction [105]. Several investigations have explored the ability of pyridinoline cross-links to detect bone resorption in periodontitis lesions [39,63,106–108], in peri-implantitis [40], and in response to periodontal therapy [40,61,66,107,109–111].

Palys et al [39] related ICTP levels to the subgingival microflora of various disease states on GCF. Subjects were divided into groups representing health, gingivitis, and chronic periodontitis, and GCF and plaque samples were collected from each subject. The samples were analyzed for ICTP levels and the presence of 40 subgingival species using checkerboard DNA-DNA hybridization techniques. ICTP levels differed significantly between health, gingivitis, and periodontitis subjects, and related modestly to several clinical disease parameters. ICTP levels were also strongly correlated with whole-subject levels of several periodontal pathogens including *Tanerella forsythensis*, *Porphyromonas gingivalis*, *Prevotella intermedia*, and *Treponema denticola*. Oringer et al [40] examined the relationship between ICTP levels and subgingival species around implants and teeth in 20 partially edentulous and 2 fully edentulous patients. No significant differences were found among ICTP levels and subgingival plaque composition between implants and teeth. Strong correlations were found between elevated ICTP levels at implant sites and colonization with organisms associated with failing implants such as *Prevotella intermedia*, *Fusobacterim nucleatum* subsp *vincentii*, and *Streptococcus gordonii* [40].

Diagnostic tools have also been applied to evaluate the response to active periodontal therapy. Golub et al [63] found that treatment of chronic periodontitis patients with scaling and root planing (SRP) and an MMP inhibitor (subantimicrobial doxycycline hyclate) resulted in a 70% reduction in GCF ICTP levels after 1 month, concomitant with a 30% reduction in collagenase levels. An investigation of periodontitis patients treated with

SRP also demonstrated significant correlations between GCF ICTP levels and clinical periodontal disease parameters, including attachment loss, pocket depth, and bleeding on probing [93]. In addition, elevated GCF ICTP levels at baseline, especially at shallow sites, were found to be predictive for future attachment loss as early as 1 month after sampling. Furthermore, treatment of a group of periodontitis subjects by SRP and locally delivered minocycline led to rapid reductions in GCF ICTP levels [63].

Studies assessing the role of GCF ICTP levels as a diagnostic marker of periodontal disease activity have produced promising results to date. ICTP has been shown to be a good predictor of future alveolar bone and attachment loss, was strongly correlated with clinical parameters and putative periodontal pathogens, and demonstrated significant reductions after periodontal therapy [92]. Controlled human longitudinal trials are needed to fully establish the role of ICTP as a predictor of periodontal tissue destruction, disease activity, and response to therapy in periodontal patients.

Osteocalcin

Osteocalcin is a calcium-binding protein of bone and is the most abundant noncollagenous protein in mineralized tissues [112]. Osteocalcin is synthesized predominantly by osteoblasts [113] and has an important role in bone formation and turnover [114,115]. Osteocalcin exhibits chemoattractive activity for osteoclast progenitor cells and monocytes [116–118], and its synthesis in vitro is stimulated by 1,25-dihydroxyvitamin D_3. It has also been shown to promote bone resorption, and stimulate differentiation of osteoclast progenitor cells [112,119]. Elevated serum osteocalcin levels have been shown during periods of rapid bone turnover (eg, osteoporosis, multiple myeloma, and fracture repair) [120,121]. Serum osteocalcin is presently a valid marker of bone turnover when resorption and formation are coupled and is a specific marker of bone formation when formation and resorption are uncoupled [115,120,122,123].

Several studies have investigated the relationship between GCF osteocalcin levels and periodontal disease [49,63,106,124–126]. Kunimatsu et al [124] reported a positive correlation between GCF osteocalcin aminoterminal peptide levels and clinical parameters in a cross-sectional study of periodontitis and gingivitis patients. The investigators also reported that osteocalcin could not be detected in patients with gingivitis. In contrast, Nakashima et al [126] reported significant GCF osteocalcin levels from periodontitis and gingivitis patients. Osteocalcin levels were also significantly correlated with pocket depth, gingival index scores, and GCF levels of alkaline phosphatase and prostaglandin E_2. In a longitudinal study of untreated periodontitis patients with ≥ 1.5 mm attachment loss during the monitoring period, GCF osteocalcin levels alone were unable to distinguish between active and inactive sites [49]. When a combination of the biochemical markers osteocalcin, collagenase, prostaglandin E_2, α_2-macro-globulin, elastase, and alkaline phosphatase was evaluated, however, increased diagnostic sensitivity and specificity values of 80% and 91%, respectively, were reported [49].

A longitudinal study using an experimental periodontitis model in beagle dogs reported a strong correlation between GCF osteocalcin levels and active bone turnover as assessed by bone-seeking radio pharmaceutical uptake [106]. Osteocalcin, however, was shown to possess only modest predictive value for future bone loss measured by computer-assisted digitizing radiography. Moreover, treatment of chronic periodontitis patients with subantimicrobial doxycycline failed to reduce GCF osteocalcin levels [63], and a cross-sectional study of periodontitis patients reported no differences in GCF osteocalcin levels between deep and shallow sites in the same patients [125]. In addition, osteocalcin levels in the GCF during orthodontic tooth movement were highly variable between subjects and lacked a consistent pattern related to the stages of tooth movement [127]. Taken together, the results of these studies show a potential role for intact osteocalcin as a bone-specific marker of bone turnover but not as a predictive indicator for periodontal disease. Greater promise appears to be in the detection of aminoterminal osteocalcin fragments for periodontal disease detection. Additional longitudinal studies may be warranted to more fully elucidate the utility of osteocalcin as a periodontal disease activity diagnostic aid.

Role of oral fluid biomarkers in periodontal diagnosis

A biomarker or biologic marker, according to the most recent definition [128], is a substance that is objectively measured and evaluated as an indicator of normal biologic processes, pathogenic processes, or pharmacologic responses to a therapeutic intervention. Because saliva and GCF are fluids easily collected and contain locally and systemically derived markers of periodontal disease, they may offer the basis for a patient-specific biomarker assessment for periodontitis and other systemic diseases [18,129].

Due to the noninvasive and simple nature of their collection, analysis of saliva and GCF may be especially beneficial in the determination of current periodontal status and a means of monitoring response to treatment [130,131]. Many studies have shown that the determination of inflammatory mediator levels in biologic fluids is a good indicator of inflammatory activity. Therefore, studies related to the pathogenesis of periodontal diseases usually examine whether biochemical and immunologic markers in saliva or GCF might reflect the extent of periodontal destruction and possibly predict future disease progression [18,129]. Oral fluid biomarkers that have been studied for periodontal diagnosis include proteins of host origin (ie, enzymes and immunoglobulins), phenotypic markers, host cells, hormones, bacteria and bacterial products, ions, and volatile compounds [18,132–135]. Table 3 lists a sample of compounds obtained by diagnostic screening of saliva or GCF.

Future directions

There is a plethora of possibilities for the future use of oral fluids in biotechnology and health care applications, especially in the field of diagnostics. A tremendous amount of research activity is currently under way to explore the role of oral fluids as a possible medium in a variety of applications.

Recent advances in HIV diagnosis have been made using oral fluids. A commercially available kit (OraSure, OraSure Technologies, Bethlehem, Pennsylvania) has an oral specimen collection device that is placed between the buccal mucosa and buccal gingiva for 2 to 5 minutes to collect HIV-1 antibodies (not the virus) from the tissues of the cheek and gingiva. OraSure HIV-1 does not collect saliva but rather a sample called oral mucosal transudate. For different fluids (oral fluid, finger-stick or venipuncture whole blood or plasma specimens), the alternative test OraQuick (OraSure Technologies) provides accurate results for HIV-1 and HIV-2 in 20 minutes. The collector pad is placed in a vial with preservative and sent to a clinical laboratory for testing with an initial "screening" assay (ELISA). If necessary, a supplementary test (Western blot assay) is performed to verify the results of the screening assay. This process is referred to as the OraSure testing algorithm [136].

Several researchers have focused on genetic single nucleotide polymorphisms in the study of periodontitis. There is a genetic susceptibility test currently available for severe chronic periodontitis (Interleukin Genetics, Waltham, Massachusetts). This system works by detection of two types of IL-1 genetic alleles, IL-1α +4845 and IL-1β +3954 [137]. Individuals identified as "genotype positive," or found to have both of these alleles, are more likely to have the phenotype of overexpression of this gene. The increased GCF and salivary IL-1 predisposes the patient to the severe form of chronic periodontitis by way of a hyperinflammatory response to bacterial challenge. In this way, genomics has been found to be applicable in the prediction of predisposition to periodontitis in certain patient populations [138]. Socransky et al [139] took a different approach in researching IL-1 gene polymorphisms in periodontitis patients. These investigators linked previous findings regarding the association of IL-1 polymorphisms and severity of adult periodontitis with microbial species found in IL-1 genotype-negative versus IL-1 genotype-positive patients. These researchers concluded that those who were IL-1 genotype positive tended to have higher levels of the more damaging microbial species (red and orange complex organisms) associated with periodontal inflammation [139].

Li et al [140] investigated the potential use of genomics in the development of salivary diagnostics. They performed microarray testing of cell-free saliva for RNA profiling. RNA was isolated from unstimulated saliva that was collected from healthy subjects. After analysis by microarray and quantitative polymerase chain reaction, they found that it was possible to profile messenger RNAs, of which there were thousands present in the saliva. More recently, the group demonstrated the potential of salivary IL-8 levels to predict patients afflicted with squamous cell carcinoma [141].

Salivary immunocomponents have also been studied at length in oral health, including immunoglobulin subclass, immunoglobulin isotypes, and antibody levels [142–148]. Other salivary constituents that have been investigated for diagnostic uses include epithelial keratins [149], occult blood [150], salivary ions such as calcium and phosphates [151,152], and serum markers such as cortisol [153–155].

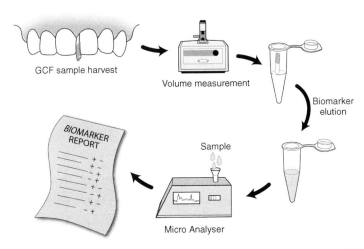

Fig. 2. Futuristic chairside diagnostic test based on GCF sampling. Considering the GCF fluid as a potential analyte for the screening of multiple biomarkers, a rapid, chairside diagnostic tool (represented in the figure as a Micro Analyser) or a "mini-lab" could be used by clinicians for risk assessment and decision making on treatment planning. The advantages of such a tool would be enhanced predictability of clinical outcomes and well-informed patients regarding personalized treatment needs. As shown, a simple clinical procedure for GCF collection could be used, followed by extraction of analytes from the test strip. The fluid present on the test strip would be subjected to volumetric quantification. After an elution procedure to "wash" and retrieve the compounds from the fluid, the sample would be analyzed. An immediate comprehensive risk report profile and biomarkers screening would enable evidence-based decision making.

Summary

Researchers in the biotechnology and medical realm are currently investigating the use of oral fluids for the diagnosis of oral and systemic diseases and for drug development. In the pharmaceutical industry, the use of biomarkers is avidly being developed for use in tailored dosing and drug metabolism studies. Professionals in seemingly unrelated arenas such as the insurance industry, the Environment Protection Agency, and Homeland Security are interested in the possible use of oral fluids to monitor biomarkers. Under investigation are possible uses of GCF and saliva in the preliminary screening for biological/chemical warfare agent exposure, environmental toxin detection, and screening for metabolites of drugs of abuse.

In the field of oral disease diagnosis, there has been a steady growing trend during the last 2 decades to develop tools to monitor periodontitis. From physical measurements such as periodontal probing to sophisticated genetic susceptibility analysis and molecular assays for the detection of biomarkers on the different stages of the disease, substantial improvements have been made on the understanding of the mediators implicated on the initiation and progression of periodontitis. At the same time, this evolutionary process has promoted the discovery of new biomarkers and the development of new therapeutic approaches mainly using host modulation. Moreover, new diagnostic technologies such as nucleic acid and protein microarrays and microfluidics are under development for risk assessment and comprehensive screening of biomarkers. These recent advances are leading to the development of more powerful diagnostic tools for practitioners to optimize their treatment predictability (Fig. 2).

References

[1] Socransky SS, Haffajee AD. The bacterial etiology of destructive periodontal disease: current concepts. J Periodontol 1992;63(4 Suppl):322–31.

[2] Genco RJ. Host responses in periodontal diseases: current concepts. J Periodontol 1992; 63(Suppl 4):338–55.

[3] Kirkwood KL, Taba M Jr, Rossa C, et al. Molecular biology of the host-microbe interaction in periodontal diseases. Selected topics: molecular signaling aspects of pathogen-mediated bone destruction in periodontal diseases. In: Newman M, Takei H, editors. Carranza's periodontology 10th edition. St. Louis (MO): Elsevier; in press.

[4] Offenbacher S. Periodontal diseases: pathogenesis. Ann Periodontol 1996;1(1):821–78.

[5] Albandar JM. Periodontal diseases in North America. Periodontol 2000 2002;29:31–69.

[6] Armitage GC. The complete periodontal examination. Periodontol 2000 2004;34:22–33.

[7] Goodson JM. Conduct of multicenter trials to test agents for treatment of periodontitis. J Periodontol 1992;63(Suppl 12):1058–63.

[8] Page RC, Martin J, Krall EA, et al. Longitudinal validation of a risk calculator for periodontal disease. J Clin Periodontol 2003;30(9):819–27.

[9] Genco RJ. Assessment of risk of periodontal disease. Compend Suppl 1994;18:678–83.

[10] Lamster IB. Current concepts and future trends for periodontal disease and periodontal therapy, part 2: classification, diagnosis, and nonsurgical and surgical therapy. Dent Today 2001;20(3):86–91.

[11] Lang NP, Tonetti MS. Periodontal diagnosis in treated periodontitis. Why, when and how to use clinical parameters. J Clin Periodontol 1996;23(3 Pt 2):240–50.

[12] Genco RJ. Current view of risk factors for periodontal diseases. J Periodontol 1996; 67(Suppl 10):1041–9.

[13] Colburn WA. Biomarkers in drug discovery and development: from target identification through drug marketing. J Clin Pharmacol 2003;43(4):329–41.

[14] Kamma JJ, Giannopoulou C, Vasdekis VG, et al. Cytokine profile in gingival crevicular fluid of aggressive periodontitis: influence of smoking and stress. J Clin Periodontol 2004; 31(10):894–902.

[15] Souza SL, Taba M Jr. Cross-sectional evaluation of clinical parameters to select high prevalence populations for periodontal disease: the site comparative severity methodology. Braz Dent J 2004;15(1):46–53.

[16] Socransky SS, Haffajee AD. Dental biofilms: difficult therapeutic targets. Periodontol 2000 2002;28:12–55.

[17] Uitto VJ. Gingival crevice fluid—an introduction. Periodontol 2000 2003;31:9–11.

[18] Kaufman E, Lamster IB. Analysis of saliva for periodontal diagnosis—a review. J Clin Periodontol 2000;27(7):453–65.

[19] Paster BJ, Boches SK, Galvin JL, et al. Bacterial diversity in human subgingival plaque. J Bacteriol 2001;183(12):3770–83.

[20] Loesche WJ, Lopatin DE, Giordano J, et al. Comparison of the benzoyl-DL-arginine-naphthylamide (BANA) test, DNA probes, and immunological reagents for ability to detect anaerobic periodontal infections due to *Porphyromonas gingivalis, Treponema denticola*, and *Bacteroides forsythus*. J Clin Microbiol 1992;30(2):427–33.

[21] Loesche WJ, Kazor CE, Taylor GW. The optimization of the BANA test as a screening instrument for gingivitis among subjects seeking dental treatment. J Clin Periodontol 1997; 24(10):718–26.

[22] Socransky SS, Haffajee AD, Cugini MA, et al. Microbial complexes in subgingival plaque. J Clin Periodontol 1998;25(2):134–44.

[23] Zambon JJ. Periodontal diseases: microbial factors. Ann Periodontol 1996;1(1):879–925.

[24] Listgarten MA, Loomer PM. Microbial identification in the management of periodontal diseases. A systematic review. Ann Periodontol 2003;8(1):182–92.

[25] Offenbacher S, Jared HL, O'Reilly PG, et al. Potential pathogenic mechanisms of periodontitis associated pregnancy complications. Ann Periodontol 1998;3(1):233–50.

[26] Muller HP, Streletz E, Muller RF, et al. Microbiologic diagnosis and treatment of periodontally involved, "hopeless" teeth. Int J Periodontics Restorative Dent 1991;11(5): 376–86.

[27] Levy D, Csima A, Birek P, et al. Impact of microbiological consultation on clinical decision making: a case-control study of clinical management of recurrent periodontitis. J Periodontol 1993;64(11):1029–39.

[28] Rosenberg ES, Torosian JP, Hammond BF, et al. Routine anaerobic bacterial culture and systemic antibiotic usage in the treatment of adult periodontitis: a 6-year longitudinal study. Int J Periodontics Restorative Dent 1993;13(3):213–43.

[29] Fine DH. Microbial identification and antibiotic sensitivity testing, an aid for patients refractory to periodontal therapy. A report of 3 cases. J Clin Periodontol 1994;21(2):98–106.

[30] Ishikawa I, Umeda M, Laosrisin N. Clinical, bacteriological, and immunological examinations and the treatment process of two Papillon-Lefevre syndrome patients. J Periodontol 1994;65(4):364–71.

[31] Ishikawa I, Kawashima Y, Oda S, et al. Three case reports of aggressive periodontitis associated with *Porphyromonas gingivalis* in younger patients. J Periodontal Res 2002; 37(5):324–32.

[32] Renvert S, Dahlen G, Wikstrom M. Treatment of periodontal disease based on microbiological diagnosis. Relation between microbiological and clinical parameters during 5 years. J Periodontol 1996;67(6):562–71.

[33] Worch KP, Listgarten MA. Treatment considerations in rapidly progressive periodontitis: a case report. Compend Contin Educ Dent 1998;19(12):1203–6.

[34] Worch KP, Listgarten MA, Korostoff JM. A multidisciplinary approach to the diagnosis and treatment of early-onset periodontitis: a case report. J Periodontol 2001;72(1): 96–106.

[35] Kamma JJ, Lygidakis NA, Nakou M. Subgingival microflora and treatment in prepubertal periodontitis associated with chronic idiopathic neutropenia. J Clin Periodontol 1998; 25(9):759–65.

[36] De Vree H, Steenackers K, De Boever JA. Periodontal treatment of rapid progressive periodontitis in 2 siblings with Papillon-Lefevre syndrome: 15-year follow-up. J Clin Periodontol 2000;27(5):354–60.

[37] Eickholz P, Kugel B, Pohl S, et al. Combined mechanical and antibiotic periodontal therapy in a case of Papillon-Lefevre syndrome. J Periodontol 2001;72(4):542–9.

[38] Pacheco JJ, Coelho C, Salazar F, et al. Treatment of Papillon-Lefevre syndrome periodontitis. J Clin Periodontol 2002;29(4):370–4.

[39] Palys MD, Haffajee AD, Socransky SS, et al. Relationship between C-telopeptide pyridinoline cross-links (ICTP) and putative periodontal pathogens in periodontitis. J Clin Periodontol 1998;25(11 Pt 1):865–71.

[40] Oringer RJ, Palys MD, Iranmanesh A, et al. C-telopeptide pyridinoline cross-links (ICTP) and periodontal pathogens associated with endosseous oral implants. Clin Oral Implants Res 1998;9(6):365–73.

[41] Novaes Junior AB, Souza SL, Taba M Jr, et al. Control of gingival inflammation in a teenager population using ultrasonic prophylaxis. Braz Dent J 2004;15(1):41–5.

[42] Madianos PN, Papapanou PN, Sandros J. *Porphyromonas gingivalis* infection of oral epithelium inhibits neutrophil transepithelial migration. Infect Immun 1997;65(10): 3983–90.

[43] Page RC, Schroeder HE. Pathogenesis of inflammatory periodontal disease. A summary of current work. Lab Invest 1976;34(3):235–49.

[44] Soder B, Jin LJ, Wickholm S. Granulocyte elastase, matrix metalloproteinase-8 and prostaglandin E2 in gingival crevicular fluid in matched clinical sites in smokers and non-smokers with persistent periodontitis. J Clin Periodontol 2002;29(5):384–91.

[45] Golub LM, Kleinberg I. Gingival crevicular fluid: a new diagnostic aid in managing the periodontal patient. Oral Sci Rev 1976;8:49–61.

[46] Golub LM, McNamara TF, Ryan ME, et al. Adjunctive treatment with subantimicrobial doses of doxycycline: effects on gingival fluid collagenase activity and attachment loss in adult periodontitis. J Clin Periodontol 2001;28(2):146–56.

[47] Cimasoni G. Crevicular fluid updated. Monogr Oral Sci 1983;12(III-VII):1–152.

[48] Estreicher A, Broggiato A, Duroux P, et al. Low molecular-weight proteins in human gingival crevicular fluid. Arch Oral Biol 1996;41(8–9):733–8.

[49] Nakashima K, Giannopoulou C, Andersen E, et al. A longitudinal study of various crevicular fluid components as markers of periodontal disease activity. J Clin Periodontol 1996;23(9):832–8.

[50] Kojima T, Andersen E, Sanchez JC, et al. Human gingival crevicular fluid contains MRP8 (S100A8) and MRP14 (S100A9), two calcium-binding proteins of the S100 family. J Dent Res 2000;79(2):740–7.

[51] Engebretson SP, Hey-Hadavi J, Ehrhardt FJ, et al. Gingival crevicular fluid levels of interleukin-1beta and glycemic control in patients with chronic periodontitis and type 2 diabetes. J Periodontol 2004;75(9):1203–8.

[52] Lamster IB, Kaufman E, Grbic JT, et al. Beta-glucuronidase activity in saliva: relationship to clinical periodontal parameters. J Periodontol 2003;74(3):353–9.

[53] Engebretson SP, Grbic JT, Singer R, et al. GCF IL-1beta profiles in periodontal disease. J Clin Periodontol 2002;29(1):48–53.

[54] Grbic JT, Lamster IB, Fine JB, et al. Changes in gingival crevicular fluid levels of immunoglobulin A following therapy: association with attachment loss. J Periodontol 1999;70(10):1221–7.

[55] Grbic JT, Lamster IB, Mitchell-Lewis D. Inflammatory and immune mediators in crevicular fluid from HIV-infected injecting drug users. J Periodontol 1997;68(3): 249–55.

[56] Gustafsson A, Asman B, Bergstrom K. Elastase and lactoferrin in gingival crevicular fluid: possible indicators of a granulocyte-associated specific host response. J Periodontal Res 1994;29(4):276–82.

[57] Lerner UH, Modeer T, Krekmanova L, et al. Gingival crevicular fluid from patients with periodontitis contains bone resorbing activity. Eur J Oral Sci 1998;106(3):778–87.

[58] Rasmussen L, Hanstrom L, Lerner UH. Characterization of bone resorbing activity in gingival crevicular fluid from patients with periodontitis. J Clin Periodontol 2000;27(1): 41–52.

[59] Shapiro L, Goldman H, Bloom A. Sulcular exudate flow in gingival inflammation. J Periodontol 1979;50(6):301–4.

[60] Novaes AB Jr, Shapiro L, Fillios LC, et al. Gingival fluid fucose to protein ratios as indicators of the severity of periodontal disease. J Periodontol 1980;51(2):88–94.

[61] Gapski R, Barr JL, Sarment DP, et al. Effect of systemic matrix metalloproteinase inhibition on periodontal wound repair: a proof of concept trial. J Periodontol 2004;75(3): 441–52.

[62] Figueredo CM, Areas A, Miranda LA, et al. The short-term effectiveness of non-surgical treatment in reducing protease activity in gingival crevicular fluid from chronic periodontitis patients. J Clin Periodontol 2004;31(8):615–9.

[63] Golub LM, Lee HM, Greenwald RA, et al. A matrix metalloproteinase inhibitor reduces bone-type collagen degradation fragments and specific collagenases in gingival crevicular fluid during adult periodontitis. Inflamm Res 1997;46(8):310–9.

[64] Kinane DF, Darby IB, Said S, et al. Changes in gingival crevicular fluid matrix metalloproteinase-8 levels during periodontal treatment and maintenance. J Periodontal Res 2003;38(4):400–4.

[65] Mantyla P, Stenman M, Kinane DF, et al. Gingival crevicular fluid collagenase-2 (MMP-8) test stick for chair-side monitoring of periodontitis. J Periodontal Res 2003;38(4):436–9.

[66] Oringer RJ, Al-Shammari KF, Aldredge WA, et al. Effect of locally delivered minocycline microspheres on markers of bone resorption. J Periodontol 2002;73(8):835–42.

[67] Ryan ME, Ramamurthy S, Golub LM. Matrix metalloproteinases and their inhibition in periodontal treatment. Curr Opin Periodontol 1996;3:85–96.

[68] Ingman T, Tervahartiala T, Ding Y, et al. Matrix metalloproteinases and their inhibitors in gingival crevicular fluid and saliva of periodontitis patients. J Clin Periodontol 1996;23(12): 1127–32.

[69] Mellanen L, Ingman T, Lahdevirta J, et al. Matrix metalloproteinases-1, -3 and -8 and myeloperoxidase in saliva of patients with human immunodeficiency virus infection. Oral Dis 1996;2(4):263–71.

[70] Teronen O, Konttinen YT, Lindqvist C, et al. Inhibition of matrix metalloproteinase-1 by dichloromethylene bisphosphonate (clodronate). Calcif Tissue Int 1997;61(1):59–61.

[71] Makela M, Salo T, Uitto VJ, et al. Matrix metalloproteinases (MMP-2 and MMP-9) of the oral cavity: cellular origin and relationship to periodontal status. J Dent Res 1994;73(8): 1397–406.

[72] Amar S, Oyaisu K, Li L, et al. Moesin: a potential LPS receptor on human monocytes. J Endotoxin Res 2001;7(4):281–6.

[73] Mogi M, Otogoto J, Ota N, et al. Interleukin 1 beta, interleukin 6, beta 2-microglobulin, and transforming growth factor-alpha in gingival crevicular fluid from human periodontal disease. Arch Oral Biol 1999;44(6):535–9.

[74] Holmlund A, Hanstrom L, Lerner UH. Bone resorbing activity and cytokine levels in gingival crevicular fluid before and after treatment of periodontal disease. J Clin Periodontol 2004;31(6):475–82.
[75] Assuma R, Oates T, Cochran D, et al. IL-1 and TNF antagonists inhibit the inflammatory response and bone loss in experimental periodontitis. J Immunol 1998;160(1):403–9.
[76] Graves DT, Delima AJ, Assuma R, et al. Interleukin-1 and tumor necrosis factor antagonists inhibit the progression of inflammatory cell infiltration toward alveolar bone in experimental periodontitis. J Periodontol 1998;69(12):1419–25.
[77] Ranney RR. Immunologic mechanisms of pathogenesis in periodontal diseases: an assessment. J Periodontal Res 1991;26(3 Pt 2):243–54.
[78] Seymour GJ, Cole KL, Powell RN. Analysis of lymphocyte populations extracted from chronically inflamed human periodontal tissues. I. Identification. J Periodontal Res 1985; 20(1):47–57.
[79] Seymour GJ, Cole KL, Powell RN. Analysis of lymphocyte populations extracted from chronically inflamed human periodontal tissues. II. Blastogenic response. J Periodontal Res 1985;20(6):571–9.
[80] Condorelli F, Scalia G, Cali G, et al. Isolation of *Porphyromonas gingivalis* and detection of immunoglobulin A specific to fimbrial antigen in gingival crevicular fluid. J Clin Microbiol 1998;36(8):2322–5.
[81] Kinane DF, Takahashi K, Mooney J. Crevicular fluid and serum IgG subclasses and corresponding mRNA expressing plasma cells in periodontitis lesions. J Periodontal Res 1997;32(1 Pt 2):176–8.
[82] Dibart S, Eftimiadi C, Socransky S, et al. Rapid evaluation of serum and gingival crevicular fluid immunoglobulin G subclass antibody levels in patients with early-onset periodontitis using checkerboard immunoblotting. Oral Microbiol Immunol 1998;13(3):166–72.
[83] Plombas M, Gobert B, De March AK, et al. Isotypic antibody response to plaque anaerobes in periodontal disease. J Periodontol 2002;73(12):1507–11.
[84] Haffajee AD, Socransky SS. Microbial etiological agents of destructive periodontal diseases. Periodontol 2000 1994;5:78–111.
[85] Courant PR, Bader H. Bacteroides melaninogenicus and its products in the gingiva of man. Periodontics 1966;4(3):131–6.
[86] Eley BM, Cox SW. Bacterial proteases in gingival crevicular fluid before and after periodontal treatment. Br Dent J 1995;178(4):133–9.
[87] Eley BM, Cox SW. Cathepsin B/L-, elastase-, tryptase-, trypsin- and dipeptidyl peptidase IV-like activities in gingival crevicular fluid: correlation with clinical parameters in untreated chronic periodontitis patients. J Periodontal Res 1992;27(1):62–9.
[88] Lamster IB. Evaluation of components of gingival crevicular fluid as diagnostic tests. Ann Periodontol 1997;2(1):123–37.
[89] Oringer RJ, Howell TH, Nevins ML, et al. Relationship between crevicular aspartate aminotransferase levels and periodontal disease progression. J Periodontol 2001;72(1): 17–24.
[90] Kamma JJ, Nakou M, Persson RG. Association of early onset periodontitis microbiota with aspartate aminotransferase activity in gingival crevicular fluid. J Clin Periodontol 2001;28(12):1096–105.
[91] Takahashi K, Mooney J, Frandsen EV, et al. IgG and IgA subclass mRNA-bearing plasma cells in periodontitis gingival tissue and immunoglobulin levels in the gingival crevicular fluid. Clin Exp Immunol 1997;107(1):158–65.
[92] Giannobile WV. C-telopeptide pyridinoline cross-links. Sensitive indicators of periodontal tissue destruction. Ann N Y Acad Sci 1999;878:404–12.
[93] Giannobile WV, Al-Shammari KF, Sarment DP. Matrix molecules and growth factors as indicators of periodontal disease activity. Periodontol 2000 2003;31:125–34.
[94] Narayanan AS, Page RC. Connective tissues of the periodontium: a summary of current work. Coll Relat Res 1983;3(1):33–64.

[95] Johnell O, Oden A, De Laet C, et al. Biochemical indices of bone turnover and the assessment of fracture probability. Osteoporos Int 2002;13(7):523–6.

[96] Calvo MS, Eyre DR, Gundberg CM. Molecular basis and clinical application of biological markers of bone turnover. Endocr Rev 1996;17(4):333–68.

[97] Eriksen EF, Charles P, Melsen F, et al. Serum markers of type I collagen formation and degradation in metabolic bone disease: correlation with bone histomorphometry. J Bone Miner Res 1993;8(2):127–32.

[98] Garnero P, Delmas PD. An immunoassay for type I collagen alpha 1 helicoidal peptide 620–633, a new marker of bone resorption in osteoporosis. Bone 2003;32(1):20–6.

[99] Risteli J, Elomaa I, Niemi S, et al. Radioimmunoassay for the pyridinoline cross-linked carboxy-terminal telopeptide of type I collagen: a new serum marker of bone collagen degradation. Clin Chem 1993;39(4):635–40.

[100] Colwell A, Russell RG, Eastell R. Factors affecting the assay of urinary 3-hydroxy pyridinium crosslinks of collagen as markers of bone resorption. Eur J Clin Invest 1993; 23(6):341–9.

[101] Black D, Marabani M, Sturrock RD, et al. Urinary excretion of the hydroxypyridinium cross links of collagen in patients with rheumatoid arthritis. Ann Rheum Dis 1989;48(8): 641–4.

[102] Uebelhart D, Gineyts E, Chapuy MC, et al. Urinary excretion of pyridinium crosslinks: a new marker of bone resorption in metabolic bone disease. Bone Miner 1990;8(1): 87–96.

[103] Garnero P, Gineyts E, Riou JP, et al. Assessment of bone resorption with a new marker of collagen degradation in patients with metabolic bone disease. J Clin Endocrinol Metab 1994;79(3):780–5.

[104] Yasumizu T, Hoshi K, Iijima S, et al. Serum concentration of the pyridinoline cross-linked carboxyterminal telopeptide of type I collagen (ICTP) is a useful indicator of decline and recovery of bone mineral density in lumbar spine: analysis in Japanese postmenopausal women with or without hormone replacement. Endocr J 1998;45(1):45–51.

[105] Giannobile WV. Crevicular fluid biomarkers of oral bone loss. Curr Opin Periodontol 1997;4:11–20.

[106] Giannobile WV, Lynch SE, Denmark RG, et al. Crevicular fluid osteocalcin and pyridinoline cross-linked carboxyterminal telopeptide of type I collagen (ICTP) as markers of rapid bone turnover in periodontitis. A pilot study in beagle dogs. J Clin Periodontol 1995;22(12):903–10.

[107] Shibutani T, Murahashi Y, Tsukada E, et al. Experimentally induced periodontitis in beagle dogs causes rapid increases in osteoclastic resorption of alveolar bone. J Periodontol 1997;68(4):385–91.

[108] Talonpoika JT, Hamalainen MM. Type I collagen carboxyterminal telopeptide in human gingival crevicular fluid in different clinical conditions and after periodontal treatment. J Clin Periodontol 1994;21(5):320–6.

[109] Perez LA, Al-Shammari KF, Giannobile WV, et al. Treatment of periodontal disease in a patient with Ehlers-Danlos syndrome. A case report and literature review. J Periodontol 2002;73(5):564–70.

[110] Williams RC, Paquette DW, Offenbacher S, et al. Treatment of periodontitis by local administration of minocycline microspheres: a controlled trial. J Periodontol 2001;72(11): 1535–44.

[111] Al-Shammari KF, Giannobile WV, Aldredge WA, et al. Effect of non-surgical periodontal therapy on C-telopeptide pyridinoline cross-links (ICTP) and interleukin-1 levels. J Periodontol 2001;72(8):1045–51.

[112] Lian JB, Gundberg CM. Osteocalcin. Biochemical considerations and clinical applications. Clin Orthop 1988;226:267–91.

[113] Bronckers AL, Gay S, Dimuzio MT, et al. Immunolocalization of gamma-carboxyglutamic acid containing proteins in developing rat bones. Coll Relat Res 1985;5(3):273–81.

[114] Ducy P, Geoffroy V, Karsenty G. Study of osteoblast-specific expression of one mouse osteocalcin gene: characterization of the factor binding to OSE2. Connect Tissue Res 1996; 35(1–4):7–14.

[115] Garnero P, Delmas PD. Biochemical markers of bone turnover. Applications for osteoporosis. Endocrinol Metab Clin N Am 1998;27(2):303–23.

[116] Chenu C, Colucci S, Grano M, et al. Osteocalcin induces chemotaxis, secretion of matrix proteins, and calcium-mediated intracellular signaling in human osteoclast-like cells. J Cell Biol 1994;127(4):1149–58.

[117] Glowacki J, Lian JB. Impaired recruitment and differentiation of osteoclast progenitors by osteocalcin-deplete bone implants. Cell Differ 1987;21(4):247–54.

[118] Mundy GR, Poser JW. Chemotactic activity of the gamma-carboxyglutamic acid containing protein in bone. Calcif Tissue Int 1983;35(2):164–8.

[119] Canalis E. Effect of growth factors on bone cell replication and differentiation. Clin Orthop 1985;193:246–63.

[120] Bataille R, Delmas P, Sany J. Serum bone gla-protein in multiple myeloma. Cancer 1987; 59(2):329–34.

[121] Slovik DM, Gundberg CM, Neer RM, et al. Clinical evaluation of bone turnover by serum osteocalcin measurements in a hospital setting. J Clin Endocrinol Metab 1984;59(2): 228–30.

[122] Brown JP, Delmas PD, Malaval L, et al. Serum bone Gla-protein: a specific marker for bone formation in postmenopausal osteoporosis. Lancet 1984;1(8386):1091–3.

[123] Delmas PD, Chatelain P, Malaval L, et al. Serum bone GLA-protein in growth hormone deficient children. J Bone Miner Res 1986;1(4):333–8.

[124] Kunimatsu K, Mataki S, Tanaka H, et al. A cross-sectional study on osteocalcin levels in gingival crevicular fluid from periodontal patients. J Periodontol 1993;64(9):865–9.

[125] Lee AJ, Walsh TF, Hodges SJ, et al. Gingival crevicular fluid osteocalcin in adult periodontitis. J Clin Periodontol 1999;26(4):252–6.

[126] Nakashima K, Roehrich N, Cimasoni G. Osteocalcin, prostaglandin E2 and alkaline phosphatase in gingival crevicular fluid: their relations to periodontal status. J Clin Periodontol 1994;21(5):327–33.

[127] Griffiths GS, Moulson AM, Petrie A, et al. Evaluation of osteocalcin and pyridinium crosslinks of bone collagen as markers of bone turnover in gingival crevicular fluid during different stages of orthodontic treatment. J Clin Periodontol 1998;25(6):492–8.

[128] Biomarkers Definitions Working Group. Biomarkers and surrogate endpoints: preferred definitions and conceptual framework. Clin Pharmacol Ther 2001;69(3):89–95.

[129] Ozmeric N. Advances in periodontal disease markers. Clin Chim Acta 2004;343(1–2):1–16.

[130] Zambon JJ, Nakamura M, Slots J. Effect of periodontal therapy on salivary enzymatic activity. J Periodontal Res 1985;20(6):652–9.

[131] Hayakawa H, Yamashita K, Ohwaki K, et al. Collagenase activity and tissue inhibitor of metalloproteinases-1 (TIMP-1) content in human whole saliva from clinically healthy and periodontally diseased subjects. J Periodontal Res 1994;29(5):305–8.

[132] Ferguson DB. Current diagnostic uses of saliva. J Dent Res 1987;66(2):420–4.

[133] Lamster IB, Grbic JT. Diagnosis of periodontal disease based on analysis of the host response. Periodontol 2000 1995;7:83–99.

[134] Mandel ID. The diagnostic uses of saliva. J Oral Pathol Med 1990;19(3):119–25.

[135] Nakamura M, Slots J. Salivary enzymes. Origin and relationship to periodontal disease. J Periodontal Res 1983;18(6):559–69.

[136] Reynolds SJ, Muwonga J. OraQuick ADVANCE Rapid HIV-1/2 antibody test. Expert Rev Mol Diagn 2004;4(5):587–91.

[137] Kornman KS, Crane A, Wang HY, et al. The interleukin-1 genotype as a severity factor in adult periodontal disease. J Clin Periodontol 1997;24(1):72–7.

[138] Greenstein G, Hart TC. Clinical utility of a genetic susceptibility test for severe chronic periodontitis: a critical evaluation. J Am Dent Assoc 2002;133(4):452–9 [quiz: 492–3].

[139] Socransky SS, Haffajee AD, Smith C, et al. Microbiological parameters associated with IL-1 gene polymorphisms in periodontitis patients. J Clin Periodontol 2000;27(11):810–8.

[140] Li Y, Zhou X, St John MA, et al. RNA profiling of cell-free saliva using microarray technology. J Dent Res 2004;83(3):199–203.

[141] St John MA, Li Y, Zhou X, et al. Interleukin 6 and interleukin 8 as potential biomarkers for oral cavity and oropharyngeal squamous cell carcinoma. Arch Otolaryngol Head Neck Surg 2004;130(8):929–35.

[142] Aufricht C, Tenner W, Salzer HR, et al. Salivary IgA concentration is influenced by the saliva collection method. Eur J Clin Chem Clin Biochem 1992;30(2):81–3.

[143] Wilton JM, Curtis MA, Gillett IR, et al. Detection of high-risk groups and individuals for periodontal diseases: laboratory markers from analysis of saliva. J Clin Periodontol 1989; 16(8):475–83.

[144] Bokor M. Immunoglobulin A levels in the saliva in patients with periodontal disease. Med Pregl 1997;50(1–2):9–11.

[145] Anil S, Remani P, Beena VT, et al. Immunoglobulins in the saliva of diabetic patients with periodontitis. Ann Dent 1995;54(1–2):30–3.

[146] Schenck K, Poppelsdorf D, Denis C, et al. Levels of salivary IgA antibodies reactive with bacteria from dental plaque are associated with susceptibility to experimental gingivitis. J Clin Periodontol 1993;20(6):411–7.

[147] Sandholm L, Tolo K, Olsen I. Salivary IgG, a parameter of periodontal disease activity? High responders to *Actinobacillus actinomycetemcomitans* Y4 in juvenile and adult periodontitis. J Clin Periodontol 1987;14(5):289–94.

[148] Nieminen A, Kari K, Saxen L. Specific antibodies against *Actinobacillus actinomycetemcomitans* in serum and saliva of patients with advanced periodontitis. Scand J Dent Res 1993; 101(4):196–201.

[149] McLaughlin WS, Kirkham J, Kowolik MJ, et al. Human gingival crevicular fluid keratin at healthy, chronic gingivitis and chronic adult periodontitis sites. J Clin Periodontol 1996; 23(4):331–5.

[150] Kopczyk RA, Graham R, Abrams H, et al. The feasibility and reliability of using a home screening test to detect gingival inflammation. J Periodontol 1995;66(1):52–4.

[151] Sewon L, Makela M. A study of the possible correlation of high salivary calcium levels with periodontal and dental conditions in young adults. Arch Oral Biol 1990;35(Suppl):211–2.

[152] Sewon LA, Karjalainen SM, Sainio M, et al. Calcium and other salivary factors in periodontitis-affected subjects prior to treatment. J Clin Periodontol 1995;22(4):267–70.

[153] Genco RJ, Ho AW, Kopman J, et al. Models to evaluate the role of stress in periodontal disease. Ann Periodontol 1998;3(1):288–302.

[154] Beck JD. Risk revisited. Community Dent Oral Epidemiol 1998;26(4):220–5.

[155] Burt BA. Risk factors, risk markers, and risk indicators. Community Dent Oral Epidemiol 1998;26(4):219.

ELSEVIER
SAUNDERS

Dent Clin N Am 49 (2005) 573–594

THE DENTAL
CLINICS
OF NORTH AMERICA

Prevention of Periodontal Diseases

Andrew R. Dentino, DDS, PhD*,
Moawia M. Kassab, DDS, MS,
Erica J. Renner, RDH, MS

Department of Surgical Sciences,
Marquette University School of Dentistry,
P.O. Box 1881, Milwaukee, WI 53201-1881, USA

Prevention of periodontal diseases, including gingivitis and periodontitis, has been defined as a multistage process with primary, secondary, and tertiary components [1]. Primary prevention involves preventing inception of disease and includes the concept of health promotion and protection strategies. These health promotion strategies, aimed at enabling groups or individuals to control and improve their health, include providing oral hygiene education and protection strategies such as fluoridation. In developed nations, dentistry has been successful in these primary prevention areas. This success is illustrated by improvements in attitudes toward the importance of oral hygiene and the provision of fluoridated water supplies [2,3]. Secondary disease prevention aims to limit the impact of disease by way of early diagnosis and treatment, thereby stopping disease progression in its earliest stages. The concept of tertiary disease prevention is focused on the rehabilitation of the functional limitations that arise due to the disabilities encountered after advanced disease and includes such things as implants and prosthetic restoration of missing teeth.

Because the ultimate goal is to maintain the dentition over a lifetime in a state of health, comfort, and function in an esthetically pleasing presentation, this article focuses on the first two stages of periodontal disease prevention as they relate to gingivitis and periodontitis. Because these diseases are biofilm mediated and oral hygiene is important in all stages of prevention, certain concepts discussed here can and should be applied to all three phases of disease prevention. This article discusses risk assessment, mechanical plaque control, chemical plaque control, current clinical recommendations for optimal prevention, and future preventive strategies.

---

* Corresponding author.

E-mail address: andrew.dentino@marquette.edu (A.R. Dentino).

0011-8532/05/$ - see front matter © 2005 Elsevier Inc. All rights reserved.
doi:10.1016/j.cden.2005.03.005
dental.theclinics.com

Risk assessment as an aid in prevention

The idea of applying risk assessment information to supportive periodontal care after thorough surgical or nonsurgical periodontal therapy is not new or untested. Axelsson and coworkers [4–6] demonstrated that this approach essentially eliminates the recurrence of caries and periodontal disease. Until recently, however, there has not been any validated and generally accepted tool for risk assessment. Through the 1960s, the concept of varying susceptibility to periodontitis was not widely accepted because early epidemiologic studies suggested that the disease was essentially pandemic in adults [7,8]. Subsequent experimental work on animals demonstrated variability in disease expression [9], and more precise human population studies showed substantially lower prevalence rates for moderate to advanced periodontitis [10]. These findings strongly suggested that differing susceptibilities for periodontal disease existed within a population. Much work has been done since that time to define local, environmental, and genetic factors that place individuals at a higher risk for developing periodontitis [11–14].

A risk factor is defined as some aspect of personal behavior or lifestyle, an environmental exposure, or an inherited characteristic that based on epidemiologic evidence is known to be hazardous to one's health and well-being [15]. The presence of a risk factor increases the probability of developing the disease and represents a possible target for prevention or therapy. Although it is beyond the scope of this article to review the evidence that has accumulated over the last 2 decades regarding identification of risk factors and their strength of association with periodontitis, there are several factors that have repeatedly been documented. Examples of such risk factors include cigarette smoking, uncontrolled diabetes, irregular dental care, and plaque in the presence of attachment loss. This article focuses on recent research efforts to quantify the risk assessment because this represents a major step forward in the attempt to tailor preventive strategies for individuals.

As dentistry and periodontics begin to transition from a repair model of oral health care to a wellness model, the need to be able to predictably quantify levels of risk is crucial. In the last World Workshop of Periodontics, the consensus report on prevention stated that the incorporation of risk assessment models for prevention of periodontal disease is an important goal. The concept of continuous multilevel risk assessment has developed and has been promoted as an important, if not essential, factor in proper patient assessment as part of treatment planning and reassessment during maintenance [16]. One of the consistent therapeutic goals in the American Academy of Periodontology's Parameters of Care is to reduce or eliminate contributing risk factors for gingivitis and periodontitis [17]. Moreover, the latest American Academy of Periodontology position paper on periodontal maintenance recommends that dental professionals should counsel people on the control of risk factors [18]. The actual assessment and application of risk levels in prevention and management of periodontitis, however, is in its infancy.

Although there are odds ratios and relative risk levels published for a variety of exposures as a crude means to assess the importance of each factor, there is currently little to no information on the interactions of these different risk factors. Clearly, not all of the relevant risk factors have been uncovered.

Recently, a few clinical risk assessment approaches or tools have been promoted in the literature. One tool is a relatively simple questionnaire [19] that provides a vague but individual risk profile for the clinician and an educational tool for communication with the patient. A more sophisticated instrument employs a continuous multilevel risk assessment that incorporates the consideration of subject, tooth, and site risk evaluations [16]. This approach generates functional diagrams that provide a more objective means of quantifying an individual's risk (Fig. 1) [16]. Depending on the area of the polygon, a patient may fall into low-, moderate-, or high-risk categories. The patient's individual periodontal risk assessment is low if all parameters fall

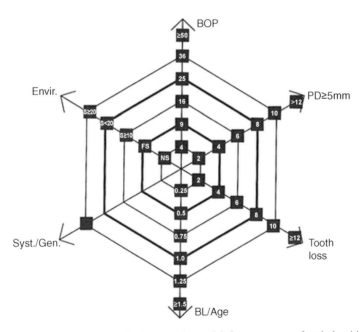

Fig. 1. Functional diagram to evaluate the patient's risk for recurrence of periodontitis. Each vector represents one risk factor or indicator with an area of relatively low risk, an area of moderate risk, and an area of high risk for disease progression. All factors have to be evaluated together; therefore, the area of relatively low risk is found within the center circle of the polygon, whereas the area of high risk is found outside the periphery of the second ring in bold. Between the two rings in bold, there is the area of moderate risk. BL, bone loss; BOP, bleeding on probing; Envir., environment; FS, frequent smoker; NS, nonsmoker; PD, pocket depth; S, smoker; Syst./Gen., systemic/general. (*From* Lang NP, Bragger U, Salvi G, et al. Supportive periodontal therapy (SPT). In: Lindhe J, Karring T, Lang NP, editors. Clinical periodontology and implantology. 4th edition. Oxford (England): Blackwell Munksgaard; 2003. p. 788; with permission.)

within the low-risk categories or if only one category in the moderate-risk range (Fig. 2). A moderate periodontal risk assessment shows at least two parameters in the moderate category, with a maximum of one parameter in the high-risk area (Fig. 3). A patient with a high periodontal risk assessment has at least two parameters in the high-risk category (Fig. 4). Although this model still needs to be validated, it provides an objective quantification of risk into three categories. This assessment could provide justification for more or less aggressive preventive care.

Using a different multifactorial model, Page and coworkers [22] developed the "Periodontal Risk Calculator" (PRC). The PRC incorporates mathematic algorithms that are based on nine known risk factors: age, smoking history, diabetes diagnosis, history of periodontal surgery, pocket depth, furcation involvements, restorations or calculus below the gingival margin, radiographic bone height, and vertical bone lesions. This Web-based instrument can be accessed at http://www.previser.com, and to the authors' knowledge, provides the first validated tool to objectively quantify risk. Because risk assessments based on subjective expert opinion have been shown

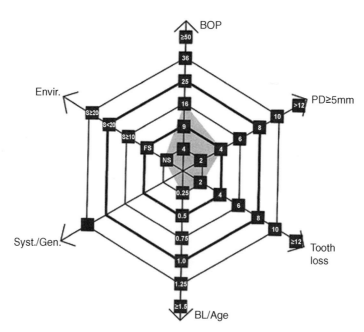

Fig. 2. Functional diagram of a low-risk maintenance patient. Bleeding on probing (BOP) is 15%, four residual pockets ≥ 5 mm are diagnosed, two teeth have been lost, the bone factor in relation to age is 0.25, no systemic factor is known, and the patient is a nonsmoker. BL, bone loss; Envir., environment; FS, frequent smoker; NS, nonsmoker; PD, pocket depth; S, smoker; Syst./Gen., systemic/general. (*From* Lang NP, Bragger U, Salvi G, et al. Supportive periodontal therapy (SPT). In: Lindhe J, Karring T, Lang NP, editors. Clinical periodontology and implantology. 4th edition. Oxford (England): Blackwell Munksgaard; 2003. p. 788; with permission.)

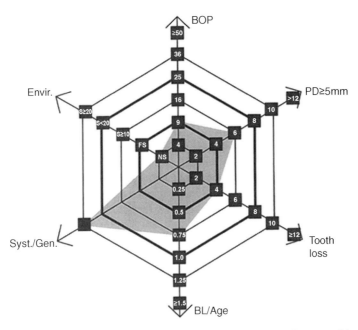

Fig. 3. Functional diagram of a medium-risk maintenance patient. Bleeding on probing (BOP) is 9%, six residual pockets ≥ 5 mm are diagnosed, four teeth have been lost, the bone factor in relation to age is 0.75, the patient has type I diabetes mellitus, and the patient is a nonsmoker. BL, bone loss; Envir., environment; FS, frequent smoker; NS, nonsmoker; PD, pocket depth; S, smoker; Syst./Gen., systemic/general. (*From* Lang NP, Bragger U, Salvi G, et al. Supportive periodontal therapy (SPT). In: Lindhe J, Karring T, Lang NP, editors. Clinical periodontology and implantology. 4th edition. Oxford (England): Blackwell Munksgaard; 2003. p. 799; with permission.)

to vary too much to be useful in everyday clinical decision making [20], the development of the PRC may well represent a major step forward in the transition from the surgical/repair model of dentistry to the wellness or medical model of patient care. Data suggest that expert clinicians in the United States and Europe appear to base most of their risk assessment on severity of disease at presentation rather than on factors such as smoking, diabetic status, and poor oral hygiene [20]. Moreover, it has been observed that "risk scores generated for individual patients by subjective expert clinician opinion are highly variable and could result in the misapplication of treatment for some patients" [21]. Overtreatment or undertreatment of periodontal diseases may be the result of subjectively forming such opinions.

Using a clinical patient data set from the VA Dental Longitudinal Study of Oral Health and Disease, Page and coworkers [22,23] retrospectively assigned risk scores to each of the 523 subjects on a 1 (lowest) to 5 (highest) risk scale using information from the baseline examination. They subsequently assessed radiographic bone loss and tooth loss over the next 15 years. The mean percentage of bone loss followed a consistent pattern from least bone loss in

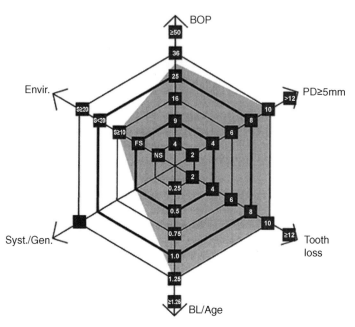

Fig. 4. Functional diagram of a high-risk maintenance patient. Bleeding on probing (BOP) is 32%, 10 residual pockets ≥5 mm are diagnosed, 10 teeth have been lost, the bone factor in relation to age is 1.25, no systemic factor is known, and the patient is an occasional smoker. BL, bone loss; Envir., environment; FS, frequent smoker; NS, nonsmoker; PD, pocket depth; S, smoker; Syst./Gen., systemic/general. (*From* Lang NP, Bragger U, Salvi G, et al. Supportive periodontal therapy (SPT). In: Lindhe J, Karring T, Lang NP, editors. Clinical periodontology and implantology. 4th edition. Oxford (England): Blackwell Munksgaard; 2003. p. 799; with permission.)

the low-risk category to greatest bone loss in the highest risk category (2<3<4<5). Several measures of tooth loss over time showed a similar relationship. Clearly, this approach to validation had weaknesses that included the retrospective nature of the study, the lack of enough low-risk subjects (periodontal risk assessment = 1) to allow for the full range of risk levels to be validated, and the lack of data on why teeth were lost. In addition, for teeth without periodontal disease at baseline, the PRC did not appear to discriminate between risk levels. This study, however, demonstrated the ability of the PRC to "predict" with accuracy and validity periodontal deterioration and even tooth loss for teeth with periodontal disease at baseline.

In addition to providing a quick and objective risk assessment, the PRC provides a periodontal diagnosis, a quantitative disease score from 1 to 100, and treatment options based on the current American Academy of Periodontology standards of care. If this technology catches on, it may have a substantial impact on the dental profession. The PRC would provide a useful tool for individual patient assessment and may help sort out cost-effective treatments and even suggest rational approaches to preventive measures. Accurate and objective risk prediction should provide dentistry the ability to make serious strides in moving toward a wellness model of patient care. It has the potential to substantially improve the allocation of health care dollars by reducing the overtreatment of low-risk patients and applying more aggressive preventive strategies to high-risk patients.

Mechanical plaque control

Successful primary or secondary prevention is based on two major factors, the first being proper, thorough treatment during active therapy and the second being patient compliance with daily plaque removal and regular professional supportive care. Because other articles in this issue of the *Dental Clinics of North America* deal with active surgical and nonsurgical treatments to eliminate disease, the current authors confine themselves to addressing current concepts in primary prevention of gingivitis and periodontitis and the personal and professional supportive methods to avoid recurrence after active therapy is finished. The authors' premise is that proper and thorough active treatment means leaving the patient with a maintainable periodontium, which can be accomplished with nonsurgical therapy in the disease control phase of treatment or after the surgical corrective phase.

There is overwhelming evidence for the direct cause-and-effect relationship between the formation and accumulation of supragingival plaque and the development of gingivitis. It is also generally accepted that the loss of attachment and alveolar bone that defines periodontitis is preceded by gingival inflammation and subgingival plaque maturation.

It has been estimated that in a periodontitis patient with a full complement of teeth (28 teeth/168 sites) only 6% or less of these sites exhibit tissue destruction at any given time [24]. Although only a small percentage of gingivitis sites may progress to periodontitis, it still cannot be discerned which inflamed sites are actively breaking down. Traditionally, the default approach has been to try to eliminate all plaque-induced inflammation, particularly in subjects who have shown a susceptibility to a destructive periodontal inflammation. The first line of defense against plaque-induced gingivitis has always been daily meticulous mechanical plaque removal supplemented by periodic professional mechanical tooth cleaning.

Toothbrushing: manual versus powered

Toothbrushing has played the major role in daily plaque control in developed nations for over 60 years. According to the Lemelson-MIT Invention Index at the Massachusetts Institute of Technology, when Americans were asked to list the five inventions that they believed they could not live without, the toothbrush was more appreciated than the car, the personal computer, the cell phone, and the microwave oven [24a].

Many novel manual toothbrush designs and methods of brushing have been described in the literature, with no one design or method showing a clear superiority. There is no consensus on the optimal frequency of toothbrushing, but it is clear that the average person is not very efficient or thorough in daily plaque removal [25]. Hawkins et al [26] and Beals et al [27] showed that most subjects spend less than a minute brushing their teeth with a manual toothbrush. It therefore seems reasonable for clinicians to ask whether it is time to start recommending powered brushes with automatic timers to moderate- and high-risk patients.

When Van der Weijden and coworkers [28,29] performed professional plaque removal on subjects for varying duration using a manual or an oscillating/rotating powered brush, they demonstrated that manual brushing, even after 6 minutes, only removed 75% of the plaque that the powered brush removed in 1 minute. Although one can argue the applicability of these particular data to direct patient use, there are additional studies that suggest that the electric toothbrush may prove advantageous for some patients. Several long-term (6 months or more) randomized controlled clinical trials have shown clinical benefits for certain powered brush designs compared with a manual brush in different populations with different levels of oral hygiene instruction [30–35]. The differences between manual and powered brushing are more evident when oral hygiene instruction is provided and reinforced during these long-term trials.

In perhaps the most comprehensive 6-month comparative clinical trial between a manual and a powered brush (oscillating/rotating type), Haffajee and coworkers [36,37] showed significantly better reduction in gingival index and attachment levels for the powered brush group, with mandibular and lingual surfaces showing the most benefit. They further demonstrated in both groups that a high level of personal supragingival plaque control had an unexpected and substantial beneficial effect on the subgingival flora. The decreased prevalence of periodontal pathogens from subgingival and supragingival plaque should lower the risk of periodontal disease initiation and recurrence. They further speculated that the lack of a significant microbiologic difference between the manual and the powered brush groups might be because the areas of greatest differences in clinical parameters (lingual and mandibular) were not the same areas that were sampled microbiologically (mesial-buccal site of each tooth).

Recently, two systematic reviews were published that addressed the comparative efficacy and safety of manual versus powered toothbrushing. Sicilia and coworkers [38] concluded that the counter-rotational and the oscillating/rotating brushes can be more beneficial than a manual toothbrush in reducing the levels of gingival bleeding. A Cochrane Review noted that no powered toothbrush designs except for the oscillating/rotating action were consistently superior to manual brushing. It was found that the oscillating/rotating brush achieves a modest reduction in plaque and gingivitis compared with manual toothbrushing and that it is safe to use [39]. The long-term implications of these findings are unknown.

There are limited data regarding the compliance of powered toothbrush use in periodontitis patients. Stalnacke and coworkers [40] found a 62% rate of daily compliance by maintenance patients at least 3 years after obtaining a powered brush. Only 3% had stopped using the powered brush altogether. In a study that specifically assessed low-compliance periodontal maintenance patients, another group showed an improved level of plaque control over 12 to 36 months in subjects using a powered brush [41]. Additional long-term studies would be useful.

More recently, McCracken et al [42] recruited a small population of untreated periodontitis patients into a short-term powered toothbrush compliance study. Using a microelectronic device within each brush to record duration and pressure, the investigators gained further insight into powered toothbrush home use. Subjects were informed that the device would measure toothbrush performance only. No details were given as to what this meant in terms of their compliance. McCracken et al [42] found that over 2 months of use, only about one third of these patients were truly compliant in using the brush for 2 minutes twice a day, nearly one third of the subjects overused the brush, and approximately one third substantially underused the brush. These data suggest that most but not all periodontitis patients using a powered brush are compliant. Patient education and motivation, as expected, play the greatest role in personal mechanical plaque control.

The plaque removal efficacy of the powered brush appears to come primarily from more efficient plaque removal on buccal and lingual ap-proximal surfaces, with the problem of interproximal plaque removal still unresolved [43]. Clearly, although powered brushes are more efficient at plaque removal, maximum benefit can only be achieved by proper instruction and patient motivation.

Interdental cleaning

Based on current knowledge, it seems reasonable to conclude that some form of regular interdental cleaning is necessary to maintain periodontal health because no toothbrush effectively disrupts true interproximal plaque, particularly in the posterior dentition. In addition, there is a clear interdental site predilection for gingivitis, periodontitis, and smooth-surface caries. Interdental areas truly are the key high-risk surfaces [44].

There are many different types of interdental cleaning aids, but the most widely recommended is dental floss or tape. Floss is most useful in the nonperiodontitis patient who has full interdental papillae and no exposed concave root surfaces. When used properly, it can penetrate the interproximal sulcus approximately 2 to 3 mm. Axelsson et al [45] recommended that flat, fluoridated dental tape be used before brushing with a fluoridated toothpaste in children and young adults. It is unfortunate that traditional manual flossing is not an easy skill for patients to learn; it has been reported that only 20% of subjects report effective flossing behavior [46]. Even in those who have been adequately trained and who can demonstrate skill retention after 1 year, there is still a substantial drop-off in daily plaque removal with time [47]. Flossing forks, superfloss and, more recently, powered flossers have been introduced to make it easier for patients to clean interproximally. The studies that have been done on these interdental devices do not have enough statistical power to show anything but equivalence.

Interproximal brushes are better alternatives for periodontitis maintenance patients who have lost interdental papillae height and who are in a secondary preventive stage [45]. Interdental brushes come in a range of sizes. It seems reasonable to assume that the largest size that fits the space being deplaqued would be the most efficacious; however, this has not been proved [48]. Considering the range of sizes needed for any given patient, it may be best to choose the size that can be used in all high-risk sites. Advantages of this type of brush include the ability to deliver topical antimicrobials or fluorides to interproximal sites while mechanically removing plaque and to provide positive stimuli to the fibroblasts in the col area. This latter benefit is speculative and is an extrapolation from recent studies in a canine model [49–51].

Fluoridated triangular toothpicks have also proved to be an excellent way to deplaque the interproximal areas up to 2 to 3 mm subgingivally and have been recommended as part of a needs-related oral hygiene regimen for patients with treated periodontitis as part of a secondary prevention program [45].

Single-tufted brushes and rubber-tipped stimulators tend to be site specific. They are most often recommended for furcations, tipped teeth, the distals of terminal molars, or tooth surfaces directly adjacent to edentulous sites.

Chemical plaque control

Mouthrinses

Chemical preventive agents have been incorporated into oral disease management for centuries; however, it is only recently that these adjunctive therapies have been scientifically studied. Recently, Addy [52] wrote a brief, informative, and rather humorous review on antiseptic use in periodontal therapy. These agents should be viewed as adjuncts and not replacements for effective mechanical plaque control. They are preventive agents, not therapeutic agents. Given that many patients cannot maintain adequate levels of plaque control using mechanical oral hygiene methods alone, chemical plaque control has become a big business. Despite some over-reaching advertisements about the efficacy of some of the currently available antiseptics for plaque control, the dental profession can be thankful for the widespread public education that is occurring on the dangers of interproximal plaque. This section emphasizes developments in the area of chemical plaque control since the last World Workshop in Periodontics [53].

The biofilm inhibitory concentrations for a given antimicrobial are generally orders of magnitude higher than the standard minimal inhibitory concentrations determined for planktonic (free-floating) organisms. A recent in vitro study compared the antimicrobial activity of three mouthrinses with planktonic bacteria and their corresponding monospecies biofilms [54]. As anticipated, the bacteria contained in biofilms were shown to have a decreased susceptibility to antimicrobial agents versus those in planktonic form. The antimicrobial mouthrinses included in the study were an essential-oil (EO)-containing mouthrinse (Listerine Antiseptic; Pfizer, Morris Plains, New Jersey), an amine fluoride/stannous fluoride–containing mouthrinse (Meridol), a triclosan and polyvinylmethyl ether/maleic acid copolymer–containing mouthrinse (Plax), and a negative control (phosphate-buffered saline). All three mouthrinses produced statistically significant (99.99%) reductions in planktonic strains compared with the control. Effects on the biofilm forms of the organisms, however, were more variable. Exposure to Listerine Antiseptic produced statistically significant reductions compared with the control, whereas Plax (Colgate Palmolive [UK] Ltd., Guildford, United Kingdom) and Meridol (Wybert GmbH, Lorrach, Germany) produced much smaller reductions that were not statistically significant. These in vitro results provide a clear demonstration of the resistance to antimicrobial agents conferred by biofilms. The results also provide additional support for employment of tests using biofilms to more accurately assess the relative activities of antiplaque agents in vitro (although when tested in vivo, there are even more obstacles to overcome).

The in vivo use of an EO-containing antiseptic mouthrinse has a long clinical history (Listerine). The active ingredient of this mouthrinse is a fixed combination of EOs (0.064% thymol, 0.092% eucalyptol, 0.060% methyl salicylate, and 0.042% menthol). Many short-term (4–6 weeks) and long-term (3–6 months) clinical studies have demonstrated the effectiveness of EO rinses in plaque and gingivitis reduction. Although the "gold standard" for antiplaque and antigingivitis mouthrinsing is still chlorhexidine [55,56], the use of an EO rinse as an adjunct to mechanical oral hygiene can be beneficial, particularly in the secondary preventive phase because it does not induce calculus formation, taste alteration, or extrinsic tooth stain like chlorhexidine [57–59].

In a 6-month supervised-use trial specifically designed to compare the antiplaque and antigingivitis efficacy of EO and chlorhexidine mouthrinses, Overholser et al [60] showed significant reduction in plaque formation and in gingivitis compared with a negative control. Although both mouthrinses had comparable antigingivitis effectiveness, the chlorhexidine mouthrinse was significantly more effective than the EO-containing mouthrinse in reducing plaque. In addition, the chlorhexidine group had more extrinsic tooth stain and calculus than the EO or the control group [60]. Charles and coworkers [61] recently presented similar results in a 6-month randomized controlled clinical study on the antiplaque and the antigingivitis effects of a chlorhexidine or EO rinse compared with control. Although the patients were randomly assigned to the groups, it is difficult to discern how the observers remained masked to the treatments, given the obvious presence of stain and calculus. The investigators also stated that there was a statistically significant difference between the chlorhexidine group and the EO group at 3 months, but toward the end of the study (6 months), there was no difference. The chlorhexidine rinse group had significantly higher calculus formation and extrinsic tooth stain compared with the EO rinse group or the control group.

Because the occurrence of extrinsic tooth stain and calculus deposits may limit patient compliance, especially for long-term use, chlorhexidine mouthrinses have greater utility when short-term plaque control is critical. This situation includes the postoperative phase following periodontal surgery, when mechanical oral hygiene is difficult. The use of an EO rinse is better suited as a long-term plaque-control adjunct for moderate- to high-risk patients for primary and secondary prevention. For patients with physical disabilities that limit their mechanical oral hygiene skills, a chlorhexidine spray may prove useful [52].

The literature presents few studies that compare the efficacy of toothbrushing with interproximal plaque control using dental flossing or interproximal dental brushing [62–64] or antimicrobial mouthrinses [57,58]. Sharma et al [58] and Bauroth et al [57] compared the efficacy of plaque removal using an EO-containing mouthrinse or dental flossing in addition to brushing. They included three groups in a parallel-arm, single-masked, randomized controlled clinical trial. The first group received the EO mouthrinse twice a day as an adjunct to the patient's regular twice daily brushing with a fluoride dentifrice, the second group was advised to floss once daily in conjunction with brushing, and the third group received a control mouthrinse to supplement brushing. The results showed significant improvement for the EO rinse and the dental floss group compared with baseline measurements. Reduction in the interproximal modified gingival index scores was "at least as good as" that provided by flossing. Although these studies were well controlled and well designed, the measurement of interproximal plaque seems problematic because the flossing group showed significantly less reduction compared with other studies that investigated the additional interproximal plaque reduction benefit comparing brushing alone to brushing and flossing [64–68]. In other words, the positive control (brushing and flossing) was not as positive as one might have expected; the reason for this is not clear in the study. Possible factors could be the length of this study compared with others. Patient compliance may have waned by the first 3-month visit, leading to poor flossing technique or a decrease in patient motivation. It should also be noted that methods for measuring true interproximal plaque are limited.

A follow-up study compared a combination of mechanical and chemical hygiene regimens. The experimental group was instructed to brush twice a day (B), floss daily (F), and rinse with the antiseptic twice daily (EO). This BFEO group represented optimal mechanical and chemical plaque control. A second group used a control mouthrinse (C) in conjunction with brushing and flossing (BFC group). A final group was assigned to brush and to use the placebo mouthrinse as a negative control (BC). A significant reduction in mean modified gingival index and plaque index was seen for the experimental group (BFEO) compared with the other two groups. The investigators suggested that the combined mechanical disruption of the interproximal plaque followed by the EO rinse provides a synergistic effect in plaque and gingivitis reduction due to better biofilm penetration. There was little comment on the low incremental reduction for interproximal mean plaque index and modified gingival index from the BC and BFC groups or on the sharp drop from 3 to 6 months in the BFC group interproximal scores.

As promising as these data are, it would be even more helpful to carry out similar studies on moderate- to high-risk patients because it has been suggested that antiseptic rinsing is not cost-effective for the general population. Recommending widespread antiseptic rinsing for the general population is essentially vast overtreatment to reduce disease only in the subpopulation of susceptible patients [52].

Toothpaste

Although the use of chlorhexidine as a mouthrinse has demonstrated significant plaque reduction, the incorporation of this agent into a dentifrice has proved difficult due to the interaction between chlorhexidine and calcium ions or anionic detergents such as sodium lauryl sulfate [69,70].

The use of antigingivitis dentifrices has been recommended for primary prevention and as a maintenance measure as part of secondary prevention in treated and maintained periodontal patients. The addition of triclosan (a broad-spectrum phenol-derived antibacterial agent) to different dentifrice formulations has been studied in various short- and long-term trials. Volpe et al [71] reviewed the use of various combinations of triclosan in reducing plaque and gingivitis in susceptible individuals.

One of the available combinations of triclosan is composed of 0.3% triclosan, 2.0% copolymer, and 0.243% sodium fluoride (Colgate Total; Colgate Palmolive Co., New York, New York). This combination was shown to alter the quality and composition of subgingival plaque [72,73].

A significant 5-year study by Cullinan et al [74] supported and expanded the previous findings. This double-blind controlled clinical trial examined the effect of the same triclosan formulation as the previous studies on the progression of periodontal disease in patients with attachment loss ≥ 2 mm. It was concluded that the use of such a dentifrice significantly slowed the progression of periodontal disease in those individuals with existing disease.

The clinical effect of a triclosan-containing dentifrice indicates that after a periodontal pocket has developed in a susceptible individual, the use of such dentifrice slows the progression of further pocket development. The effectiveness of triclosan dentifrice as a primary preventive measure against periodontitis has not been demonstrated; however, it has been used to prevent gingivitis, which is the necessary precursor to periodontitis.

One of the side effects of a triclosan dentifrice is tooth staining. A similar problem has been noted with more recent stable formulations of a stannous fluoride–containing dentifrice with proven antiplaque effects [75,76].

Irrigation

The effect of supragingival oral irrigation in periodontal therapy is to flush away loosely attached bacteria present in the gingival crevice, thereby diminishing the potential for developing gingivitis. There is contradictory evidence about the usefulness of supragingival irrigation in reducing plaque formation. Although a few studies have shown some benefits of oral irrigation (professionally applied and as a part of a home care program), the benefits have been unimpressive [77]. Recently, an improvement was demonstrated using this therapy at the clinical and subclinical level in a short-term daily home use study in periodontal patients. These results suggest that oral irrigation with water as part of a regular oral hygiene program can decrease the concentration of pro-inflammatory cytokines in gingival fluids [78]. Although these are promising findings, more work needs to be done before a strong recommendation can be made to add such a regimen to daily home care for these patients. One must weigh the benefit against the cost of the therapy. There is also the possibility of poor long-term compliance.

Clinical considerations for optimal prevention

For patients having resistance to periodontitis and who would thus be classified as low risk based on currently available risk prediction instruments, it is not clear how much mechanical and chemical preventive therapy represents overtreatment. Likewise, for primary or secondary prevention in moderate- to high-risk "susceptible" patients, there is very little understanding of what may constitute the minimal effective therapy. The best available evidence compels us to continue to try to achieve "complete" plaque control by whatever means are best suited for the patient. For a toothbrushing population such as in the United States, this means there is more need for education and motivation in needs-related personal and professional gingival plaque removal (supra- and subgingivally), with an emphasis on interproximal plaque removal in high-risk sites. Axelsson and colleagues [44,45] suggest that encouraging patients to perform interproximal plaque control on the posterior "key risk teeth" before toothbrushing may be adequate in achieving prevention because the behavior is linked with an already well-established brushing habit. In high-risk patients in a secondary prevention program, the authors believe it is wise to consider a powered toothbrush for home use. When there are no allergies or other contraindications, a personal chemical plaque control regimen with a triclosan-containing toothpaste and perhaps an EO-containing mouthrinse twice daily would provide a cost-effective, evidence-based approach to prevention. Other adjunctive home care approaches for the high-risk patient include a dilute sodium hypochlorite solution (1 teaspoon household bleach/250 mL tap water) for subgingival irrigation as recommended by Slots et al [79]. As an adjunct to the professional supportive periodontal therapy, the use of a 1:9 ratio of povidone-iodine to water in the ultrasonic unit has also proved useful, particularly for advanced chronic or aggressive periodontitis cases [79]. When implants are present, plastic-tipped ultrasonics are preferred and metal instruments must be avoided.

Continuous multilevel risk assessment and management is now the standard of care. Clinicians must counsel patients on their risk profile and help them take decisive steps to reduce risk at each level [16]. Perhaps the one area that could have the greatest overall public health benefit immediately is smoking cessation counseling.

Every dentist should be well familiar with the five "A's" of smoking cessation (Box 1) and the five first-line pharmacotherapies approved by the Food and Drug Administration for smoking cessation (Table 1). Clinicians must be willing to guide patients through this process. There is a new current dental terminology code (D1320) that is available for reimbursement, and each year more insurance plans are reimbursing for this service. Because the prevalence for adolescent smoking has risen dramatically since 1990, clinicians need to be proactive in discouraging adolescent and preadolescent patients from starting smoking. It is estimated that over 3000 additional teens and preteens become regular tobacco users each day [80]. It certainly makes

---

Box 1. The five "A's" for brief intervention

1. Ask about tobacco use. Identify and document tobacco use status for every patient at every visit.
2. Advise to quit. In a clear, strong, and personalized manner, urge every tobacco user to quit.
3. Assess willingness to make a quit attempt. Is the tobacco user willing to make a quit attempt at this time?
4. Assist in quit attempt. For the patient willing to make a quit attempt, use counseling and pharmacotherapy to help him or her quit.
5. Arrange follow-up. Schedule follow-up contact, preferably within the first week after the quit date.

Table 1
Suggestions for the clinical use of first-line pharmacotherapies approved for smoking cessation by the Food and Drug Administration

Pharmacotherapy	Precautions/ contraindications	Side effects	Dosage	Duration	Availability	Cost/d[a]
Bupropion SR	History of seizure or history of eating disorder	Insomnia, dry mouth	Begin treatment 1–2 wk prequit 150 mg 1×/morning for 3 d then 150 mg 2×/d	7–12 wk (up to 6 mo)	Zyban (prescription only)	$3.33
Nicotine gum	—	Mouth soreness, dyspepsia	1–24 cigs/d: 2 mg gum (≤24 pcs/d) 25+ cigs/d: 4 mg gum (≤24 pcs/d)	≤12 wk	Nicorette/Nicorette Mint (OTC only)	$6.25 for 10 (2-mg) pieces, $6.87 for 10 (4-mg) pieces
Nicotine inhaler	—	Local irritation of mouth and throat	6–16 cartridges/d	≤6 mo	Nicotrol Inhaler (prescription only)	$10.94 for 10 cartridges
Nicotine nasal spray	—	Nasal irritation	8–40 doses/d	3–6 mo	Nicotrol NS (prescription only)	$5.40 for 12 doses
Nicotine patch	—	Local skin reaction, insomnia	21 mg/24 h then 14 mg/24 h then 7 mg/24 h	4 wk then 2 wk then 2 wk	Nicoderm CQ (OTC only) and generic patches (prescription and OTC)	Brand name: $4.00–$4.50[b]
			15 mg/16 h	8 wk	Nicotrol (OTC only)	

Abbreviations: cigs, cigarettes; OTC, over the counter; pcs, pieces.

[a] Costs are based on retail prices of medication purchased in April 2000 at a national chain pharmacy located in Madison, Wisconsin.

[b] Generic brands of the patch recently became available and may be less expensive.

Information contained within this table is not comprehensive. Please see package insert for additional information.

sense for dental professionals to take a leading role in combating this chronic addiction because they see these patients more frequently than physicians.

Finally, dental care providers must assess the patient's disease status each time he or she returns for supportive periodontal therapy. Clinicians must use the data available from the medical history review, risk assessment, and clinical examination, including radiographs when taken. As part of the supportive periodontal therapy rotations at Marquette University School of Dentistry, the students are given a laminated card that lists some specific criteria they should employ to assess the stability or instability of their maintenance patients. These criteria are listed in Box 2. Application of objective criteria such as these in the general practitioner's office may provide

---

Box 2. Site- and patient-level criteria to consider in assessing the stability of periodontal maintenance patients

Inflammation as measured by bleeding on probing
Full mouth bleeding on probing >15% suggests instability
Sites that consistently show bleeding on probing over time
    may be unstable
Sites that consistently show no bleeding on probing are likely
    stable

Probing depth measurements
Sites with a probing depth increase of ≥2 mm from baseline or
    previous visit are considered unstable
Number of significant periodontal pocket depths (10 or more
    sites with ≥4 mm probing depth are considered unstable)
Probing depth ≥6 mm at any site is considered unstable
Progressive gingival recession from baseline or previous
    charting

Radiographic considerations
Loss of crestal bone height based on vertical bite wings is
    considered unstable
Consistent presence of crestal lamina dura suggests stability

Patient-level considerations
Poor hygiene in the presence of attachment loss plaque index
    >30% is considered unstable
Smoking more than one-half pack per day is considered
    unstable
Diabetes mellitus with HBA1c ≥9 is considered
    unstable
High-stress events, divorce, loss of a loved one,
    and unemployment are considered unstable

a more rational approach to appropriate referrals to the periodontist. Based on a recent retrospective survey of changes in referral patterns to periodontal offices over the past 20 years, it seems that some guidelines are needed if the goal of helping the public to keep their teeth in a state of health, comfort, and function in an esthetically pleasing presentation [81] is to be reached.

Future preventive strategies

Vaccine development for periodontitis is a possible protection strategy for primary prevention. Different groups have been developing vaccines that target important surface structures of certain periodontopathogens. These surface structures include the fimbrial protein and hemagglutinating subunits necessary for adhesion and colonization of *Porphyromonas gingivalis* and the surface cysteine proteinases Arg- and Lys-gingipains that allow *P gingivalis* to bind to and degrade host tissues, causing destruction by way of a prostaglandin E_2–dependent mechanism [82–85].

New drug delivery systems are also in development that should provide more cost-effective, slow-release antimicrobials and anti-inflammatory agents for primary prevention in high-risk subjects and secondary prevention in more moderate- to low-risk cases. The possibility of using these systems to deliver antimicrobial, anti-inflammatory, or immune-modulating agents is currently being tested [86,87].

Another somewhat futuristic approach to primary or secondary prevention involves introducing nonpathogenic bacterial competitor strains (bacterial replacement therapy) as a means to prevent the colonization and establishment of pathogenic strains of bacteria. To date, most work done in this area has been geared toward dental caries rather than periodontal disease; however, progress has been made in construction of a nonpathogenic *Streptococcus mutans* strain that can colonize the oral cavity but has no ability to produce acid due to a lactate dehydrogenase deletion mutation [88–90]. These are just a few of the biologic therapies making their way into clinics. Considering how far we have come in 50 years, it is truly an exciting time to be a dentist.

Acknowledgments

The authors thank Julayne Erz for her expert assistance and Timothy Creamer, MD, for his helpful comments in the preparation of this manuscript.

References

[1] Andersen R, Marcus M, Mahshigan M. A comparative systems perspective on oral health promotion and disease prevention. In: Cohen LK, Gift HC, editors. Disease prevention and oral health promotion. Copenhagen (Denmark): Munksgaard; 1995. p. 307–40.

[2] Baehni PC, Bourgeois DM. Epidemiology of periodontal health and disease. Paper presented at the Proceedings of the European Workshop on Mechanical Plaque Control. Berne (Switzerland), May 9–12, 1998.

[3] Petersson HG, Bratthall D. The caries decline: a review of reviews. Eur J Oral Sci 1996;104: 436–43.

[4] Axelsson P, Lindhe J. Effect of controlled oral hygiene procedures on caries and periodontal disease in adults. Results after 6 years. J Clin Periodontol 1981;8(3):239–48.

[5] Axelsson P, Lindhe J, Nystrom B. On the prevention of caries and periodontal disease. Results of a 15-year longitudinal study in adults. J Clin Periodontol 1991;18(3):182–9.

[6] Axelsson P, Nystrom B, Lindhe J. The long-term effect of a plaque control program on tooth mortality, caries and periodontal disease in adults. Results after 30 years of maintenance. J Clin Periodontol 2004;31(9):749–57.

[7] Marshall-Day CD, Stephens RG, Quigley LF. Periodontal disease: prevalence and incidence. J Periodontol 1955;26:185–203.

[8] Page RC. Periodontal diseases: a new paradigm. J Dent Educ 1998;62(10):812–21.

[9] Lindhe J, Hamp SE, Loe H. Plaque induced periodontal disease in beagle dogs. A 4-year clinical, roentgenographical and histometrical study. J Periodontal Res 1975;10(5):243–55.

[10] Brown LJ, Loe H. Prevalence, extent, severity and progression of periodontal disease. Periodontol 2000 1993;2:57–71.

[11] Haber J, Wattles J, Crowley M, et al. Evidence for cigarette smoking as a major risk factor for periodontitis. J Periodontol 1993;64(1):16–23.

[12] Grossi SG, Zambon JJ, Ho AW, et al. Assessment of risk for periodontal disease. I. Risk indicators for attachment loss. J Periodontol 1994;65(3):260–7.

[13] Oliver RC, Tervonen T. Diabetes–a risk factor for periodontitis in adults? J Periodontol 1994;65(Suppl 5):530–8.

[14] Meisel P, Siegemund A, Grimm R, et al. The interleukin-1 polymorphism, smoking, and the risk of periodontal disease in the population-based SHIP study. J Dent Res 2003;82(3): 189–93.

[15] Last JM. A dictionary of epidemiology. 4th edition. Oxford (England): Oxford University Press; 2001.

[16] Lang NP, Bragger U, Salvi G, et al. Supportive periodontal therapy (SPT). In: Lindhe J, Karring T, Lang NP, editors. Clinical periodontology and implantology. 4th edition. Oxford (England): Blackwell Munksgaard; 2003. p. 781–802.

[17] Parameters of care. American Academy of Periodontology. J Periodontol 2000;71(5 Suppl): i–ii, 847–83.

[18] Position paper periodontal maintenance. J Periodontol 2003;74(9):1395–401.

[19] Schutte DW, Donley TG. Determining periodontal risk factors in patients presenting for dental care. J Dent Hyg 1996;70(6):230–4.

[20] Persson GR, Attstrom R, Lang NP, et al. Perceived risk of deteriorating periodontal conditions. J Clin Periodontol 2003;30(11):982–9.

[21] Persson GR, Mancl LA, Martin J, et al. Assessing periodontal disease risk: a comparison of clinicians' assessment versus a computerized tool. J Am Dent Assoc 2003;134(5):575–82.

[22] Page RC, Krall EA, Martin J, et al. Validity and accuracy of a risk calculator in predicting periodontal disease. J Am Dent Assoc 2002;133(5):569–76.

[23] Page RC, Martin J, Krall EA, et al. Longitudinal validation of a risk calculator for periodontal disease. J Clin Periodontol 2003;30(9):819–27.

[24] Greenwell H, Bissada NF. Emerging concepts in periodontal therapy. Drugs 2002;62(18): 2581–7.

[24a] Legon J. Toothbrush trounces car as top invention. Available at: http://www.cnn.com/ 2003/TECH/ptech/01/22/toothbrush.king. Accessed May 6, 2005.

[25] Jepsen S. The role of manual toothbrushes in effective plaque control. Paper presented at the Proceedings of the European Workshop on Mechanical Plaque Control. Berne (Switzerland), May 9–12, 1998.

[26] Hawkins BF, Kohout FJ, Lainson PA, et al. Duration of toothbrushing for effective plaque control. Quintessence Int 1986;17(6):361–5.

[27] Beals D, Ngo T, Feng Y, et al. Development and laboratory evaluation of a new toothbrush with a novel brush head design. Am J Dent 2000;13(Spec No):5A–14A.

[28] Van der Weijden GA, Timmerman MF, Nijboer A, et al. A comparative study of electric toothbrushes for the effectiveness of plaque removal in relation to toothbrushing duration.Timerstudy. J Clin Periodontol 1993;20(7):476–81.

[29] Van der Weijden GA, Timmerman MF, Snoek I, et al. Toothbrushing duration and plaque removal efficacy of electric toothbrushes. Am J Dent 1996;9:31–6.

[30] Baab DA, Johnson RH. The effect of a new electric toothbrush on supragingival plaque and gingivitis. J Periodontol 1989;60(6):336–41.

[31] Wilson S, Levine D, Dequincey G, et al. Effects of two toothbrushes on plaque, gingivitis, gingival abrasion, and recession: a 1-year longitudinal study. Compend Suppl 1993;(16): S569–79.

[32] Yukna RA, Shaklee RL. Evaluation of a counter-rotational powered brush in patients in supportive periodontal therapy. J Periodontol 1993;64(9):859–64.

[33] Van der Weijden GA, Timmerman MF, et al. The long-term effect of an oscillating/rotating electric toothbrush on gingivitis. An 8-month clinical study. J Clin Periodontol 1994;21(2): 139–45.

[34] Ainamo J, Xie Q, Ainamo A, et al. Assessment of the effect of an oscillating/rotating electric toothbrush on oral health. A 12-month longitudinal study. J Clin Periodontol 1997;24(1): 28–33.

[35] Dentino AR, Derderian G, Wolf M, et al. Six-month comparison of powered versus manual toothbrushing for safety and efficacy in the absence of professional instruction in mechanical plaque control. J Periodontol 2002;73(7):770–8.

[36] Haffajee AD, Smith C, Torresyap G, et al. Efficacy of manual and powered toothbrushes (II). Effect on microbiological parameters. J Clin Periodontol 2001;28(10):947–54.

[37] Haffajee AD, Thompson M, Torresyap G, et al. Efficacy of manual and powered toothbrushes (I). Effect on clinical parameters. J Clin Periodontol 2001;28(10):937–46.

[38] Sicilia A, Arregui I, Gallego M, et al. A systematic review of powered vs manual tooth-brushes in periodontal cause-related therapy. J Clin Periodontol 2002;29(Suppl 3):39–54 [discussion: 90–1].

[39] Heanue M, Deacon SA, Deery C, et al. Manual versus powered toothbrushing for oral health. Cochrane Database Syst Rev 2003;1:CD002281.

[40] Stalnacke K, Soderfeldt B, Sjodin B. Compliance in use of electric toothbrushes. Acta Odontol Scand 1995;53(1):17–9.

[41] Hellstadius K, Asman B, Gustafsson A. Improved maintenance of plaque control by electrical toothbrushing in periodontitis patients with low compliance. J Clin Periodontol 1993;20(4):235–7.

[42] McCracken GI, Janssen J, Steen N, et al. A clinical evaluation of a novel data logger to determine compliance with the use of powered toothbrushes. J Clin Periodontol 2002;29(9): 838–43.

[43] Van der Weijden GA, Timmerman MF, Danser MM, et al. The role of electric toothbrushes: advantages and limitations. Paper presented at the Proceedings of the European Workshop on Mechanical Plaque Control. Berne (Switzerland), May 9–12, 1998.

[44] Axelsson P. Needs-related plaque control measures based on risk prediction. Paper presented at the Proceedings of the European Workshop on Mechanical Plaque Control. Berne (Switzerland), May 9–12, 1998.

[45] Axelsson P, Albandar JM, Rams TE. Prevention and control of periodontal diseases in developing and industrialized nations. Periodontol 2000 2002;29:235–46.

[46] Lang WP, Farghaly MM, Ronis DL. The relation of preventive dental behaviors to periodontal health status. J Clin Periodontol 1994;21(3):194–8.

[47] Stewart JE, Wolfe GR. The retention of newly-acquired brushing and flossing skills. J Clin Periodontol 1989;16(5):331–2.

[48] Kinane DF. The role of interdental cleaning in effective plaque control: need for interdental cleaning in primary and secondary prevention. Paper presented at the Proceedings of the European Workshop on Mechanical Plaque Control. Berne (Switzerland), May 9–12, 1998.

[49] Sakamoto T, Horiuchi M, Tomofuji T, et al. Spatial extent of gingival cell activation due to mechanical stimulation by toothbrushing. J Periodontol 2003;74(5):585–9.

[50] Tomofuji T, Morita M, Horiuchi M, et al. The effect of duration and force of mechanical toothbrushing stimulation on proliferative activity of the junctional epithelium. J Periodontol 2002;73(10):1149–52.

[51] Tomofuji T, Ekuni D, Yamamoto T, et al. Optimum force and duration of toothbrushing to enhance gingival fibroblast proliferation and procollagen type I synthesis in dogs. J Periodontol 2003;74(5):630–4.

[52] Addy M. The use of antiseptics in periodontal therapy. In: Lindhe J, Karring T, Lang NP, editors. Clinical periodontology and implantology. 4th edition. Oxford (England): Blackwell Munksgaard; 2003. p. 464–93.

[53] Hancock EB. Periodontal diseases: prevention. Ann Periodontol 1996;1(1):223–49.

[54] Fine DH, Furgang D, Barnett ML. Comparative antimicrobial activities of antiseptic mouthrinses against isogenic planktonic and biofilm forms of Actinobacillus actinomycetemcomitans. J Clin Periodontol 2001;28(7):697–700.

[55] Lang NP, Hotz P, Graf H, et al. Effects of supervised chlorhexidine mouthrinses in children. A longitudinal clinical trial. J Periodontal Res 1982;17(1):101–11.

[56] Ernst CP, Prockl K, Willershausen B. The effectiveness and side effects of 0.1% and 0.2% chlorhexidine mouthrinses: a clinical study. Quintessence Int 1998;29(7):443–8.

[57] Bauroth K, Charles CH, Mankodi SM, et al. The efficacy of an essential oil antiseptic mouthrinse vs. dental floss in controlling interproximal gingivitis: a comparative study. J Am Dent Assoc 2003;134(3):359–65.

[58] Sharma NC, Charles CH, Qaqish JG, et al. Comparative effectiveness of an essential oil mouthrinse and dental floss in controlling interproximal gingivitis and plaque. Am J Dent 2002;15(6):351–5.

[59] Sharma N, Charles CH, Lynch MC, et al. Adjunctive benefit of an essential oil-containing mouthrinse in reducing plaque and gingivitis in patients who brush and floss regularly: a six-month study. J Am Dent Assoc 2004;135(4):496–504.

[60] Overholser CD, Meiller TF, DePaola LG, et al. Comparative effects of 2 chemotherapeutic mouthrinses on the development of supragingival dental plaque and gingivitis. J Clin Periodontol 1990;17(8):575–9.

[61] Charles CH, Mostler KM, Bartels LL, et al. Comparative antiplaque and antigingivitis effectiveness of a chlorhexidine and an essential oil mouthrinse: 6-month clinical trial. J Clin Periodontol 2004;31(10):878–84.

[62] Bergenholtz A, Bjorne A, Vikstrom B. The plaque-removing ability of some common interdental aids. An intraindividual study. J Clin Periodontol 1974;1(3):160–5.

[63] Graves RC, Disney JA, Stamm JW. Comparative effectiveness of flossing and brushing in reducing interproximal bleeding. J Periodontol 1989;60(5):243–7.

[64] Kiger RD, Nylund K, Feller RP. A comparison of proximal plaque removal using floss and interdental brushes. J Clin Periodontol 1991;18(9):681–4.

[65] Finkelstein P, Grossman E. The effectiveness of dental floss in reducing gingival inflammation. J Dent Res 1979;58(3):1034–9.

[66] Fischman SL. The history of oral hygiene products: how far have we come in 6000 years? Periodontol 2000;1997(15):7–14.

[67] Anderson NA, Barnes CM, Russell CM, et al. A clinical comparison of the efficacy of an electromechanical flossing device or manual flossing in affecting interproximal gingival bleeding and plaque accumulation. J Clin Dent 1995;6(1):105–7.

[68] Lobene RR, Soparkar PM, Newman MB. Use of dental floss. Effect on plaque and gingivitis. Clin Prev Dent 1982;4(1):5–8.

[69] Barkvoll P, Rolla G, Svendsen K. Interaction between chlorhexidine digluconate and sodium lauryl sulfate in vivo. J Clin Periodontol 1989;16(9):593–5.

[70] Gjermo P, Rolla G. The plaque-inhibiting effect of chlorhexidine-containing dentifrices. Scand J Dent Res 1971;79(2):126–32.

[71] Volpe AR, Petrone ME, De Vizio W, et al. A review of plaque, gingivitis, calculus and caries clinical efficacy studies with a fluoride dentifrice containing triclosan and PVM/MA copolymer. J Clin Dent 1996;7(Suppl):S1–14.

[72] Ellwood RP, Worthington HV, Blinkhorn AS, et al. Effect of a triclosan/copolymer dentifrice on the incidence of periodontal attachment loss in adolescents. J Clin Periodontol 1998;25(5):363–7.

[73] Rosling B, Wannfors B, Volpe AR, et al. The use of a triclosan/copolymer dentifrice may retard the progression of periodontitis. J Clin Periodontol 1997;24(12):873–80.

[74] Cullinan MP, Westerman B, Hamlet SM, et al. The effect of a triclosan-containing dentifrice on the progression of periodontal disease in an adult population. J Clin Periodontol 2003;30(5):414–9.

[75] Boyd RL. Long-term evaluation of a SnF2 gel for control of gingivitis and decalcification in adolescent orthodontic patients. Int Dent J 1994;44(1 Suppl 1):119–30.

[76] White DJ. A "return" to stannous fluoride dentifrices. J Clin Dent 1995;6(Spec No):29–36.

[77] Greenstein G. The role of supra- and subgingival irrigation in the treatment of periodontal diseases. Chicago: American Academy of Periodontology; 1995.

[78] Cutler CW, Stanford TW, Abraham C, et al. Clinical benefits of oral irrigation for periodontitis are related to reduction of pro-inflammatory cytokine levels and plaque. J Clin Periodontol 2000;27(2):134–43.

[79] Slots J, Jorgensen MG. Effective, safe, practical and affordable periodontal antimicrobial therapy: where are we going, and are we there yet? Periodontol 2000 2002;28:298–312.

[80] Fiore MC, Bailey WC, Cohen SJ, et al. Treating tobacco use and dependence. Rockville (MD): US Department of Health and Human Services; 2000.

[81] Cobb CM, Carrara A, El-Annan E, et al. Periodontal referral patterns, 1980 versus 2000: a preliminary study. J Periodontol 2003;74(10):1470–4.

[82] Page RC. Vaccination and periodontitis: myth or reality. J Int Acad Periodontol 2000;2(2): 31–43.

[83] Vasel D, Sims TJ, Bainbridge B, et al. Shared antigens of *Porphyromonas gingivalis* and *Bacteroides forsythus*. Oral Microbiol Immunol 1996;11(4):226–35.

[84] Bainbridge BW, Page RC, Darveau RP. Serum antibodies to *Porphyromonas gingivalis* block the prostaglandin E2 response to lipopolysaccharide by mononuclear cells. Infect Immun 1997;65(11):4801–5.

[85] Roberts FA, Houston LS, Lukehart SA, et al. Periodontitis vaccine decreases local prostaglandin E2 levels in a primate model. Infect Immun 2004;72(2):1166–8.

[86] AntonyRaj P, Rajkumar L, Dentino AR. New and novel technology for intra-oral delivery of antimicrobials. J Dent Res 2004;83(Spec Iss A):1468.

[87] AntonyRaj P, Dentino AR. A novel bifunctional molecule targets oral pathogens. J Dent Res 2002;82(Spec Iss A):3935.

[88] Hillman JD, Chen A, Duncan M, et al. Evidence that L-(+)-lactate dehydrogenase deficiency is lethal in *Streptococcus mutans*. Infect Immun 1994;62(1):60–4.

[89] Hillman JD. Genetically modified *Streptococcus mutans* for the prevention of dental caries. Antonie Van Leeuwenhoek 2002;82(1–4):361–6.

[90] Hillman JD, Duncan MJ, Stashenko KP. Cloning and expression of the gene encoding the fructose-1, 6-diphosphate-dependent L-(+)-lactate dehydrogenase of *Streptococcus mutans*. Infect Immun 1990;58(5):1290–5.

ELSEVIER
SAUNDERS

THE DENTAL
CLINICS
OF NORTH AMERICA

Dent Clin N Am 49 (2005) 595–610

Nutrition and Periodontal Disease

Robert E. Schifferle, DDS, MMSc, PhD

*Departments of Periodontics & Endodontics and Oral Biology, School of Dental Medicine,
University at Buffalo, State University of New York, 318 Foster Hall, 3435 Main Street,
Buffalo, NY 14214-3092, USA*

The role of diet in the etiology of dental caries is well established. The role of diet in the development and progression of periodontal disease, however, is less well understood. Recent studies have noted that as people lose teeth, there is a trend toward the presence of a poorer diet [1,2]. A person's diet can exert a topical or a systemic effect on the body and its tissues. Before tooth eruption, foods provide a nutritional or systemic effect during tooth development and in the maturation of dentine and enamel. After the tooth erupts, foods play a topical or dietary role in the maintenance of tooth structure. It is well known that the caries process can be modified through dietary (food selection and eating habit changes) rather than nutritional changes. For example, during growth and development, nutritional fluoride provides a systemic effect, making the tooth more resistant to decalcification by incorporation into the structure of the tooth. After the tooth has formed and erupted into the oral cavity, dietary fluoride provides a topical effect by modification of the surface layer of exposed enamel, cementum, and dentin. In this review, general concepts of nutrition are discussed first, followed by an overview of the current understanding of the relationship between nutrition and periodontal disease.

Nutrients can be considered major or minor as determined by the amounts consumed in our diets. Major nutrients are consumed in gram quantities. These include protein, carbohydrates, lipids, and water. Adults need approximately 0.8 g of protein per kilogram of body weight, whereas infants require 2.0 g of protein per kilogram of body weight to support their growth and development. Adults need about 130 g of carbohydrate per day to provide sufficient glucose for the brain and erythrocytes to function. In adults, about 20 to 30 g of essential fatty acids are needed daily for hormone

E-mail address: res@buffalo.edu

production. Minor nutrients are required in milligram to microgram quantities and include vitamins and minerals.

The Food and Nutrition Board of the National Academy of Sciences has defined the quantitative intake of some nutrients [3]. The recommended dietary allowance (RDA) is defined as the amount of a nutrient that meets the needs of 97% to 98% of all people of a given age and sex. When there is insufficient information available to determine an average requirement for a specific nutrient, an adequate intake (AI) is assigned. This value is the amount that should be adequate to maintain a defined nutrition state. The current standards for the United States also apply to Canada because a committee of scientists from both countries established the values. The daily value (DV) is a generic standard developed by the Food and Drug Administration that can be used on food packaging without regard to age or sex differences. The DV is generally set at the highest nutrient recommendation and often exceeds the RDA or AI. The main purpose of the DV is to help provide a guide for nutrient content on food labels.

Protein, carbohydrates, and lipids

Protein provides us with amino acids, the building blocks of our bodies. Protein is the most common substance in the body after water, making up about 50% of the body's dry weight. Proteins can be structural proteins such as collagen, a major organic component of bone, teeth, periodontal ligament, and muscle. Proteins also make up the enzymes, which are used to support bodily functions. When protein is eaten, it is broken down to its component amino acids, which can be used for protein synthesis and repair. Twenty-two amino acids are needed for protein synthesis, 9 of which are considered essential amino acids. These 9 essential amino acids—histidine, isoleucine, leucine, lysine, methionine, phenylalanine, threonine, tryptophan, and valine—must be provided by the diet for protein synthesis to occur. Excess amino acids not used in protein synthesis or repair are used for energy. Protein provides 4 kcal of energy per gram. The RDA for protein for adults is 0.8 g of protein per day per kg body weight. Major sources of dietary protein are milk, meat, eggs, and legumes.

The main role of carbohydrates is to provide the body with energy. Carbohydrates are primarily used as a source of energy but they also aid in fat metabolism. Carbohydrates provide 4 kcal of energy per gram. Carbohydrates are found within the body as glycoprotein and glycosaminoglycans. They are essential for synthesis of the ground substance of the connective tissues, such as chondroiton, keratin, and dermatan sulfates. Glucose is also essential for erythrocyte and brain function. The body stores carbohydrates as glycogen (polysaccharides composed of α-linked glucose molecules). Carbohydrates are protein sparing, in that when inadequate amounts of dietary carbohydrates are ingested, the body breaks down protein to provide glucose. The RDA for carbohydrate is 130 g/d for adults. Major sources of carbohydrates are sugars and starches. Dietary fiber is also carbohydrate in nature, with soluble and insoluble forms. Diets high in fiber have been shown in some studies to lead to a decrease in intestinal disorders and several forms of colon cancer [4]. Wheat bran, a form of insoluble fiber, is composed of β-linked glucose molecules, which are not digestible by humans. Insoluble fiber helps retain fluid and provides bulk in the gastrointestinal system. Oat bran is a form of soluble fiber. Soluble fiber helps bind cholesterol molecules and can play a role in a cholesterol-lowering diet [5]. The AI for fiber for adults is 25 g/d for women and 38 g/d for men.

The main role of lipids is to provide energy, energy storage, and thermal insulation. The average diet in the United States provides about one third of all calories from fat. In a 2400-kcal diet, this amount is 800 kcal or about 100 g of lipid. The body requires two essential fatty acids: linoleic and linolenic acid. Fats are also needed for the body to absorb the fat-soluble vitamins A, D, E, and K. There is no RDA for lipids, but to meet AI recommendations, about 5% of our total energy must be obtained from plant oils. Lipids are a more concentrated source of energy than carbohydrates or proteins, providing 9 kcal of energy per gram.

Vitamins

Vitamins are organic substances present in small quantities in food and are required for the body to maintain appropriate metabolic reactions. Vitamins are not made (or are made in inadequate amounts) by the body and must therefore be supplied by food or made from a provitamin. Vitamins are used in milligram to microgram quantities. Vitamins can be grouped as fat-soluble or water-soluble. Vitamins A, D, E, and K are fat-soluble, whereas the B vitamins and vitamin C are water-soluble. Except for vitamin K, fat-soluble vitamins are not readily excreted and can accumulate in the body. Excess amounts of the water-soluble vitamins are generally excreted by way of the kidneys; howver, vitamins B_{12} and B_6 can accumulate in the body. The functions of the fat-soluble vitamins are reviewed first, followed by the B vitamins and vitamin C (Table 1).

Vitamin A, a fat-soluble vitamin, is required for vision, as a component of visual purple (essential for night vision), and for the maturation of epithelial tissues. Preformed vitamin A is present in foods (primarily animal fats and fish oils) as retinoids, which are toxic in high doses. Carotenoids are present in food and can be precursors of vitamin A, functioning as a provitamin. β-carotene is the main carotenoid found in foods. β-carotene is nontoxic in high doses and can function as an antioxidant. Preformed vitamin A does not function as an antioxidant. The RDA is 900 μg/d of retinol equivalents for men and 700 μg/d of retinol equivalents for women.

Vitamin D is a fat-soluble vitamin that can be considered a conditional vitamin—it can be obtained from the diet and synthesized in the body with adequate exposure to sunlight. In the northern latitudes, sunlight is often

Table 1
National Academy of Sciences recommended dietary allowances or adequate intakes of vitamins for men and women aged 19 to 50 years

Vitamin	Men	Women
A	900 μg/d	700 μg/d
Thiamin (B$_1$)	1.2 mg/d	1.1 mg/d
Riboflavin (B$_2$)	1.3 mg/d	1.1 mg/d
Niacin	16 mg/d	14 mg/d
B$_6$	1.3 mg/d	1.3 mg/d
Folate	400 μg/d	400 μg/d
B$_{12}$	2.4 μg/d	2.4 μg/d
Panothenic acid	5 mg/d[a]	5 mg/d[a]
Biotin	30 μg/d[a]	30 μg/d[a]
C	90 mg/d	75 mg/d
D	5 μg/d[a]	5 μg/d[a]
E	15 mg/d	15 mg/d
K	120 μg/d[a]	120 μg/d[a]

[a] Adequate intake.

Reprinted with permission from (Dietary reference intakes for vitamin C, vitamin E, selenium, and carotenoids) © (2000) by the National Academy of Sciences. Courtesy of the National Academies Press, Washington, DC.

inadequate, especially during the winter months, necessitating the dietary intake of vitamin D. Vitamin D functions to maintain blood calcium levels and the metabolism of osseous tissues. Vitamin D enhances the absorption of calcium from the intestines. When levels of blood calcium are inadequate, there is inadequate calcification of the osseous tissues, resulting in rickets or osteomalacia. High doses of vitamin D can lead to toxicity. The AI for adults <51 years old is 5 μg/d, 10 μg/d for those aged 51 to 70 years, and 15 μg/d for those older than 70 years. A major source of dietary vitamin D is fortified milk.

Vitamin E is a fat-soluble vitamin whose primary role is to function as an antioxidant. It is composed of eight related compounds called tocopherols or tocotrienols. The most active form is α-tocopherol, which is incorporated into the lipid membrane of cells helping to quench free radicals, thus protecting the fatty acids in the lipid bilayer. The RDA for vitamin E is 15 mg/d. It has a much greater margin of safety than that observed for vitamins A and D. Most of the vitamin E in our diets comes from plant oils. Animal fats contain very little vitamin E.

Vitamin K is required for blood clotting. The "K" is derived from the Danish word *koagulation*. Vitamin K is needed for the carboxylation of glutamic acid to allow for the synthesis of seven clotting factors produced in the liver. The drug warfarin (Coumadin) is a vitamin K antagonist that functions by inhibiting the production of the clotting factors. Vitamin K is also needed for the production of osteonectin and "matrix gla protein," which are present in bone [6]. The vitamin K–mediated carboxylation of glutamic acid to γ-carboxyglutamic acid results in calcium-binding function by these proteins. Low levels of vitamin K have been associated with decreased bone density measurements. Vitamin K can be obtained from the diet, but there is also a significant amount produced by intestinal bacteria. The AI for vitamin K is 90 μg/d for women and 120 μg/d for men.

Vitamin B complex is a group of related substances that are involved in energy production from carbohydrate and fats, in red blood cell formation, and in protein and amino acid metabolism. In the early twentieth century, the deficiency disease beriberi was cured by "vitamin B," which was later found to be a complex of many vitamins. As vitamin B complex was isolated, the individual vitamins were assigned numbers. B_1 was named thiamine, B_2 riboflavin, and so forth. Except for vitamins B_6 and B_{12}, most B vitamins are presently designated by their chemical names. Because the level of B vitamins is reduced during the refining of grains, flour has been supplemented with thiamin, riboflavin, and niacin since the 1940s to approximate the levels seen in whole grains. Folate was added in 1998.

Thiamin (B_1) has a primary role in energy production. It is required for the metabolism of carbohydrates and branched-chain amino acids. The classic disease of thiamin deficiency is beriberi. This nutritional disease affects the muscular, nervous, cardiovascular, and gastrointestinal systems. It can develop in 7 to 10 days from eating a diet that is severely deficient in thiamin. The RDA for thiamin is 1.1 mg/d for women and 1.2 mg/d for men. Fortified bread, pork, and orange juice are major sources of thiamin.

Riboflavin (B_2) is also important for energy production. It is involved in redox reactions within the body. There is no known primary deficiency disease associated with riboflavin. A riboflavin deficiency often results in an oral presentation of glossitis, angular cheilosis, or stomatitis [7]. The RDA for riboflavin is 1.1 mg/d for women and 1.3 mg/d for men. Milk is a major source of riboflavin.

Niacin is present in food as two forms, niacin (nicotinic acid) and niacinamide (nicotinamide). Niacin is involved in over 200 cellular pathways, primarily those responsible for energy production and synthesis and metabolism of fatty acids. In addition to being available from food, niacin can also be synthesized from tryptophan. The primary deficiency disease of niacin is pellagra, which has symptoms including dermatitis, dementia, and diarrhea. About 10,000 people died annually from pellagra in the United States during the earlier parts of the twentieth century. The enrichment of refined flour with niacin in the early 1940s led to the disappearance of pellagra in the United States. Niacin can also be used to moderate elevated cholesterol levels. Pharmacologic doses of niacin (50–100 times the RDA) can lower low-density lipoprotein cholesterol and raise high-density lipoprotein cholesterol. Adverse effects of these higher doses include flushing and itching of the skin, nausea, and possible liver damage. The RDA for niacin is 14 mg/d for women and 16 mg/d for men.

Pantothenic acid is part of coenzyme A. This enzyme is required for ATP production from protein, carbohydrates, lipids, and alcohol. The AI for pantothenic acid is 5 mg/d.

Biotin is an essential cofactor for different carboxylase enzymes. Three of these carboxylases are involved with amino acid metabolism and energy production. A fourth enzyme is involved in fatty acid synthesis. In addition to food, intestinal bacteria help provide biotin. The AI for biotin is 30 µg/d.

Vitamin B_6 consists of three compounds: pyridoxal, pyridoxine, and pyridoxamine. Vitamin B_6 is involved in over 100 cellular reactions. It is needed for amino acid, lipid, and homocysteine metabolism and for the synthesis of heme. Vitamin B_6 is also required for the conversion of tryptophan to niacin. Vitamin B_6 has also been used to treat carpal tunnel syndrome, with varying results [8,9]. The RDA of vitamin B_6 for adults is 1.3 to 1.7 mg/d. Vitamin B_6 is stored in the body, and long-term use of higher doses (>200 mg/d) has been shown to lead to irreversible nerve damage.

Folate is also called folic acid and folacin. It is involved in DNA synthesis and amino acid metabolism. It has a close relationship with vitamin B_{12}, which is needed for regeneration of a folate coenzyme. When folate levels are low, DNA synthesis is impaired. This impairment can lead to an inability of erythrocyte precursor cells to divide, leading to megloblastic anemia with large immature blood cells noted. This form of anemia is also observed with a vitamin B_{12} deficiency. Neural tube defects may arise during early pregnancy if maternal folate levels are low. It is estimated that 70% of neural tube defects could be prevented if all women entered pregnancy with optimal levels of folate [10]. Flour has been fortified with folate since 1998. The RDA for folate is 400 µg/d. The level of folate in nonprescription vitamins is limited to 400 µg/d by the Food and Drug Administration because high doses of folate could mask the anemia associated with a vitamin B_{12} deficiency.

Vitamin B_{12} is also known as cyanocobalamin. Vitamin B_{12} is not found in plant foods but found only in foods from animal sources. To obtain adequate levels of vitamin B_{12}, strict vegetarians must eat eggs or dairy products, eat foods fortified with vitamin B_{12}, or take supplemental vitamins. Vitamin B_{12} is needed for folate and homocysteine metabolism. It is associated with enzymes that transfer carbon units and is involved in proper functioning of the nervous system. The primary disease associated with vitamin B_{12} deficiency is pernicious anemia. This disease is due to a genetic defect that leads to deficient absorption of vitamin B_{12} from the small intestine. In pernicious anemia, patients present not only with a megaloblastic (macrocytic) anemia similar to that observed with folate deficiency but also with neurologic symptoms that without treatment, could lead to death within 2 to 5 years. Early signs of B_{12} deficiency are numbness of the extremities and difficulty walking. People who frequently eat meat can maintain stores of vitamin B_{12} that could last for 5 years. The RDA for vitamin B_{12} is 2.4 µg/d for adults. Because absorption of vitamin B_{12} generally declines as people age, high-dose oral supplementation or monthly injections may be required to maintain adequate stores.

Vitamin C is also known as ascorbic acid. It was named for its ability to cure scurvy. All plants and most animals synthesize ascorbic acid. Only humans, nonhuman primates, and a few other animals do not make ascorbic acid. Vitamin C is involved in many cellular functions. It is needed for the hydroxylation of proline and lysine during collagen production and functions as an antioxidant. The classic vitamin C deficiency disease is scurvy, a hemorrhagic disease, which presents with muscle weakness, lethargy, diffuse tissue bleeding, painful and swollen joints, ecchymoses, increased fractures, poor wound healing, gingivitis, and loss of integrity of the periodontal ligament. In 1753, Dr. James Lind, a Royal Navy surgeon, performed an experiment with British sailors who had symptoms of scurvy. He studied six groups of sailors. For each group, he added different components to the typical ship's diet: (1) cider; (2) vinegar; (3) sulfuric acid, ethanol, ginger, cinnamon; (4) sea water; (5) garlic, mustard, and herbs; and (6) two oranges and a lemon. Those receiving the oranges and lemon recovered in about 1 week and those receiving cider recovered after more than 2 weeks. There was no improvement seen with the other four supplement regimens [11]. Finally, in 1795, more than 40 years after Lind's discovery, rations for British sailors were made to include citrus fruits.

The RDA for vitamin C is 75 mg/d for women and 90 mg/d for men, with an additional 35 mg/d for smokers. The additional 35 mg/d for smokers is thought to counter the oxidative effects of smoking. Average body stores of vitamin C are 1 to 2 g.

Water

The average human contains about 40 L of water, with about 25 L of intracellular water and about 15 L of extracellular water. About 75% by weight of a newborn baby is water, whereas adult men are about 60% and adult women are about 50% water. Water acts as a solvent and reactive medium for cellular function in the body. A person can live about 8 weeks without food but only days without water because the human body cannot conserve, store, or synthesize water as it can for some of the other nutrients.

Minerals

Minerals make up about 4% of body weight. Important minerals are found in the skeleton and in enzymes, hormones, and vitamins. Minerals help provide structure for bones and teeth and maintain normal heart rhythm, muscle contraction, nerve conduction, and acid-base balance. They can be integral parts of enzymes and hormones. Minerals are classified as major minerals (nutritional need >100 mg/d) or trace minerals (nutritional need <100 mg/d). The major minerals are sodium, potassium, calcium, magnesium, phosphorus, and sulfur. The trace minerals are iron, zinc, iodine, selenium, fluoride, copper, cobalt, chromium, manganese, and molybdenum.

Major minerals

   Sodium is the major cation in extracellular fluid; it is the key electrolyte. Sodium helps maintain fluid balance in the body and plays an essential role in nerve conduction. Almost all dietary sodium is absorbed in the intestinal tract. The average person has 250 g of salt (sodium chloride) in their body, 125 g in extracellular fluid, 90 g in mineralized tissues, and less than 30 g in intracellular fluid. The Food and Nutrition Board has set 500 mg/d as a minimum requirement for sodium, but this is presently being evaluated [12]. The DV for sodium is 2400 mg/d. The typical daily adult intake is 3–7 g (Table 2).

   Potassium is the major cation in intracellular fluid. It is involved in many of the same functions as sodium, but intracellularly. It has been associated with decreased blood pressure and risk of stroke. Potassium deficiency is more likely than sodium deficiency because we do not usually add potassium to our foods. A low potassium plasma level can be life threatening, presenting with muscle cramps, confusion, and an irregular heartbeat. A deficiency may be seen with the use of diuretics that waste potassium. The minimum requirement for potassium is set at 2 g/d, whereas the DV is 3.5 g/d.

   Calcium is a major mineral. The body contains about 1200 g of calcium (about 40% of the total body mineral), of which about 99% is in the skeleton. Bone is about 50% mineral, 20% protein, 5% fat, and about 25% water. Most of the mineral is present as hydroxyapatite. Calcium plays a major role in nerve conduction and blood clotting. Calcium is in equilibrium between bone, extracellular water, and soft tissue, with about

Table 2
National Academy of Sciences recommended dietary allowances or adequate intakes of minerals for men and women aged 19 to 50 years

Mineral	Men	Women
Calcium	1000 mg/d[a]	1000 mg/d[a]
Chromium	35 μg/d[a]	25 μg/d[a]
Copper	900 μg/d	900 μg/d
Fluoride	3.8 mg/d[a]	3.1 mg/d[a]
Iodine	150 μg/d	150 μg/d
Iron	8 mg/d	18 mg/d
Magnesium	400–420 mg/d	310–320 mg/d
Manganese	2.3 mg/d[a]	1.8 mg/d[a]
Molybdenum	45 μg/d	45 μg/d
Phosphorous	700 mg/d	700 mg/d
Selenium	55 μg/d	55 μg/d
Zinc	11 mg/d	8 mg/d

   [a] Adequate intake.

   Reprinted with permission from (Dietary reference intakes for vitamin C, vitamin E, selenium, and carotenoids) © (2000) by the National Academy of Sciences. Courtesy of the National Academies Press, Washington, DC.

0.7 g absorbed and redeposited daily. Calcium is regulated by parathyroid hormone, calcitonin, and vitamin D. The AI for adults is 1000 to 1200 mg/d.

Phosphorus is found in all plant and animal cells. A primary dietary deficiency of phosphorous is not known. About 600 to 900 g of phosphorus is present in bone in hydroxyapatite. It was once thought that phosphate intake could influence calcium absorption, but it is now known that phosphate intake has little consequence for calcium absorption at normal levels of intake. The RDA for phosphorous is 700 mg/d, and the DV is 1000 mg/d.

Magnesium is present in all tissues. The average person has about 25 g, with most stored in bone and about 25% found in soft tissues. After potassium, magnesium is the second most prominent intracellular cation. It is concentrated in mitochondria and involved in energy transfer. In plants, it is found in chloroplasts. The RDA for magnesium is 310 mg/d for women and 400 mg/d in men.

Sulfur is found mainly in proteins. It is present in the amino acids methionine and cysteine, and the active sites of coenzyme A and glutathione contain sulfur residues. Sulfur is present in heparin and chondroitin sulfates. The vitamins thiamin and biotin contain sulfur, and vitamin D may be present as a sulfate salt. There is no RDA for sulfur because most sulfur in the diet is derived from protein.

Trace minerals

The trace minerals are iron, zinc, iodine, selenium, fluoride, copper, cobalt, chromium, manganese, and molybdenum. Trace minerals are those with a daily nutritional need less than 100 mg. The total amount of trace minerals in the body is about 15 g.

Iron is important as a functional component of hemoglobin and it aids immune function. The typical person has about 4 g of iron: 2.5 g in hemoglobin, 0.3 g in myoglobin and cytochromes, and about 1 g in iron stores (ferritin). Most iron is used to make red blood cells in the bone marrow. Iron deficiency leads to anemia, which is seen more in women during their reproductive years and in children due to their rapid growth. Typical iron intake is about 10 mg/d, but only about 10% is absorbed. Meat (heme) iron is better absorbed than vegetable (nonheme) iron. Absorption is increased with vitamin C, in the presence of meat, and from gastric acidity. The RDA is 18 mg/d for adult women and 8 mg/d for men.

Zinc is a cofactor for over 50 enzymes (eg, carbonic anhydrase, alkaline phosphatase, alcohol dehydrogenase, and superoxide dismutase). About 2 g of zinc is stored in the body, with most present in bone. A zinc deficiency can lead to small stature, mild anemia, and impaired wound healing. Good sources of zinc are meats, whole grains, and legumes. The RDA is 8 mg/d for women and 11 mg/d for adult men.

Iodine was first discovered in 1811 and used to treat goiter in 1820. Iodine is present in thyroxine and triiodothyronine and helps maintain an appropriate metabolism. Body stores are about 20 to 50 mg, with about 8 mg being concentrated in the thyroid. A major source of iodine in the diet is from iodized salt. The RDA for iodine is 150 µg/d.

Fluoride functions to decrease the solubility of calcified tissues. Teeth having fluorapatite crystals have an increased resistance to decalcification. In some studies, fluoride has been shown to increase bone density, and is sometimes used to treat osteoporosis [13]. The fluoride present in saliva can help promote remineralization of enamel. The AI of fluoride is 3.1 mg/d for adult women and 3.8 mg/d for adult men.

Selenium can function as an antioxidant like vitamins C and E and β-carotene. Selenium is present in the glutathione peroxidase system and helps minimize oxidative damage to lipid membranes. This enzyme system may help to spare vitamin E. The RDA for selenium is 55 µg/d for adult men and women.

Copper and iron are required for the formation of hemoglobin. Copper is stored bound to ceruloplasmin, a copper-dependent ferroxidase that helps to oxidize iron. Ceruloplasmin is required for optimal use of ferritin. Copper is found in two members of the superoxide dismutase family, which help quench superoxide free radicals. The RDA for copper is 900 µg/d.

Chromium is present in all tissues, but the total body content is low (<6 mg). It helps maintain normal sugar and fat metabolism. Chromium plays a role in the uptake of glucose into cells, possibly through a chromium-binding protein, which may upregulate insulin receptors. A chromium deficiency can lead to increased serum cholesterol levels and poor glucose tolerance. The AI for chromium is 25 µg/d for women and 35 µg/d for men. The DV is 120 µg/d. Good sources of this element are brewers yeast, liver, cheese, and whole grains.

Manganese is a cofactor for enzymes involved in the synthesis of proteoglycans. Some manganese-containing enzymes are present in mito-chondria. The AI of manganese is 1.8 mg/d for women and 2.3 mg/d for men.

Molybdenum is a constituent of xanthine oxidase, aldehyde oxidase, and sulfite oxidase. No deficiency disorder has been recognized. The RDA for adults is 45 µg/d and the DV is 75 µg/d.

Five ultratrace minerals may have a role in human nutrition, but there are no RDA or AI values for them [12]. These ultratrace minerals include boron, nickel, silicon, arsenic, and vanadium [14]. Boron appears to interact with calcium and magnesium and to have a role in ion transport within cellular membranes. Nickel may function as a cofactor in amino acid and fatty acid metabolism. Silicon may play a role in bone metabolism with the organic bony matrix in some animals, but no conclusive evidence is available for humans. Arsenic is probably involved in the metabolism of methionine and in some nucleic acid synthesis. Vanadium may have a role in insulin metabolism.

Role of nutrition in periodontal disease

Periodontal diseases are a group of bacterial inflammatory disorders that result in destruction of the supporting tissues of the teeth. They include chronic periodontitis, aggressive periodontitis, and necrotizing ulcerative gingivitis and periodontitis. Periodontal diseases result from bacterial infections. Therapy to reduce oral microbial levels can reduce gingivitis and stabilize periodontitis. Although dietary components play a major role in the pathogenesis of dental caries, diet plays primarily a modifying role in the progression of periodontal disease. A periodontal lesion is essentially a wound, and sufficient host resources must be available for optimal healing. The effect of nutrition on the immune system and its role in periodontal disease has been recently reviewed [15,16]. Neiva et al [17] recently reviewed the literature on the use of specific nutrients to prevent or treat periodontal diseases. These investigators concluded that although the treatment of periodontal disease by nutritional supplementation has minimal side effects, the data on its efficacy are limited.

Protein and other nutrients are needed to provide adequate host defenses. The periodontal defenses include cell-mediated immunity, antibody or humoral immunity, the complement system, and innate immunity. The crevicular and junctional epithelium provide an epithelial barrier function. This epithelial surface provides a major defensive barrier to invasion by antigens, noxious products, and bacteria. It undergoes a rapid turnover and is therefore dependent on sufficient protein, zinc, folic acid, iron, vitamin A, and vitamin C. When patients are undernourished, their nutritionally deficient status could result in a reversible loss of barrier function.

Calcium is the major mineral present in osseous tissues. Deficiency can lead to a decrease in serum calcium, resulting in mobilization from host tissues. Calcium is needed for normal bone metabolism, with an interplay between the osteoblasts, osteocytes, and osteoclasts. Calcium homeostasis is controlled by parathyroid hormone and calcitonin.

Dietary calcium has long been a candidate to modulate periodontal disease. Animal and human studies of calcium intake, bone mineral density, and tooth loss provide a rationale for hypothesizing that low dietary intake of calcium is a risk factor for periodontal disease. A recent epidemiologic study by Nishida et al [18] suggested that low dietary intake of calcium results in more severe periodontal disease. In this study, data from the Third National Health and Nutrition Examination Survey (NHANES III) were analyzed. Low levels of dietary calcium were found to be associated with periodontal disease in young men and women and in older men. Further studies are needed to better define the role of calcium in periodontal disease and to determine the extent to which calcium supplementation can modulate periodontal disease and tooth loss.

Excess vitamin A can lead to gingival pathology. In a case report, a 20-year-old woman presented with gingival erosions, ulcerations, bleeding, swelling, and a loss of keratinization. Headache, dry mouth, and loss of hair were also noted. She reported a history of taking 200,000 IU of vitamin A daily for 6 months to reduce acne. When the vitamin supplementation was stopped, gingival improvement was noted within 1 week. At 2 months, the appearance of the oral tissues was found to be normal [19]. This case report has excellent clinical photographs.

Several studies and case reports have evaluated the role of vitamin C in periodontitis. Vitamin C has long been a candidate for modulating periodontal disease. Studies of scorbutic gingivitis and the effects of vitamin C on extracellular matrix and immunologic and inflammatory responses provide a rationale for hypothesizing that vitamin C is a risk factor for periodontal disease. Collagen is a major component of the periodontium, being one of the major proteins in the gingival connective tissues and bone. For collagen maturation to occur, adequate vitamin C must be available within the body for the hydroxylation of lysine and proline.

Vogel et al [20] evaluated the role of megadoses of vitamin C on polymorphonuclear chemotaxis and on the progression of experimental gingivitis. Four months of daily vitamin C (500 mg three times a day) supplementation resulted in a significant increase in plasma ascorbate levels but did not increase host resistance during 4 weeks of experimental gingivitis as evaluated by clinical parameters, by polymorphonuclear chemotaxis, and by changes in crevicular fluid enzyme levels.

Leggott et al [21] evaluated the effect of controlled ascorbic acid depletion and supplementation on periodontal health. Eleven men ate a diet low in vitamin C (<5 mg/d) and received supplementation of 60 mg/d during weeks 1 and 2; 0 mg/d during weeks 3, 4, 5, and 6; 600 mg/d during weeks 7, 8, 9, and 10; and 0 mg/d during weeks 11, 12, 13, and 14. Ascorbic acid depletion, with good oral hygiene, led to a decrease in plasma ascorbate levels and an increase in gingival inflammation and bleeding but did not result in severe periodontal disease or changes in pocket depth. This study showed that a vitamin C deficiency influenced the early stages of gingival inflammation but did not lead to a loss of attachment during the time frame of this study.

A diet low in vitamin C can lead to the development of scurvy. In one case report, a 48-year-old man presented with the sudden development of scurvy. His gingiva was bright red, inflamed, and edematous. Acute leukemia and diabetes were ruled out. He was screened for a vitamin deficiency, and a low plasma level of ascorbic acid was determined. After completing a 5-day diet history, nutritional analysis revealed deficiencies in several nutrients. A typical daily diet for this patient was coffee, a peanut butter sandwich, tuna noodle casserole, and one-half case of beer. His average daily consumption of vitamin C was less than 1 mg/d. Treatment consisted of vitamin C and vitamin B complex supplementation, a diversified diet, and periodontal scaling and root planing. His general health and his periodontal condition showed rapid improvement [22]. Excellent photos are presented showing the progression of disease.

Cessation of chronic vitamin C intake can also result in oral scurvy. In this case report, a 49-year-old man presented with "sore gums." His gingiva showed the presence of petechial hemorrhages, crevicular bleeding, and mucosal ulcerations. He reported a daily intake of 1 g of vitamin C for 1 year, which was stopped about 10 days previously. Taking 1 g of vitamin C for 2 weeks allowed for the regression of the lesions. He stopped for 1 week and the lesions returned. He was gradually reduced to 100 mg/d over a 7-week period and remained free of oral symptoms [23]. This condition is known as rebound or conditional scurvy.

Nishida et al [24] evaluated the effect of dietary intake of vitamin C and the presence of periodontal disease. Dietary intake of vitamin C showed a weak but statistically significant relationship to periodontal disease in current and former smokers as measured by clinical attachment. The greatest clinical effect on periodontal tissues was shown in smokers who took the lowest levels of vitamin C.

Low serum levels of vitamin D have been linked with a loss of periodontal attachment. NHANES III data from over 11,000 subjects were analyzed for serum vitamin D levels and attachment loss [25]. In subjects less than 50 years of age, there was no significant association noted between vitamin D levels and attachment loss. In patients 50 years or older, serum vitamin D levels were inversely associated with attachment loss for men and women. It was concluded that the increased risk for periodontal disease might be attributable to low levels of vitamin D, which would reduce bone mineral density, or to an immunomodulatory effect.

Intake of tomato products has also been shown to be associated with a reduced risk of congestive heart failure in patients with periodontitis [26]. Data from NHANES III were evaluated for monthly tomato consumption, serum lycopene (a phytochemical found in tomatoes) levels, and congestive heart failure. Subjects with periodontitis have an increased risk of congestive heart failure, and increased tomato consumption appears to reduce this risk.

Herbal and nutritional supplements

Various herbal and nutritional supplements have been touted as being beneficial for the prevention and treatment of periodontal disease. Few cross-sectional studies exist, however, and there are no randomized longitudinal studies. Coenzyme Q_{10} is distributed throughout all human tissues. It is involved in the electron transport functions of the mitochondria. It has also been proposed as a modulator of periodontal disease. In vivo and in vitro reports in the literature suggest that patients with periodontal disease may have a deficiency of coenzyme Q_{10} and that treatment with this coenzyme may improve a patient's periodontal disease status [27–33]. Most studies showed that in gingival biopsy samples, periodontally diseased tissues had lower levels of coenzyme Q_{10} than periodontally healthy gingival tissues.

With only a limited number of reports in the literature, it is premature to recommend coenzyme Q_{10} for the treatment of periodontal disease, although its use would appear to have a minimal risk of side effects.

In Africa, Asia, and the Middle East, some populations have long used chewing sticks to clean their teeth. The chewing stick, or miswak, is usually made from the *Salvadora persica* plant. These sticks are usually chewed and rubbed against the teeth to remove plaque. Use of the miswak generally was equivalent to and sometimes better than the use of a toothbrush in reducing plaque and gingivitis scores [34,35]. The miswak has also been shown to have a selective antimicrobial effect against various oral microorganisms [34,36–38]. This effect is attributable to the natural antimicrobial agents that the plant uses to fight microbial infection. In response to chewing, these agents leach out from the miswak into the oral cavity and interact with the oral flora. Other plants have also been used as chewing sticks. The rural and urban people of Namibia use *Diospyros lycioides* for oral hygiene. This plant contains antimicrobial compounds that can inhibit the growth of *Streptococcus mutans*, *Porphyromonas gingivalis*, and *Prevotella intermedia* [39]. Other plant-derived agents used for oral hygiene practices include mango leaf in India [40] and *Massularia acuminata* and *Distemonanthus benthamianus* in Nigeria [41]. The polyphenols extracted from green tea have been shown to inhibit the metabolism of *Porphyromonas gingivalis*, leading to a reduction of toxic products [42]. Many other natural products have been used throughout the world in an attempt to improve the oral health of the resident population. Some are without merit but others have shown promise in the quest for better dental health.

Clinical implications

Although it is reasonable to consume a nutritionally adequate diet to maintain host resistance and maintain the integrity of the periodontal tissues, insufficient evidence is available to justify treatment with vitamin and mineral supplementation in the adequately nourished individual. Periodontal disease is an infectious disease caused by bacterial infection and can be treated and prevented by the elimination of bacterial plaque in the adequately nourished individual. In patients who have inadequate nutrition, it may be reasonable to suggest a vitamin or mineral supplement.

References

[1] Marshall TA, Warren JJ, Hand JS, et al. Oral health, nutrient intake and dietary quality in the very old. J Am Dent Assoc 2002;133(10):1369–79.
[2] Hung HC, Willett W, Ascherio A, et al. Tooth loss and dietary intake. J Am Dent Assoc 2003;134(9):1185–92.

[3] Trumbo P, Schlicker S, Yates AA, et al. Dietary reference intakes for energy, carbohydrate, fiber, fat, fatty acids, cholesterol, protein and amino acids. J Am Diet Assoc 2002;102(11): 1621–30.

[4] Slattery ML, Curtin KP, Edwards SL, et al. Plant foods, fiber, and rectal cancer. Am J Clin Nutr 2004;79(2):274–81.

[5] Liu S. Intake of refined carbohydrates and whole grain foods in relation to risk of type 2 diabetes mellitus and coronary heart disease. J Am Coll Nutr 2002;21(4):298–306.

[6] Bugel S. Vitamin K and bone health. Proc Nutr Soc 2003;62(4):839–43.

[7] Blanck HM, Bowman BA, Serdula MK, et al. Angular stomatitis and riboflavin status among adolescent Bhutanese refugees living in southeastern Nepal. Am J Clin Nutr 2002; 76(2):430–5.

[8] Kasdan ML, Janes C. Carpal tunnel syndrome and vitamin B6. Plast Reconstr Surg 1987; 79(3):456–62.

[9] Keniston RC, Nathan PA, Leklem JE, et al. Vitamin B6, vitamin C, and carpal tunnel syndrome. A cross-sectional study of 441 adults. J Occup Environ Med 1997;39(10): 949–59.

[10] Green NS. Folic acid supplementation and prevention of birth defects. J Nutr 2002; 132(Suppl 8):2356S–60S.

[11] Sutton G. Putrid gums and 'dead men's cloaths': James Lind aboard the Salisbury. J R Soc Med 2003;96(12):605–8.

[12] Wardlaw G, Hampl J, DiSilvestro R. Perspectives in nutrition. 6th edition. New York: McGraw-Hill; 2004.

[13] Ringe JD, Setnikar I. Monofluorophosphate combined with hormone replacement therapy in postmenopausal osteoporosis. An open-label pilot efficacy and safety study. Rheumatol Int 2002;22(1):27–32.

[14] Uthus EO, Seaborn CD. Deliberations and evaluations of the approaches, endpoints and paradigms for dietary recommendations of the other trace elements. J Nutr 1996; 126(Suppl 9):2452S–9S.

[15] Boyd LD, Madden TE. Nutrition, infection, and periodontal disease. Dent Clin N Am 2003; 47(2):337–54.

[16] Enwonwu CO, Phillips RS, Falkler WA Jr. Nutrition and oral infectious diseases: state of the science. Compend Contin Educ Dent 2002;23(5):431–8 [quiz: 448].

[17] Neiva RF, Steigenga J, Al-Shammari KF, et al. Effects of specific nutrients on periodontal disease onset, progression and treatment. J Clin Periodontol 2003;30(7):579–89.

[18] Nishida M, Grossi SG, Dunford RG, et al. Calcium and the risk for periodontal disease. J Periodontol 2000;71(7):1057–66.

[19] de Menezes AC, Costa IM, El-Guindy MM. Clinical manifestations of hypervitaminosis A in human gingiva. A case report. J Periodontol 1984;55(8):474–6.

[20] Vogel RI, Lamster IB, Wechsler SA, et al. The effects of megadoses of ascorbic acid on PMN chemotaxis and experimental gingivitis. J Periodontol 1986;57(8):472–9.

[21] Leggott PJ, Robertson PB, Rothman DL, et al. The effect of controlled ascorbic acid depletion and supplementation on periodontal health. J Periodontol 1986;57(8):480–5.

[22] Charbeneau TD, Hurt WC. Gingival findings in spontaneous scurvy. A case report. J Periodontol 1983;54(11):694–7.

[23] Siegel C, Barker B, Kunstadter M. Conditioned oral scurvy due to megavitamin C withdrawal. J Periodontol 1982;53(7):453–5.

[24] Nishida M, Grossi SG, Dunford RG, et al. Dietary vitamin C and the risk for periodontal disease. J Periodontol 2000;71(8):1215–23.

[25] Dietrich T, Joshipura KJ, Dawson-Hughes B, et al. Association between serum concentrations of 25-hydroxyvitamin D3 and periodontal disease in the US population. Am J Clin Nutr 2004;80(1):108–13.

[26] Wood N, Johnson RB. The relationship between tomato intake and congestive heart failure risk in periodontitis subjects. J Clin Periodontol 2004;31(7):574–80.

[27] Hansen IL, Iwamoto Y, Kishi T, et al. Bioenergetics in clinical medicine. IX. Gingival and leucocytic deficiencies of coenzyme Q10 in patients with periodontal disease. Res Commun Chem Pathol Pharmacol 1976;14(4):729–38.

[28] Iwamoto Y, Nakamura R, Folkers K, et al. Study of periodontal disease and coenzyme Q. Res Commun Chem Pathol Pharmacol 1975;11(2):265–71.

[29] Littarru GP, Nakamura R, Ho L, et al. Deficiency of coenzyme Q 10 in gingival tissue from patients with periodontal disease. Proc Natl Acad Sci U S A 1971;68(10):2332–5.

[30] Nakamura R, Littarru GP, Folkers K, et al. Deficiency of coenzyme Q in gingiva of patients with periodontal disease. Int J Vitam Nutr Res 1973;43(1):84–92.

[31] Nakamura R, Littarru GP, Folkers K, et al. Study of CoQ10-enzymes in gingiva from patients with periodontal disease and evidence for a deficiency of coenzyme Q10. Proc Natl Acad Sci U S A 1974;71(4):1456–60.

[32] Tsunemitsu A, Matsumura T. Effect of coenzyme Q administration on hypercitricemia of patients with periodontal disease. J Dent Res 1967;46(6):1382–4.

[33] Wilkinson EG, Arnold RM, Folkers K. Bioenergetics in clinical medicine. VI. Adjunctive treatment of periodontal disease with coenzyme Q10. Res Commun Chem Pathol Pharmacol 1976;14(4):715–9.

[34] al-Otaibi M. The miswak (chewing stick) and oral health. Studies on oral hygiene practices of urban Saudi Arabians. Swed Dent J Suppl 2004;167:2–75.

[35] Darout IA, Albandar JM, Skaug N. Periodontal status of adult Sudanese habitual users of miswak chewing sticks or toothbrushes. Acta Odontol Scand 2000;58(1):25–30.

[36] Darout IA, Albandar JM, Skaug N, et al. Salivary microbiota levels in relation to periodontal status, experience of caries and miswak use in Sudanese adults. J Clin Periodontol 2002;29(5):411–20.

[37] Kemoli AM, van Amerongen WE, de Soet JJ. Antimicrobial and buffer capacity of crude extracts of chewing sticks (Miswaki) from Kenya. ASDC J Dent Child 2001;68(3):152, 183–8.

[38] Wu CD, Darout IA, Skaug N. Chewing sticks: timeless natural toothbrushes for oral cleansing. J Periodontal Res 2001;36(5):275–84.

[39] Cai L, Wei GX, van der Bijl P, et al. Namibian chewing stick, *Diospyros lycioides*, contains antibacterial compounds against oral pathogens. J Agric Food Chem 2000;48(3):909–14.

[40] Bairy I, Reeja S, Siddharth, et al. Evaluation of antibacterial activity of *Mangifera indica* on anaerobic dental microglora based on in vivo studies. Indian J Pathol Microbiol 2002;45(3): 307–10.

[41] Aderinokun GA, Lawoyin JO, Onyeaso CO. Effect of two common Nigerian chewing sticks on gingival health and oral hygiene. Odontostomatol Trop 1999;22(87):13–8.

[42] Sakanaka S, Okada Y. Inhibitory effects of green tea polyphenols on the production of a virulence factor of the periodontal-disease-causing anaerobic bacterium *Porphyromonas gingivalis*. J Agric Food Chem 2004;52(6):1688–92.

ELSEVIER
SAUNDERS

THE DENTAL
CLINICS
OF NORTH AMERICA

Dent Clin N Am 49 (2005) 611–636

Nonsurgical Approaches for the Treatment of Periodontal Diseases

Maria Emanuel Ryan, DDS, PhD

*Department of Oral Biology and Pathology, School of Dental Medicine,
Stony Brook University, State University of New York,
South Campus, Stony Brook, NY 11794-8702, USA*

Periodontal diseases are the most common dental conditions. Gingivitis is gingival inflammation associated with plaque and calculus accumulation. Gingivitis may or may not progress to more advanced forms of the disease known as periodontitis, which is associated with alveolar bone loss and diagnosed by increases in probing depths, loss of clinical attachment, and radiographic evidence of bone loss. Periodontitis is chronic and progressive and there is no known cure. Periodontal disease, however, is treatable and may even be prevented. Risk for periodontal disease and lack of treatment of periodontitis have been linked to the systemic health of the patient. Periodontitis is a complex interaction between an infection and a susceptible host.

Periodontal disease is initiated by an infection; however, it appears to behave not like a classic infection but more like an opportunistic infection. As a biofilm-mediated disease, periodontal disease is inherently difficult to treat. One of the greatest challenges in treatment arises from the fact that there is no way to eliminate bacteria from the oral cavity, so bacteria will always be present in the periodontal milieu. In addition, the bacteria within the biofilm are more resistant to antimicrobial agents and various components of the host response. When certain, more virulent species exist in an environment that allows them to be present in greater proportions, there is the opportunity for periodontal destruction to occur. Although it is apparent that plaque is essential for the development of the disease, the

The author is a consultant, serves on a number of advisory boards, and is named on patents as an inventor of therapeutic applications of tetracyclines discussed in this article. These patents have been fully assigned to the research foundation of Stony Brook University, State University of New York, Stony Brook, New York, and have been licensed exclusively to CollaGenex Pharmaceuticals, Newtown, Pennsylvania.

E-mail address: maria.ryan@stonybrook.edu

doi:10.1016/j.cden.2005.03.010
dental.theclinics.com

severity and pattern of the disease are not explained solely by the amount of plaque present.

In the 1980s, research began to focus on the relationship between the bacteria in the oral cavity and the response of the individual challenged by these bacteria or the bacterial host [1]. As a result of multiple studies, it was recognized that although there is evidence that specific bacterial pathogens initiate the pathogenesis of periodontal disease, the host response to these pathogens is equally if not more important in mediating connective tissue breakdown including bone loss. It has become clear that certain host-derived enzymes known as the matrix metalloproteinases (MMPs) and changes in bone resorptive osteoclast cell activity driven by factors known as cytokines and other inflammatory mediators such as prostanoids cause most of the tissue destruction in the periodontium (Fig. 1) [2].

Risk factors

It has been recognized that the severity of periodontal disease, its rate of progression, and its response to therapy vary from patient to patient. Bacteria are essential for the initiation of the disease but insufficient by themselves to cause the disease. The host must be susceptible, and it is the patient's risk factors that determine susceptibility to the disease. Risk factors are patient characteristics associated with the development of a disease.

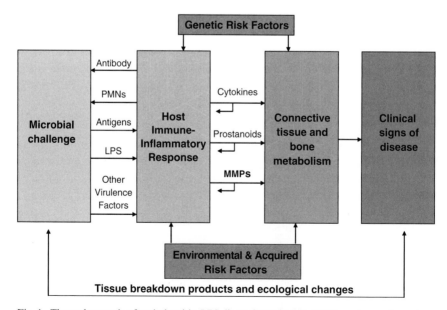

Fig. 1. The pathogenesis of periodontitis. LPS, lipopolysaccharide; PMNs, polymorphonuclear neutrophils. (*Adapted from* Page RC, Kornman KS. The pathogenesis of human periodontitis: an introduction. Periodontol 2000 1997;14:10; with permission.)

Risk assessment in the patient with periodontitis

There are a number of environmental and acquired risk factors that play a major role in the host response and can increase a patient's susceptibility to periodontitis. Listed in Box 1 [3–5] are the risk factors that should be

---

Box 1. Risk assessment for periodontitis

1. Heredity as determined by genetic testing and family history
2. Smoking including frequency, current use, and history
3. Hormonal variations such as those seen in
    a. pregnancy in which there are increased levels of estradiol and progesterone that may change the environment and permit the virulent organisms to become more destructive
    b. menopause in which the reductions in estrogen levels lead to osteopenia and eventually osteoporosis
4. Systemic diseases such as
    a. diabetes (the duration and level of control are important)
    b. osteoporosis
    c. immune system disorders such as HIV
    d. hematologic disorders such as neutropenias
    e. connective tissue disorders such as Marfan's and Ehlers-Danlos syndromes
5. Stress as reported by the patient
6. Nutritional deficiencies that may require a dietary analysis
7. Medications such as
    a. calcium channel blockers
    b. immunomodulatory agents
    c. anticonvulsants
    d. those known to cause dry mouth or xerostomia
8. Faulty dentistry such as overhangs and subgingival margins
9. Excessive occlusal loads
10. Poor oral hygiene resulting in excessive plaque and calculus
11. History of periodontal disease
12. Additional risk factors including hyperlipidemia and possibly arthritis

---

Data from Refs. [3–5].

assessed because they can affect the onset, rate of progression, and severity of periodontal disease and response to therapy.

It is important to document and determine the patient's risk and to convey to the patient that these risk factors can be more than additive. The value of risk assessment is that it can help the practitioner to establish an accurate diagnosis, provide an optimal treatment plan, and determine appropriate maintenance programs. Risk assessment may help to explain variability in treatment responses. In patients with multiple risk factors, the practitioner may proceed with caution with regard to invasive surgical procedures and may aggressively use pharmacologic adjuncts such as antimicrobials and host modulatory therapy in addition to mechanical therapy. When considering a risk-based approach to therapy, there is less watching and waiting to see what will happen and more frequent active treatment and maintenance therapy. It is also important to note that risk assessment is an ongoing process because a patient's risk changes throughout his or her life.

Risk modification

Some of these risk factors can be modified to reduce a patient's susceptibility to periodontitis. In addition to more frequent dental visits, including active treatment and maintenance visits, risk reduction may include the strategies listed in Box 2. The field of "perioceutics," or the use of pharmacologic agents specifically developed to better manage periodontitis, is emerging to aid in the management of susceptible patients who develop periodontal disease. When patients are unable to effectively reduce risk—such as the risk presented by the patient's genetics, smokers who are unable to kick the habit, patients who are unable to maintain adequate oral hygiene, the inability to reduce stress, diabetics who are poorly controlled despite the physician's best efforts, and the inability or unwillingness of the physician to alter medications—patients may require the use of perioceutics. Perioceutics includes antimicrobial therapies that can be used to address changes in the microflora and host modulatory therapy that can be used to address a host response consisting of excessive levels of enzymes, cytokines, and prostanoids and excessive osteoclast function that may be related to certain risk factors.

The antimicrobial approach

The antimicrobial approach to periodontal therapy has been used for many years, recognizing that the prevalence and severity of these diseases can be reduced by mechanical plaque removal or by the use of a variety of systemic or topically applied antimicrobial agents aimed at inhibiting pathogenic bacteria.

Box 2. Risk reduction strategies

1. More frequent visits for those with a genetic predisposition and the use of perioceutics (use of pharmacotherapeutics for the management of periodontitis)
2. Smoking cessation using one or more of the six approved regimens; these regimens rarely are successful as sole therapies (multiple forms of therapy often are used in combination with counseling to achieve success)
3. Hormonal variations such as those seen in
    a. pregnancy require good oral care before pregnancy to prevent complications during pregnancy; treatment of women during pregnancy may be necessary to prevent adverse pregnancy outcomes
    b. menopause may require hormonal supplements, calcium, and other medications and supplements prescribed by the physician to prevent osteopenia
4. Systemic diseases that require consultation with the physician include
    a. diabetes (for improved glycemic control)
    b. osteoporosis (requiring calcium supplements, bisphosphonates)
    c. immune system and hematologic disorders
    d. connective tissue disorders
5. Stress management; possible referral to a psychologist or psychiatrist
6. Nutritional supplementation; possible referral to a nutritionist
7. Medications can be changed in consultation with the physician
8. Corrective dentistry
9. Occlusal adjustments
10. Improved oral hygiene

Mechanical therapy

Brushing and flossing, as part of an oral hygiene routine, is the first-line approach to microbial reduction. The American Dental Association (ADA) recommends brushing for 2 minutes twice a day and flossing once a day. Many patients also use interproximal brushes, stimudents, and other mechanical aids to reduce plaque levels. Proper oral hygiene can effectively reduce gingivitis and aid in the treatment of periodontitis. Oral hygiene instructions should be given to all patients undergoing periodontal therapy. The unfortunate reality is that despite clinicians' best efforts, many patients do not spend a sufficient amount of time brushing and most cannot or will not floss on a daily basis [6]. These circumstances result in a population in which more than 50% of adults have gingivitis [7]. Studies have demonstrated that powered toothbrushes, particularly those that work with rotation oscillation action, are safe and often more effective than manual toothbrushes at reducing plaque and gingivitis in the long- and short-term [8]. Powered brushes with timers help patients to comply with the recommended 30 seconds per quadrant of toothbrushing twice a day. Despite attempts to encourage plaque removal solely by mechanical means, adjuncts to existing home care routines have been developed to aid in the removal of plaque.

Tooth scaling by the dental care provider is also a key component in treating and preventing gingivitis. Aggressive subgingival debridement includes scaling and root planing (SRP) by manual instrumentation or with sonic or ultrasonic scalers. SRP has become the "gold standard" nonsurgical treatment of periodontitis, with multiple clinical studies demonstrating that it effectively reduces the microbial load and leads to reductions in bleeding on probing and probing depths and allows for gains in clinical attachment. A review of nonsurgical mechanical pocket therapy by Cobb [9] reveals mean probing depth reductions and clinical attachment level gains of 1.29 mm and 0.55 mm, respectively, for initial probing depths of 4 to 6 mm before treatment and 2.16 mm and 1.19 mm, respectively, for initial probing depths of >6 mm before treatment. Conventional non-surgical periodontal therapy involves performing SRP in single or multiple quadrants or sextants per visit and is usually completed in 2 to 6 weeks. The new concept of full-mouth disinfection for the prevention of reinfection from bacterial reservoirs has recently been introduced and shows promising results but requires further investigation [10]. In addition, the use of lasers within the periodontal pocket is being investigated and may emerge as a new technical modality for nonsurgical therapy in the near future [11].

Mechanical removal of plaque and calculus (nonsurgical and with surgical access) is time-consuming, operator and patient dependent, and difficult to master [12]. Although mechanical and surgical interventions continue to be the most widely used methods of controlling disease progression, instrumentation inevitably leaves behind significant numbers of microorganisms, including putative pathogens. Recolonization of these pathogens can occur within 60 days of SRP, resulting in the need for regular maintenance visits. The need for chemotherapeutic agents as adjuncts to mechanical and surgical debridement is compelling.

Antiseptics

Antiseptics can be used topically or subgingivally. They are agents that kill oral microorganisms that cause gingivitis, periodontitis, and caries. Antiseptics are not antibiotics or disinfectants and do not cause bacterial resistance.

Rinses and irrigation

Antiseptic mouthrinses have been used to aid in controlling plaque build-up. They have been used to complement, not replace mechanical therapy. Two clinically proven ADA-accepted antiseptic mouthrinses are Peridex (Zila, Inc., Phoenix, Arizona; chlorhexidine gluconate) and Listerine Antiseptic Mouthrinse (four essential oils; Pfizer, Inc., Morris Plains, New Jersey), studied in clinical trials of at least 6 months' duration. Both of these rinses have demonstrated an extremely broad spectrum of kill *in vitro* and *in vivo*. In a number of randomized, double-blinded, controlled 6-month clinical studies, these two agents demonstrated comparable efficacy for improving reductions in plaque and gingivitis compared with brushing alone [13,14]. Clinical studies have demonstrated additional benefits with the use of these antiseptic mouthrinses, such as control of oral malodor [15,16], enhancement of the benefits of oral irrigation [17,18], improvement in the gingival health around dental implants [19], reductions in plaque and gingivitis in orthodontic patients [20], reductions in bacteria in saliva and dental aerosols when used preprocedurally [21], and support of early healing after gingival flap surgery [22,23].

Chlorhexidine gluconate. Chlorhexidine gluconate is available at 0.12% in the United States and has strong substantivity [24]. Chlorhexidine is available only by prescription and is partly to fully covered by some prescription plans. Chorhexidine can stain teeth, the tongue, and aesthetic restorations. It can promote supragingival calculus formation and may alter taste perception [25]. When prescribed, it is recommended that patients rinse twice a day for 30 seconds with 15 mL after brushing and flossing and after toothpaste has been completely rinsed out of the mouth.

Listerine. Listerine is available over-the-counter and is composed of a fixed combination of essential oils: thymol (0.064%), eucalyptol (0.092%), methyl salicylate (0.060%), and menthol (0.042%). Some patients complain of a transient tingling sensation. Listerine's comparable efficacy in reducing interproximal plaque and gingivitis to the "gold standard" of flossing was demonstrated in a recent study in which 611 subjects rinsed twice daily or flossed once daily as an adjunct to brushing for 6 months [26,27]. In addition, the incremental benefit (with regard to plaque and gingivitis reduction) of Listerine in patients who were already brushing and flossing was demonstrated in a brush, floss, and rinse study [28]. The recommendation for use is rinse twice a day for 30 seconds with 20 mL after brushing and flossing.

Toothpaste

Triclosan. Triclosan is present in a toothpaste (Colgate Total; Colgate Palmolive, Piscataway, New Jersey) currently available in the United States. Triclosan is a substantive antibacterial agent that adheres to the oral mucosa, hard, and soft tissues for up to 12 hours. Colgate Total is approved by the

Food and Drug Administration (FDA) and accepted by the ADA for treatment of gingivitis, plaque, caries, calculus, and oral malodor. Placebo-controlled studies in smokers [29] and in subjects with recurrent periodontitis [30] suggest that an oral hygiene regimen including a triclosan/copolymer dentrifice may sustain the short-term effect of nonsurgical therapy in smokers and improve on healing after nonsurgical treatment of recurrent periodontitis as measured by improvements in gingival inflammation, probing depths, and probing attachment levels. Triclosan *in vitro* has anti-inflammatory effects, inhibiting cytokine-stimulated (interleukin 1β and tumor necrosis factor α) production of prostanoids (prostaglandin E$_2$) from monocytes, reducing the activity of the enzyme cyclooxygenase 2 responsible for the production of prostanoids in culture, and inhibiting bone resorption in a parathyroid hormone–induced release of calcium from bone cultures [31].

Locally applied antiseptic
Periochip. Periochip (Dexcel Pharmaceuticals, Israel) is an orange-brown, biodegradable, rectangular chip rounded at one end that has an active ingredient of chlorhexidine gluconate (2.5 mg) that is released into the pocket over a period of 7 to 10 days. It has been found to suppress the pocket flora for up to 11 weeks post application [32]. In a 9-month randomized, blinded, and controlled parallel arm study, Periochip, as an adjunct to SRP, significantly reduced probing depths and maintained clinical attachment levels relative to baseline at 9 months compared with controls with repeated application of the Periochip up to three applications per site over 9 months [33]. Periochip effects on alveolar bone were demonstrated in a 9-month randomized, blinded, and placebo-controlled study. After 9 months of adjunctive treatment with Periochip, no sites exhibited bone loss and 25% of the sites experienced bone gain as measured through subtraction radiography [34]. In contrast, 15% of periodontal sites treated with SRP alone experienced bone loss. Periochip has a documented safety profile and does not cause any visible staining. The most frequently observed adverse event in the clinical trials was mild to moderate toothache, which often resolved spontaneously and required no further treatment. This adverse event occurred less frequently with subsequent Periochip placements. Periochip is the only locally applied nonantibiotic antimicrobial approved by the FDA as an adjunct to SRP procedures for the reduction of probing pocket depth or as part of a routine periodontal maintenance program. The recommendation for use adjunctive to SRP involves isolation of the periodontal pocket of 5 mm or more, drying the surrounding area, and grasping the Periochip with a forceps and inserting the chip, curved end first, into the pocket to its maximum depth. The chip can be maneuvered further into position with a plastic instrument. One site can be treated per chip.

Antibiotics

Locally applied antimicrobials

To have a therapeutic effect on the microflora, antimicrobial agents must reach adequate concentrations to kill or inhibit the growth of target organisms. The drug of choice has to reach the site where the organisms exist, stay there long enough to get the job done, and not cause harm. Mouthrinses do not reach the depths of periodontal pockets, whereas irrigation can deliver drugs to the base of the pocket. Because the gingival crevicular fluid (GCF) in the pocket is replaced about every 90 seconds, the duration of exposure during subgingival irrigation is short, and topically applied subgingival agents are rapidly washed out. With regard to the systemic administration of antibiotics to patients with periodontitis, early research suggested that doxycycline administered systemically [35,36] was highly concentrated in the GCF at levels 5 to 10 times greater than found in serum. Furthermore, tetracyclines show substantivity because they bind to the tooth structure and are slowly released as still-active agents. Even this supposed hyperconcentration of the drug in the GCF resulted in a level of antibiotic to which many organisms were not susceptible. More recent work has challenged earlier findings of hyperconcentration of tetracyclines in the GCF. In the 2 hours after the administration of a single dose of tetracycline (250 mg), minocycline (100 mg), or doxycycline (100 mg), the concentration of these tetracyclines was found to be highest in the plasma, intermediate in the GCF (doxycycline achieving the highest levels), and lowest in the saliva [37]. Further experimentation may be required to resolve this issue because there was a great deal of variability in the average GCF concentrations (0–8 µg/mL) in this study, and steady-state levels of the drug were never achieved. To address the issue of reaching adequate concentrations at the base of the pocket with adequate duration, controlled local delivery of antimicrobials was developed (Table 1).

Dental research has provided us with a better understanding of the microbial etiology and the nature of periodontitis. Periodontitis, initiated by bacteria, frequently appears in localized areas in the patient's mouth or is confined to localized areas by treatment. These infected localized areas lend themselves well to treatment with a controlled local delivery system using an antimicrobial [38]. Antimicrobial agents may be applied directly to the pocket, thereby eliminating many of the adverse side effects associated with

Table 1
Periodontal antimicrobial delivery systems

Objective	Mouthrinse or toothpaste	Local irrigation	Systemic delivery	Controlled delivery
Reach the pocket >4 mm	Poor	Good	Good	Excellent
Adequate concentration	Poor	Good	Fair	Excellent
Adequate duration	Poor	Poor	Fair	Good

systemic delivery of antibiotics. Nonresorbable and resorbable intrapocket delivery systems have been used. There is evidence that local delivery of sustained-release antimicrobials may lead to improvements in periodontal health, although a few side effects such as transient discomfort, erythema, recession, transient resistance, and allergy have been reported. Oral candidiasis has been reported in a small number of cases with local tetracycline delivery.

Systems have been developed for the release of all three commercially available tetracyclines at high doses and at a regular rate over a 10- to 14-day period. The first such FDA-approved system, Actisite, was developed by Dr. Max Goodson in 1983 [39]. Actisite consisted of a nonresorbable polymer fiber of ethyl vinyl acetate, 25% saturated with tetracycline hydrochloride. Use of this product resulted in substantially higher doses of tetracycline in the pocket (1590 μg/mL in the GCF and 43 μg/mL in the tissue) than could be achieved by systemic dosing (2–8 μg/mL). A local concentration of 30 μg/mL eliminates most pathogenic bacteria associated with periodontal diseases. When using locally applied antimicrobials, the area being treated is saturated with doses of the therapeutic agent that can be sustained for prolonged periods. Despite the high doses of drug that are achieved locally, serum levels of the drug do not exceed 0.1 μg/mL. The use of a singly applied tetracycline fiber as an adjunct to SRP proved to be more effective than scaling alone at reducing bleeding on probing, pocket depth, and achieving attachment gain as early as 60 days after placement, with additional improvements at 6 months. At 6 months after a single application of Actisite, the respective average results for SRP plus tetracycline fiber therapy versus SRP only were 1.81 mm versus 1.08 mm for pocket depth, 1.56 mm versus 1.08 mm for attachment gain, and 63% versus 50% for bleeding on probing reductions [40]. Subsequent studies concluded that SRP combined with full-mouth Actisite therapy versus SRP alone resulted in increased bone density (+2.43 computer-assisted densitometric image analysis [CADIA] versus −2.13 CADIA) and increased alveolar bone height (+0.24 mm versus −0.29 mm) at 6 months after therapy [41]. Despite its demonstrated efficacy, this product is no longer marketed to the dental community. Actisite was difficult to use, requiring considerable operator skill, and because it was not resorbed, a second visit had to be scheduled to remove it. In attempts to improve on ease of placement of local antimicrobials into the pocket and to obviate the need for a second visit to remove the product, bioabsorbable delivery systems were developed.

Atridox. The second FDA-approved locally delivered tetracycline to be developed was Atridox (Atrix Laboratories, Inc., Fort Collins, Colorado), a 10% formulation of doxycycline in a bioabsorbable, "flowable" poly-DL-lactide and N-methyl-2-pyrrolidone mixture delivery system that allows for controlled release over 7 days. This system is supplied in two prefilled syringes to be mixed at chairside and applied subgingivally to the base of the pocket through a cannula. The flowable polymer gel of Atridox fills and conforms to pocket morphology, then solidifies to a waxlike substance after contact with GCF. Significant reductions (60%) in anaerobic pathogens are sustained for up to 6 months after placement of Atridox [42]. In subjects with chronic adult periodontitis, the application of this doxycycline gel at baseline and 4 months later resulted in reductions in probing depths (1.3 mm) and gains in clinical attachment (0.8 mm) equivalent to SRP alone at 9 months after baseline [43]. An important finding of these studies was that for the Atridox treatment group, smoking status did not seem to affect the outcome of clinical parameters such as probing depth reductions and clinical attachment level gains, whereas smokers and even former smokers did not respond as well to mechanical therapy alone [44]. A recent study supports these findings, indicating that locally applied Atridox improves the healing following nonsurgical therapy in smokers [45]. The side effect profile was equivalent to placebo. Despite the results of the initial phase III studies, it is likely that this agent will be used not as a monotherapy for the management of periodontal disease but as an adjunct to mechanical therapy.

Removal of the offending plaque and calculus deposits by SRP has proved to be effective. Disruption of the biofilm improves on the efficacy of antimicrobial agents. Phase IV studies conducted to support improved outcomes by using Atridox as an adjunct to scaling have demonstrated incremental benefits of use [46]. One arm of a 6-month study involved initiating therapy with ultrasonic scaling combined with Atridox, followed at 3 months by SRP alone in those sites with pocket depths that remained >5 mm. Results showed that this approach was at least as effective in improving probing depths and clinical attachment levels as the second arm of the study that involved SRP alone followed at 3 months by ultrasonic scaling and Atridox in those sites with pocket depths that remained >5 mm. The main difference between the two arms of this study was that the response was far more dramatic at 3 months for the combination therapy than the SRP alone, but the addition of either therapy at the 3-month interval allowed for equivalence to be achieved by 6 months.

Atridox is the only resorbable site-specific locally applied antibiotic proven to promote clinical attachment gains and reduce pocket depths, bleeding on probing, and levels of pathogenic bacteria. Clinical use of the product involves twisting and locking together two syringes—one with a purple stripe containing Atrigel and the second containing 50 mg of doxycycline hyclate—and pushing the contents of one into the other, back and forth, mixing for about 90 seconds (or about 100 times). After completion of mixing, all contents are placed into the syringe with the purple stripe and a blunt metal or plastic cannula is screwed on to the end and bent to resemble a periodontal probe. The cannula tip is placed into the base of the pocket and the Atridox is expressed, withdrawing the syringe as the pocket begins to fill. When the pocket is filled, the product is separated from the cannula by pressing the tip up against the tooth. A wet plastic instrument may be used to tap the product lightly into the pocket if it is desirable to place additional Atridox into the site. A single syringe of Atridox can be used to treat multiple sites (approximately 8–12), the number of sites depending on the severity of the disease.

Arestin. With regard to minocycline, there is a non–FDA-cleared ointment product of 2% (wt/wt) minocycline hydrochloride known as Dentamycine (Wyeth, United Kingdom) or PerioCline (Sunstar, Japan) and marketed in a number of countries. In a four-center double-blinded randomized trial conducted in Belgium, the minocycline ointment was applied once every 2 weeks for four applications due to insufficient sustained-release properties. Probing depth reductions were significantly greater in the SRP plus minocycline group versus SRP alone, whereas there was only a trend toward improvement in clinical attachment levels and bleeding indices in the SRP plus minocycline treatment group [47]. In a long-term 15-month study, after placement of the gel subgingivally at baseline, at 2 weeks, and at 1, 3, 6, 9, and 12 months, results showed a statistically significant improvement for all clinical and microbiologic parameters for adjunctive minocycline ointment [48].

A minocycline microsphere system (Arestin; Johnson and Johnson, New Brunswick, New Jersey) has been approved by the FDA. The Arestin microspheres are bioadhesive, bioresorbable, allow for sustained release, and are administered as a powder with a proven safety record. Arestin is indicated as an adjunct to SRP procedures for reduction of pocket depth in patients with adult periodontitis. Arestin may be used as part of a periodontal maintenance program, which includes good oral hygiene and SRP. In subjects with chronic adult periodontitis, the application of minocycline microspheres three times over the course of 9 months (at baseline and at 3 and 6 months) resulted in an average of 0.25 mm improvement above average probing depth reductions seen with SRP alone at month 9 [49]. When the data are stratified in accordance with severity of baseline probing depths, there are 20% improvements in mild sites, 40% in moderately diseased sites, and 100% in severely diseased sites compared with SRP alone. SRP plus Arestin resulted in a greater percentage of pockets showing a change of pocket depth ≥ 2 mm and ≥ 3 mm compared with SRP alone at 9 months. The data also show that for pockets of 5 to 7 mm at baseline, greater reductions in pocket depths occurred in pockets that were deeper at baseline. In smokers, the mean reduction in pocket depths at 9 months was less in all treatment groups than in nonsmokers; however, SRP plus Arestin produced significantly greater pocket depth reductions than SRP alone at 6 and 9 months [49].

Arestin is delivered to sites of 5 mm or greater through a cartridge (containing 1 mg of minocycline hydrochloride) attached to a handle. The tip is removed from the cartridge and placed subgingivally, and the handle is depressed to express the Arestin from the cartridge. A single site can be treated with a single cartridge.

Periochip. For information on Periochip, see the section "Locally applied antiseptic."

Systemic antimicrobials

For the most part, systemic antimicrobial therapy has been reserved for advanced cases of periodontitis: (1) for sites that have not responded as expected to debridement with or without locally applied chemotherapeutic agents and/or host modulatory agents, and (2) for patients diagnosed with aggressive forms of periodontitis that demonstrate progressive periodontal destruction. Systemic antibiotics may be recommended as adjuncts to conventional mechanical therapy, but strong evidence for their use as a monotherapy has not been developed. There appears to be a consensus that systemic antimicrobial therapy should be reserved for situations that cannot be managed with mechanical therapy alone (with or without locally applied antimicrobials or antiseptics), such as severe or acute infections, early-onset periodontal diseases, aggressive types of periodontitis, and recurrent or refractory cases [50]. For these special situations, randomized double-blinded clinical trials and longitudinal assessments of patients indicate that systemic antimicrobials may be useful in slowing disease progression [51]. Acute necrotizing ulcerative gingivitis can be cured with metronidazole [52], and aggressive adolescent periodontitis associated with *Actinobacillus actinomycetemcomitans* can be controlled or eradicated with metronidazole-amoxicillin combination therapy [53].

Systemic antibiotic therapy has the advantage of simple, easy administration of a drug or combination of drugs to multiple periodontal sites and extradental oral sites that may harbor periodontal pathogens. The disadvantages include uncertain patient compliance, the inability of the drugs to achieve adequate concentration at the site of infection, increased risk of adverse drug reactions, the potential for the selection of multiple antibiotic-resistant organisms, and the overgrowth of opportunistic pathogens [50]. Microbial analysis can be used to determine the specific antimicrobial susceptibility pattern of the suspected pathogens, can help to choose the appropriate antibiotics, and may be followed-up with additional testing to verify the elimination or suppression of the putative pathogens. For some clinicians, microbial analysis may be reserved for cases that are refractory to an initial course of antimicrobial therapy. Common antibiotic therapies for the treatment of periodontitis include metronidazole, 500 mg, three times a day for 8 days; clindamycin, 300 mg, three times a day for 8 days; doxycycline or minocycline, 100 to 200 mg, every day for 21 days; ciprofloxacin, 500 mg, twice a day for 8 days; azithromycin, 500 mg, every day for 4 to 7 days; metronidazole and amoxicillin, 250 mg of each drug, three times a day for 8 days; and metronidazole and ciprofloxacin, 500 mg of each drug, twice a day for 8 days [54]. For adult patients with acute periodontal abscesses, an antibiotic regimen as an adjunct to incision and drainage is amoxicillin (1 g loading dose followed by 500 mg, three times a day for

3 days), with patient follow-up re-evaluation. For patients with allergies to β-lactam drugs, antibiotic regimens include azithromycin (1 g loading dose followed by 500 mg, every day for 2 days) or clindamycin (600 mg loading dose followed by 300 mg, four times a day for 3 days).

The host modulatory approach

Host modulation is a new term that has been incorporated into dental jargon and has not been well defined. The definition of *host* from a medical dictionary reads "the organism from which a parasite obtains its nourishment or in the transplantation of tissue, the individual who receives the graft" [55]. The definition for the term *modulation* is "the alteration of function or status of something in response to a stimulus or an altered chemical or physical environment" [55]. In diseases of the periodontium that are initiated by bacteria, it is clear that the host is the individual who harbors these pathogens; however, it was not clear for many years that it was possible to modulate the host response to these pathogens. Host modulation with chemotherapeutics or drugs is an exciting new adjunctive therapeutic option for the management of periodontal diseases. The concept of host modulation is fairly new to the field of dentistry but is universally understood by most physicians who routinely apply the principals of host modulation to the management of a number of chronic progressive disorders including arthritis and osteoporosis.

A number of host modulatory agents have been investigated in clinical trials for their potential use as adjuncts to mechanical nonsurgical periodontal therapy. These agents have included the systemic (flurbiprofen) and topical (ketoprofen) use of nonsteroidal anti-inflammatory drugs, the systemic use of subantimicrobial-dose doxycycline (SDD; Periostat [Colla-Genex Pharmaceuticals, Newtown, Pennsylvania]), and the systemic use of bisphosphonates (Fosamax). The only systemic host modulatory agent approved by the FDA for adjunctive use in conjunction with nonsurgical periodontal procedures is Periostat. The points of intervention of these agents in the host response can be seen in Fig. 2. In addition, a number of local host modulatory agents have been investigated in clinical trials for their potential use as adjuncts to surgical procedures not only to improve on wound healing but also to stimulate regeneration of lost bone, periodontal ligament, and cementum, restoring the complete periodontal attachment apparatus. These agents have included enamel matrix proteins (Emdogain), bone morphogenetic proteins 2 and 7, growth factors (platelet-derived growth factor and insulin-like growth factor), and tetracyclines. The initial local host modulatory agent approved by the FDA for adjunctive use during surgery was Emdogain; platelet-derived growth factor combined with a resorbable synthetic bone matrix (GEM 21S) was approved recently by the FDA. Emdogain has also been studied as an adjunct to nonsurgical therapy. The results of a 3-month double-blinded, split-mouth, controlled

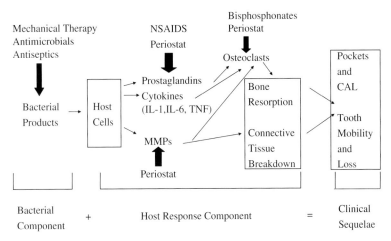

Fig. 2. Points of intervention for nonsurgical therapy. CAL, clinical attachment loss; IL, interleukin; NSAIDS, nonsteroidal anti-inflammatory drugs; TNF, tumor necrosis factor.

and randomized study do not support the use of Emdogain during routine nonsurgical debridement of periodontal pockets as measured 3 months post SRP [56]. Histologic evaluation of human intrabony defects following nonsurgical periodontal therapy with and without application of Emdogain failed to show periodontal regeneration with subgingival application of Emdogain [57]. The clinical utility of host modulation for nonsurgical procedures in clinical practice is limited in the remainder of this article to the use of SDD (Periostat).

SDD is a 20-mg dose of doxycycline (Periostat) that is FDA approved and ADA accepted. It is indicated as an adjunct to SRP in the treatment of chronic periodontitis. It has been evaluated as taken twice daily for up to 9 months of continuous dosing in clinical trials. The duration of use may vary from patient to patient. A risk factor assessment in addition to clinical evaluation of patients can help guide the practitioner with regard to length of use and need for repeat use. A minimum of 3 months of host modulatory therapy is suggested for reasons described later. Current clinical studies in susceptible patient populations such as osteopenic women are investigating extended continuous use of up to 2 years. The 20-mg twice per day dose exerts its therapeutic effect by enzyme, cytokine, and osteoclast inhibition, rather than by any antibiotic effect. Research studies have found no evidence of any detectable antimicrobial effect on the oral flora or the bacterial flora in other regions of the body and have identified clinical benefit when SDD is used as an adjunct to SRP. At the present time, SDD is the only FDA-approved, ADA-accepted host modulatory therapy specifically indicated for the treatment of chronic periodontitis.

SDD works so well as a host modulatory agent because of its pleiotropic effects on multiple components of the host response (see Fig. 2). The only enzyme (MMP) inhibitors that have been tested for the treatment of periodontitis are members of the tetracycline family of compounds. In an early study using these different tetracyclines, Golub et al [58] reported that the semisynthetic compounds (ie, doxycycline) were more effective than tetracycline in reducing excessive collagenase activity in the GCF of adult periodontitis patients. Recent clinical trials have focused on doxycycline because it was found to be a more effective inhibitor of collagenase than minocycline or tetracycline [59,60] and because of its safety profile, pharmacokinetic properties, and systemic absorption. In an effort to eliminate the side effects of long-term tetracycline therapy (especially the emergence of tetracycline-resistant organisms), SDD capsules were prepared and tested [61]. Each capsule contained 20 mg of doxycycline compared with the commercially available 50- and 100-mg antimicrobially effective capsules. In multiple clinical studies conducted using SDD, there has not been a difference in the composition or resistance level of the oral flora [62,63], and recent studies demonstrate no appreciable differences in fecal or vaginal microflora samples [63]. In addition, these studies have demonstrated no overgrowth of opportunistic pathogens such as *Candida* in the oral cavity, gastrointestinal, or genitourinary systems.

With regard to MMP inhibition, Golub et al [64] reported that a 2-week regimen of SDD reduced collagenase in GCF and in the adjacent gingival tissues surgically excised for therapeutic purposes. Subsequent studies using SDD therapy adjunctive to routine scaling and prophylaxis indicated that after 1 month of treatment, there were continued reductions in the excessive levels of collagenase in the GCF but after cessation of SDD administration, there was a rapid rebound of collagenase activity to placebo levels, suggesting that a 1-month treatment regimen with this host modulatory agent was insufficient to produce a long-term benefit [65]. In contrast, during the same study, a 3-month regimen produced a prolonged drug effect without a rebound in collagenase levels to baseline during the no-treatment phase of the study. The mean levels of GCF collagenase were significantly reduced (47.3% from baseline levels) in the SDD-treated group versus the placebo group, which received scaling and prophylaxis alone (29.1% from baseline levels). Accompanying these reductions in collagenase levels were gains in the relative attachment levels in the SDD-treated group [65,66]. Continuous drug therapy over a period of several months appears to be necessary for maintaining near normal collagenase levels over prolonged periods. It is reasonable to speculate, however, that these MMPs will eventually reappear in susceptible patients, and those individuals having the most risk factors and the greatest microbial challenge will require more frequent host modulatory therapy than other patients.

A series of double-blinded placebo-controlled studies of 3, 6, and 9 months' duration showed clinical efficacy based on the reduction of pocket depth, gains in clinical attachment levels, biochemical efficacy based on the inhibition of collagenase activity, and protection of serum alpha$_1$-antitrypsin (a naturally occurring protective mediator) from collagenase attack in the periodontal pocket [59,67,68]. Golub et al [69] showed that a 2-month regimen of SDD significantly decreased the level of bone-type collagen breakdown products (pyridinoline cross-linked carboxyterminal telopeptide of type I collagen) and MMP-8 and MMP-13 enzyme levels (neutrophil and bone-type collagenase) in adult periodontitis subjects, providing biochemical evidence of reduction of bone resorption to support computer-assisted subtraction radiography data [70,71], the latter providing evidence of a reduction in the loss of alveolar bone height after 12 months of therapy with SDD.

A 9-month randomized, double-blinded placebo-controlled trial conducted at five dental centers demonstrated clinical efficacy and safety of SDD versus placebo as an adjunct to SRP, the "gold standard" of periodontal therapy. Again, the benefits of host modulatory therapy in addition to mechanical therapy were seen, with statistically significant reductions in probing depths, bleeding on probing, gains in clinical attachment levels, and the prevention of disease progression [72,73]. In a discontinuation study in which SDD administration was discontinued after 9 months of continuous therapy, the incremental improvements demonstrated in the SDD group were maintained for at least 3 months post treatment. There was no rebound effect in pocket depth reductions or clinical attachment level gains; in fact, there appeared to be slight continued improvements in both of these clinical parameters [72,73], presumably due to the enhanced clinical status of the patients who benefited from adjunctive Periostat and the known persistence of doxycycline in the bone and soft tissue of the periodontium. The clinical relevance of such findings confirms the utility of an MMP inhibitor in the management of adult periodontitis.

Recent phase IV clinical studies have been performed that have revealed clinical and biochemical success using SDD in different populations of susceptible individuals, including subjects who are genetically susceptible [74]; subjects who have severe generalized periodontitis [75], diabetes [76,77], or osteoporosis [78]; subjects who are institutionalized geriatric patients [79]; and smokers [80]. The use of SDD in these at-risk patient populations significantly improved clinical response to SRP, and in the case of smokers, the subjects who were treated with SRP plus SDD experienced probing depth reductions and clinical attachment level gains equivalent to, and in some studies superior to, the response seen in nonsmokers who were treated with SRP alone [80]. In addition, it becomes apparent that the use of systemic host modulatory therapy by the dentist may not only improve the patient's periodontal condition but also provide systemic benefits for other inflammatory disorders with related tissue destruction, such as arthritis, cardiovascular disease, dermatologic conditions, diabetes, osteoporosis, and so forth. Dental studies have reported dramatic reductions in hemoglobin A$_{1c}$ levels (a long-term marker of glycemic control) in addition to improvements in clinical parameters in diabetic subjects treated with SDD plus SRP compared with SRP alone [76,77]. Dental studies in osteoporotic women have reported reductions in the loss of alveolar bone height and bone density (as measured by computer-assisted densitometric image analyses) in addition to clinical attachment level gains and no attachment loss in subjects treated with SDD plus SRP compared with subjects treated with SRP alone who experienced no attachment level gains and loss of attachment in a number of sites over the 12 months of the study [78]. Another assumption that can be made is that patients who are currently being prescribed host modulatory agents by their physicians, such as nonsteroidal anti-inflammatory drugs, bisphosphonates, or tetracyclines, and newer agents targeting specific cytokines for the management of medical conditions may be experiencing periodontal benefits from these systemically administered medications.

In the clinical trials of SDD (20-mg dose), the drug was well tolerated, and the profile of unwanted effects was virtually identical in the SDD and placebo groups [73,75,81,82]. SDD is indicated in the management of chronic periodontitis [68,73,83,84]. SDD should not be used in conditions such as gingivitis or periodontal abscess, or whenever an antibiotic is indicated. SDD can be used in aggressive periodontitis cases that are being treated nonsurgically [75]. Furthermore, emerging studies have supported the efficacy of SDD as an adjunct to periodontal surgery [85]. SDD may also be of benefit in cases that are refractory to treatment or in patients with risk factors such as smoking or diabetes in whom the treatment response might be somewhat limited. SDD is contraindicated in anyone with a history of allergy or hypersensitivity to tetracyclines. It should not be given to pregnant or lactating females or children less than 12 years old (because of the potential for discoloration of the developing dentition). Doxycycline may reduce the efficacy of oral contraceptives, so advice should be given to use alternative forms of birth control, if necessary. There is a risk of increased sensitivity to sunlight (manifested by an exaggerated sunburn) seen with higher doses of doxycycline, but this has not been reported in any of the clinical trials at the subantimicrobial dose. A typical prescription for Periostat (20-mg doxycycline tablets) is for at least 3 months (180 tablets, 1 tablet twice a day until complete), and refills may be provided for longer courses of therapy.

SDD treatment can also be combined with the local delivery of antibiotics to the periodontal pocket by way of sustained delivery systems. The two treatments target different aspects of the pathogenic process: local delivery systems deliver antimicrobial concentrations of an antibacterial agent directly to the site of the pocket, whereas SDD is a systemic host response modulator. Thus, combining these two complementary treatment strategies is another example of how antibacterial therapy (ie, SRP plus locally applied antibiotics) can be combined with host modulatory therapy (SDD) to maximize the clinical benefit for patients. Preliminary results from a 6-month 180-patient clinical trial designed to evaluate the safety and efficacy of SDD combined with a locally applied antimicrobial (Atridox) plus SRP versus SRP alone demonstrated that patients receiving the combination of treatment experienced more than a 2-mm improvement in mean attachment level gain and pocket depth reduction, which was highly statistically significant ($P < 0.0001$) compared with SRP alone.

Clinical application

The author has implemented a three-pronged approach to periodontal therapy in her clinical practice (Fig. 3). The initial visit by a patient includes a medical and dental history, a risk assessment profile, periodontal charting, and radiographic analysis. The patient must be made aware of the fact that periodontal disease is not curable but that it can be treated and well controlled with constant monitoring by the dentist/hygienist and good patient compliance. The patient must also be informed of the need for periodontal therapy, which should not be considered optional or elective but necessary to promote not only good oral health but also good general health, as recent studies have suggested.

Initial therapy consists of risk reduction strategies (see Box 2). Modification of any risk factors such as smoking, nutrition, stress, contributing

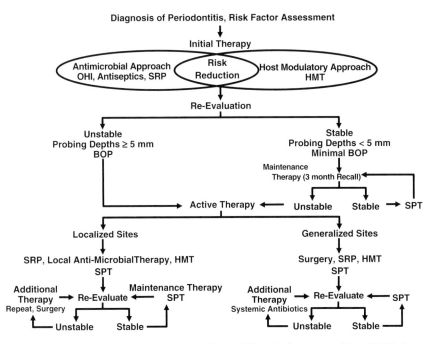

Fig. 3. Periodontal therapy treatment algorithm. BOP, bleeding on probing; HMT, host modulatory therapy; OHI, oral hygiene instruction; SPT, supportive periodontal therapy (reinforce OHI, scaling, antiseptics).

medications, faulty restorations, poor oral hygiene, and poor diabetic control should be addressed at this time. Oral hygiene instructions are extremely important and must be reinforced continuously over the course of therapy; the use of adjunctive antiseptic agents is often employed. SRP is the core of nonsurgical therapy, with anesthesia administered as needed. At-home oral hygiene and in-office SRP approaches are designed to reduce the bacterial load. In addition, an initial course of host modulatory therapy (Periostat) may be prescribed to reduce excessive levels of enzymes, cytokines, and prostanoids, especially in susceptible patients as identified by risk assessment. A patient's refusal or inability to modify contributing risk factors is an important consideration for treatment planning and evaluation of therapeutic responses. In the case of adjunctive chemotherapies, the more risk factors and the poorer the hygiene, the greater the need for antiseptics, antibiotics, and host modulation of longer duration or repeat therapy in the future.

After completion of initial therapy, re-evaluation is the next step (see Fig. 3). At this point, the decision is made to continue with active (additional) therapy or to place the patient in the maintenance phase of therapy. If all probing depths are <5 mm and there is minimal bleeding on probing and gingival inflammation, then the decision is made to place the patient in the maintenance phase of therapy. The patient is typically maintained on the host modulatory agent through the first maintenance visit. If the treated sites remain stable for this 3-month period, then the patient is removed from the host modulatory agent and placed in the typical maintenance program (3- to 4-month visits) until the need for additional active therapy is required. If there are probing depths ≥5 mm at re-evaluation, then the therapeutic approach may differ depending on the number of sites per quadrant and radiographic assessment of the sites.

Typically for isolated sites with probing depths ≥5 mm at re-evaluation, a nonsurgical approach may include rescaling the sites and placement of a locally applied antimicrobial agent (ie, Atridox, Arestin, or Peiochip), with the continued adjunctive use of the host modulatory agent. Sites treated with locally applied antimicrobials should be re-evaluated at 3 months and a decision can be made by the clinician as to whether an additional application of the same locally applied antimicrobial may be used or another locally applied antimicrobial may be administered, and so forth. Clinicians must use their clinical judgment. If this treatment is insufficient to achieve adequate pocket depth reduction or if there are multiple sites in a quadrant with probing depths ≥5 mm, then a surgical approach may be indicated to reduce the probing depths through resective or regenerative techniques. After all probing depths are <5 mm, the patient is placed in the maintenance phase of therapy as described earlier.

In certain patients with aggressive periodontitis or in those truly refractory to the therapy described previously, the use of systemic antimicrobials or additional host modulatory agents in a polypharmacologic approach can be considered. Microbial and antibiotic susceptibility testing may be helpful in these situations. Examples of additional host modulatory approaches have included low doses of nonsteroidal anti-inflammatory drugs (flurbiprofen), which demonstrated incremental benefits in a small clinical study [86] or low doses of bisphosphonates, which have not yet been investigated in combination in human clinical studies but have shown incremental benefits in animal studies of osteoporosis. Patients who are difficult to manage, who are most susceptible with multiple risk factors, or who present with moderate to severe disease requiring comprehensive periodontal treatment planning should be referred to the periodontal specialist for care and close monitoring.

To improve our ability to make appropriate treatment decisions for patients undergoing periodontal therapy, it would be extremely useful to have access to the types of diagnostic tests that are available to our medical colleagues. Therapeutic technologies have surpassed our ability to adequately diagnose active versus inactive lesions, identify subtle changes in the tissues and, thereby, prevent additional loss of attachment and bone. Studies have shown that SRP alone, although effective at improving clinical parameters such as probing depths that are routinely used to assess the outcome of periodontal procedures, may not be sufficient to reduce excessive levels of many of the underlying destructive mediators, particularly in susceptible patients. In the future, dental diagnostics currently being developed to aid in clinical assessment of patients may be performed in a centralized diagnostic laboratory facility rather than at chairside. Oral samples and perhaps even blood samples collected from patients and sent to a centralized diagnostic laboratory will include plaque samples for microbial assessments, buccal cheek swabs for genetic testing, and GCF (single or multiple sites or full-mouth rinse collections) and saliva for analysis of host response mediators such as enzymes, cytokines, and prostanoids. The information gained from improved quantitative diagnostics will be used to create a profile of the patient's risk—not only for oral disease but also potentially for systemic disorders—to determine the patient's level of periodontal disease activity, aid in treatment planning decisions, and better monitor the patient's response to therapy. Until such diagnostic techniques are made available, clinicians have no choice but to rely on clinical judgment to determine the most appropriate course of therapy.

Summary

Periodontal pathogens and destructive host responses are involved in the initiation and progression of periodontitis in the individual at risk for disease. Therefore, the successful long-term management of this disease may require a treatment strategy that integrates therapies that address all of these components. There is now overwhelming evidence for the role of bacterial pathogens and host-derived MMPs, cytokines, and other mediators in the destructive processes of periodontal disease, distinguishing them as viable targets for chemotherapeutic adjunctive approaches. The introduction of novel adjunctive therapies to enhance the efficacy of existing mechanical procedures has contributed favorably to an integrated approach for the long-term clinical management of periodontitis.

Finally, as the era of periodontal medicine evolves, the additional benefits of adjunctive local and systemic antimicrobials and systemic host modulatory approaches need to be considered. In particular, host modulators used to manage periodontal disease by inhibiting mediators of host tissue destruction such as MMPs, cytokines, and prostanoids may have additional beneficial effects on systemic diseases such as cardiovascular disease, diabetes, and osteoporosis. The surgeon general's report [87] recognizes "the mouth as a mirror of health or disease, as a sentinel or early warning system, as an accessible model for the study of other tissues and organs, and as a potential source of pathology affecting other systems and organs." The findings discussed in this article with regard to the use of therapeutics to better manage chronic periodontal disease may have applications to other associated systemic diseases such as diabetes, cardiovascular disease, stroke, respiratory disease, and adverse pregnancy outcomes. The proper management of periodontitis may prove to have an impact on general health, making a significant contribution to human welfare.

Acknowledgments

The author would like to acknowledge Laura Bertolotti for her assistance in the organization of this manuscript.

References

[1] Maynard J. Eras in periodontics. In: Periodontal disease management: a conference for the dental team. Boston: American Academy of Periodontology; 1993. p. 3–10.
[2] Offenbacher S. Periodontal diseases: pathogenesis. Ann Periodontol 1996;1(1):821–78.
[3] Genco RJ. Host responses in periodontal diseases: current concepts. J Periodontol 1992; 63(Suppl 4):338–55.
[4] Grossi SG, Zambon JJ, Ho AW, et al. Assessment of risk for periodontal disease. I. Risk indicators for attachment loss. J Periodontol 1994;65(3):260–7.
[5] Salvi GE, Lawrence HP, Offenbacher S, et al. Influence of risk factors on the pathogenesis of periodontitis. Periodontol 2000 1997;14:173–201.
[6] Bader HI. Floss or die: implications for dental professionals. Dent Today 1998;17(7):76–82.
[7] Oliver RC, Brown LJ, Loe H. Periodontal diseases in the United States population. J Periodontol 1998;69(2):269–78.
[8] Heanue M, Deacon SA, Deery C, et al. Manual versus powered toothbrushing for oral health. Cochrane Database Syst Rev 2003;1:CD002281.
[9] Cobb CM. Non-surgical pocket therapy: mechanical. Ann Periodontol 1996;1(1):443–90.
[10] Koshy G, Corbet EF, Ishikawa I. A full-mouth disinfection approach to nonsurgical periodontal therapy—prevention of reinfection from bacterial reservoirs. Periodontol 2000 2004;36:166–78.

[11] Aoki A, Sasaki KM, Watanabe H, et al. Lasers in nonsurgical periodontal therapy. Periodontol 2000 2004;36:59–97.

[12] Greenstein G. Periodontal response to mechanical non-surgical therapy: a review. J Periodontol 1992;63(2):118–30.

[13] Overholser CD, Meiller TF, DePaola LG, et al. Comparative effects of 2 chemotherapeutic mouthrinses on the development of supragingival dental plaque and gingivitis. J Clin Periodontol 1990;17(8):575–9.

[14] Mankodi S, Mostler K, Charles CH, et al. Comparative antiplaque/antigingivitis efficacies of two antiseptic mouthrinses. J Dent Res 1990;69(special):246.

[15] Pitts G, Brogdon C, Hu L, et al. Mechanism of action of an antiseptic, anti-order mouthwash. J Dent Res 1983;62(6):738–42.

[16] De Boever EH, Loesche WJ. Assessing the contribution of anaerobic microflora of the tongue to oral malador. J Am Dent Assoc 1995;126(10):1384–93.

[17] Ciancio SG, Mather ML, Zambon JJ, et al. Effect of a chemotherapeutic agent delivered by an oral irrigation device on plaque, gingivitis, and subgingival microflora. J Periodontol 1989;60(6):310–5.

[18] Flemmig TF, Newman MG, Nachnani S, et al. Chlorhexidine and irrigation in gingivitis: 6 months correlative clinical and microbiological findings. J Dent Res 1989; 68[San Francisco, CA]:383.

[19] Ciancio SG, Lauciello F, Shibly O, et al. The effect of an antiseptic mouthrinse on implant maintenance: plaque and peri-implant gingival tissues. J Periodontol 1995;66(11):962–5.

[20] Brightman LJ, Terezhalmy GT, Greenwell H, et al. The effects of a 0.12% chlorhexidine gluconate mouthrinse on orthodontic patients aged 11 through 17 with established gingivitis. Am J Orthod Dentofacial Orthop 1991;100(4):324–9.

[21] Fine DH, Yip J, Furgang D, et al. Reducing bacteria in dental aerosols: pre-procedural use of an antiseptic mouthrinse. J Am Dent Assoc 1993;124(5):56–8.

[22] Zambon JJ, Ciancio SG, Mather ML, et al. The effect of an antimicrobial mouthrinse on early healing of gingival flap surgery wounds. J Periodontol 1989;60(1):31–4.

[23] Sanz M, Newman MG, Anderson L, et al. Clinical enhancement of post-periodontal surgical therapy by a 0.12% chlorhexidine gluconate mouthrinse. J Periodontol 1989;60(10):570–6.

[24] Fine DH. Mouthrinses as adjuncts for plaque and gingivitis management. A status report for the American Journal of Dentistry. Am J Dent 1988;1(6):259–63.

[25] Ciancio SG. Antiseptics and antibiotics as chemotherapeutic agents for periodontitis management. Compend Contin Educ Dent 2000;21(1):59–66.

[26] Sharma NC, Charles CH, Qaqish JG, et al. Comparative effectiveness of an essential oil mouthrinse and dental floss in controlling interproximal gingivitis and plaque. Am J Dent 2002;15(6):351–5.

[27] Bauroth K, Charles CH, Mankodi SM, et al. The efficacy of an essential oil antiseptic mouthrinse vs. dental floss in controlling interproximal gingivitis: a comparative study. J Am Dent Assoc 2003;134(3):359–65.

[28] Sharma N, Charles CH, Lynch MC, et al. Adjunctive benefit of an essential oil-containing mouthrinse in reducing plaque and gingivitis in patients who brush and floss regularly: a six-month study. J Am Dent Assoc 2004;135(4):496–504.

[29] Kerdvongbundit V, Wikesjo UM. Effect of triclosan on healing following non-surgical periodontal therapy in smokers. J Clin Periodontol 2003;30(12):1024–30.

[30] Furuichi Y, Rosling B, Volpe AR, et al. The effect of a triclosan/copolymer dentifrice on healing after non-surgical treatment of recurrent periodontitis. J Clin Periodontol 1999; 26(2):63–6.

[31] Xu T, Deshmukh M, Barnes VM, et al. Effectiveness of a triclosan/copolymer dentifrice on microbiological and inflammatory parameters. Compend Contin Educ Dent 2004; 25(7 Suppl 1):46–53.

[32] Stabholz A, Sela MN, Friedman M, et al. Clinical and microbiological effects of sustained release chlorhexidine in periodontal pockets. J Clin Periodontol 1986;13(8):783–8.

[33] Jeffcoat MK, Bray KS, Ciancio SG, et al. Adjunctive use of a subgingival controlled-release chlorhexidine chip reduces probing depth and improves attachment level compared with scaling and root planing alone. J Periodontol 1998;69(9):989–97.

[34] Jeffcoat MK, Palcanis KG, Weatherford TW. Use of a biodegradable chlorhexidine chip in the treatment of adult periodontitis: clinical and radiographic findings. J Periodontol 2000; 71(2):256–62.

[35] Gordon JM, Walker CB, Murphy JC, et al. Tetracycline: levels achievable in gingival crevice fluid and in vitro effect on subgingival organisms. Part I. Concentrations in crevicular fluid after repeated doses. J Periodontol 1981;52(10):609–12.

[36] Pascale D, Gordon J, Lamster I, et al. Concentration of doxycycline in human gingival fluid. J Clin Periodontol 1986;13(9):841–4.

[37] Sakellari D, Goodson JM, Kolokotronis A, et al. Concentration of 3 tetracyclines in plasma, gingival crevice fluid and saliva. J Clin Periodontol 2000;27(1):53–60.

[38] Killoy WJ, Cobb CM. Controlled local delivery of tetracycline in the treatment of periodontitis. Compendium 1992;13(12):1150–4.

[39] Goodson JM, Holborow D, Dunn RL, et al. Monolithic tetracycline-containing fibers for controlled delivery to periodontal pockets. J Periodontol 1983;54(10):575–9.

[40] Goodson JM, Cugini MA, Kent RL, et al. Multicenter evaluation of tetracycline fiber therapy: II. Clinical response. J Periodontal Res 1991;26(4):371–9.

[41] Fourmousis I, Tonetti MS, Mombelli A, et al. Evaluation of tetracycline fiber therapy with digital image analysis. J Clin Periodontol 1998;25(9):737–45.

[42] Walker CB, Godowski KC, Borden L, et al. The effects of sustained release doxycycline on the anaerobic flora and antibiotic-resistant patterns in subgingival plaque and saliva. J Periodontol 2000;71(5):768–74.

[43] Garrett S, Johnson L, Drisko CH, et al. Two multi-center studies evaluating locally delivered doxycycline hyclate, placebo control, oral hygiene, and scaling and root planing in the treatment of periodontitis. J Periodontol 1999;70(5):490–503.

[44] Ryder MI, Pons B, Adams D, et al. Effects of smoking on local delivery of controlled-release doxycycline as compared to scaling and root planing. J Clin Periodontol 1999;26(10):683–91.

[45] Tomasi C, Wennstrom JL. Locally delivered doxycycline improves the healing following non-surgical periodontal therapy in smokers. J Clin Periodontol 2004;31(8):589–95.

[46] Wennstrom JL, Newman HN, MacNeill SR, et al. Utilisation of locally delivered doxycycline in non-surgical treatment of chronic periodontitis. A comparative multi-centre trial of 2 treatment approaches. J Clin Periodontol 2001;28(8):753–61.

[47] van Steenberghe D, Bercy P, Kohl J, et al. Subgingival minocycline hydrochloride ointment in moderate to severe chronic adult periodontitis: a randomized, double-blind, vehicle-controlled, multicenter study. J Periodontol 1993;64(7):637–44.

[48] van Steenberghe D, Rosling B, Soder PO, et al. A 15-month evaluation of the effects of repeated subgingival minocycline in chronic adult periodontitis. J Periodontol 1999;70(6): 657–67.

[49] Williams RC, Paquette DW, Offenbacher S, et al. Treatment of periodontitis by local administration of minocycline microspheres: a controlled trial. J Periodontol 2001;72(11): 1535–44.

[50] Slots J. Systemic antibiotics in periodontics. J Periodontol 2004;75(11):1553–65.

[51] Haffajee AD, Socransky SS, Dzink JL, et al. Clinical, microbiological and immunological features of subjects with refractory periodontal diseases. J Clin Periodontol 1988;15(6): 390–8.

[52] Duckworth R, Waterhouse JP, Britton DE, et al. Acute ulcerative gingivitis. A double-blind controlled clinical trial of metronidazole. Br Dent J 1966;120(12):599–602.

[53] van Winkelhoff AJ, Rodenburg JP, Goene RJ, et al. Metronidazole plus amoxycillin in the treatment of *Actinobacillus actinomycetemcomitans* associated periodontitis. J Clin Periodontol 1989;16(2):128–31.

[54] Slots J, van Winkelhoff AJ. Antimicrobial therapy in periodontics. J Calif Dent Assoc 1993; 21(11):51–6.

[55] Thomas C, editor. Taber's medical dictionary. Philadelphia: F.A. Davis Company; 2004.

[56] Gutierrez MA, Mellonig JT, Cochran DL. Evaluation of enamel matrix derivative as an adjunct to non-surgical periodontal therapy. J Clin Periodontol 2003;30(8):739–45.

[57] Sculean A, Windisch P, Keglevich T, et al. Histologic evaluation of human intrabony defects following non-surgical periodontal therapy with and without application of an enamel matrix protein derivative. J Periodontol 2003;74(2):153–60.

[58] Golub LM, Wolff M, Lee HM, et al. Further evidence that tetracyclines inhibit collagenase activity in human crevicular fluid and from other mammalian sources. J Periodontal Res 1985;20(1):12–23.

[59] Golub LM, Evans RT, McNamara TF, et al. A non-antimicrobial tetracycline inhibits gingival matrix metalloproteinases and bone loss in *Porphyromonas gingivalis*-induced periodontitis in rats. Ann N Y Acad Sci 1994;732:96–111.

[60] Burns FR, Stack MS, Gray RD, et al. Inhibition of purified collagenase from alkali-burned rabbit corneas. Invest Ophthalmol Vis Sci 1989;30(7):1569–75.

[61] Golub LM, Sorsa T, Lee HM, et al. Doxycycline inhibits neutrophil (PMN)-type matrix metalloproteinases in human adult periodontitis gingiva. J Clin Periodontol 1995;22(2): 100–9.

[62] Thomas J, Walker C, Bradshaw M. Long-term use of subantimicrobial dose doxycycline does not lead to changes in antimicrobial susceptibility. J Periodontol 2000;71(9): 1472–83.

[63] Walker C, Thomas J, Nango S, et al. Long-term treatment with subantimicrobial dose doxycycline exerts no antibacterial effect on the subgingival microflora associated with adult periodontitis. J Periodontol 2000;71(9):1465–71.

[64] Golub LM, Ciancio S, Ramamamurthy NS, et al. Low-dose doxycycline therapy: effect on gingival and crevicular fluid collagenase activity in humans. J Periodontal Res 1990;25(6): 321–30.

[65] Ashley RA. Clinical trials of a matrix metalloproteinase inhibitor in human periodontal disease. SDD Clinical Research Team. Ann N Y Acad Sci 1999;878:335–46.

[66] Golub LM, McNamara TF, Ryan ME, et al. Adjunctive treatment with subantimicrobial doses of doxycycline: effects on gingival fluid collagenase activity and attachment loss in adult periodontitis. J Clin Periodontol 2001;28(2):146–56.

[67] Crout RJ, Lee HM, Schroeder K, et al. The "cyclic" regimen of low-dose doxycycline for adult periodontitis: a preliminary study. J Periodontol 1996;67(5):506–14.

[68] Lee HM, Golub LM, Chan D, et al. Alpha 1-Proteinase inhibitor in gingival crevicular fluid of humans with adult periodontitis: serpinolytic inhibition by doxycycline. J Periodontal Res 1997;32(1 Pt 1):9–19.

[69] Golub LM, Lee HM, Greenwald RA, et al. A matrix metalloproteinase inhibitor reduces bone-type collagen degradation fragments and specific collagenases in gingival crevicular fluid during adult periodontitis. Inflamm Res 1997;46(8):310–9.

[70] Caton J, Blieden T. Subantimicrobial doxycycline therapy for periodontitis. J Periodontol 1997;76:177.

[71] Ciancio S, Ashley R. Safety and efficacy of sub-antimicrobial-dose doxycycline therapy in patients with adult periodontitis. Adv Dent Res 1998;12(2):27–31.

[72] Caton JG. Evaluation of Periostat for patient management. Compend Contin Educ Dent 1999;20(5):451–62.

[73] Caton JG, Ciancio SG, Blieden TM, et al. Treatment with subantimicrobial dose doxycycline improves the efficacy of scaling and root planing in patients with adult periodontitis. J Periodontol 2000;71(4):521–32.

[74] Ryan ME, Lee HM. Treatment of genetically susceptible patients with a subantimicrobial dose of doxycycline. J Dent Res 2000;79:3719.

[75] Novak MJ, Johns LP, Miller RC, et al. Adjunctive benefits of subantimicrobial dose doxycycline in the management of severe, generalized, chronic periodontitis. J Periodontol 2002;73(7):762–9.

[76] Al-Chazi MN, Ciancio SG, Aljada A, et al. Evaluation of efficacy of administration of subantimicrobial-dose doxycycline in the treatment of generalized adult periodontitis in diabetics. J Dent Res 2003;82(special issue A):1752a.

[77] Engebretson SP, Hey-Hadavi J, Celenti R, et al. Low-dose doxycycline treatment reduces glycosylated hemoglobin in patients with type 2 diabetes: a randomized controlled trial. J Dent Res 2003;82(special issue A):1445a.

[78] Payne JB, Reinhardt RA. Potential application of low-dose doxycycline to treat periodontitis in post-menopausal women. Adv Dent Res 1998;12(2):166–9.

[79] Mohammad AR, Preshaw PM, Hefti AF, et al. Subantimicrobial-dose doxycycline for treatment of periodontitis in an institutionalized geriatric population. J Dent Res 2003; 82(special issue B):2701a.

[80] Preshaw PM, Bradshaw MH, Hefti AF, et al. Adjunctive subantimicrobial-dose doxycycline for treatment of smokers with periodontitis. J Dent Res 2003;82(special issue B):1739a.

[81] Emingil G, Atilla G, Sorsa T, et al. The effect of adjunctive low-dose doxycycline therapy on clinical parameters and gingival crevicular fluid matrix metalloproteinase-8 levels in chronic periodontitis. J Periodontol 2004;75(1):106–15.

[82] Preshaw PM, Hefti AF, Novak MJ. Subantimicrobial dose doxycycline enhances the efficacy of scaling and root planing in chronic periodontitis: a multicenter trial. J Periodontol 2004; 75(8):1068–76.

[83] Bezerra MM, de Lima V, Alencar VB, et al. Selective cyclooxygenase-2 inhibition prevents alveolar bone loss in experimental periodontitis in rats. J Periodontol 2000;71(6):1009–14.

[84] Mercado FB, Marshall RI, Bartold PM. Inter-relationships between rheumatoid arthritis and periodontal disease. A review. J Clin Periodontol 2003;30(9):761–72.

[85] Choi DH, Moon IS, Choi BK, et al. Effects of sub-antimicrobial dose doxycycline therapy on crevicular fluid MMP-8, and gingival tissue MMP-9, TIMP-1 and IL-6 levels in chronic periodontitis. J Periodontal Res 2004;39(1):20–6.

[86] Lee HM, Ciancio SG, Tuter G, et al. Subantimicrobial dose doxycycline efficacy as a matrix metalloproteinase inhibitor in chronic periodontitis patients is enhanced when combined with a non-steroidal anti-inflammatory drug. J Periodontol 2004;75(3):453–63.

[87] US Department of Health and Human Services. Oral health in America: a report of the surgeon general—executive summary. Rockville (MD): US Department of Health and Human Services, NIDCR, NIH; 2000. p. 1–13.

THE DENTAL
CLINICS
OF NORTH AMERICA

ELSEVIER
SAUNDERS

Dent Clin N Am 49 (2005) 637–659

Periodontal Regeneration Techniques for Treatment of Periodontal Diseases

Hom-Lay Wang, DDS, MSD*, Jason Cooke, DDS

Department of Periodontics/Prevention/Geriatrics, School of Dentistry, University of Michigan, 1011 North University Avenue, Ann Arbor, MI 48109-1078, USA

Two techniques with the most successful documentation of periodontal regeneration are osseous grafting and guided tissue regeneration (GTR) [1–3]. Although some regeneration may occur following regenerative procedures [4,5], it is not always predictable and complete regeneration may be an unrealistic goal for many clinical situations. This article describes the biologic basis and clinical applicability of osseous grafting and GTR and the newly developed biologic modifiers that show promising results in periodontal regeneration.

Definitions

- *Regeneration* refers to the reproduction or reconstitution of a lost or injured tissue [6].
- *Periodontal regeneration* is defined as the restoration of lost periodontium or supporting tissues and includes formation of new alveolar bone, new cementum, and new periodontal ligament.
- *Repair* describes healing of a wound by tissue that does not fully restore the architecture or the function of the part [6].
- *New attachment* is defined as the union of connective tissue or epithelium with a root surface that has been deprived of its original attachment apparatus. This new attachment may be epithelial adhesion or connective tissue adaptation or attachment and may include new cementum.

This study was supported partially by the University of Michigan, Periodontal Graduate Student Research Fund.

* Corresponding author.
E-mail address: homlay@umich.edu (H.-L. Wang).

doi:10.1016/j.cden.2005.03.004

- *Reattachment* describes the reunion of epithelial and connective tissue with a root surface [6].
- *GTR* describes procedures attempting to regenerate lost periodontal structures through differential tissue responses and typically refers to regeneration of periodontal attachment [6]. Barrier techniques are used for excluding connective tissue and gingiva from the root in the belief that they interfere with regeneration [6].
- *Bone fill* is defined as the clinical restoration of bone tissue in a treated periodontal defect. Bone fill does not address the presence or absence of histologic evidence of new connective tissue attachment or the formation of new periodontal ligament [6].
- *Open probing clinical attachment* is used to describe the tissue seen at re-entry surgery after regeneration procedures [7]. This term has not been commonly used because the clinical attachment cannot be probed in the open environment.

Biologic foundation

Surgical debridement and resective procedures are the traditional surgical treatments used to improve clinical disease parameters and arrest its progression [8–11]. Few reports of minimal regeneration of bone and the tooth-supporting structures after these therapeutic treatments have been described [12]. These methods typically heal by repair, forming a combination of connective tissue adhesion/attachment or forming a long junctional epithelium [13,14].

The concept of "compartmentalization," in which the connective tissues of the periodontium are divided into four compartments—the lamina propria of the gingiva (gingival corium), the periodontal ligament, the cementum, and the alveolar bone—was developed by Melcher in 1976 [15]. From this concept of compartmentalization, GTR procedures developed and barrier membranes were used to accomplish the objectives of epithelial exclusion: cell/tissue repopulation control, space maintenance, and clot stabilization [3,16,17]. GTR is based on the exclusion of gingival connective tissue cells and the prevention of epithelial downgrowth into the wound. By exclusion of these tissues, cells with regenerative potential (periodontal ligament [PDL], bone cells, and possibly cementoblasts) can enter the wound site first and promote regeneration.

Wound healing principles

Research confirms that periodontal surgical wounds go through the same sequence of healing events as all incisional wounds: the formation of a fibrin clot between the flap margin and the root surface and replacement of this fibrin clot by a connective tissue matrix attached to the root surface [18]. When the "fibrin linkage" is maintained, it allows for a new connective tissue attachment to the root surface. In the case of the fibrin linkage being disrupted, a long junctional epithelium–type attachment results [19]. Regenerative failures may be a direct result of the tensile strength of the fibrin clot being exceeded, resulting in a tear [19]. A potential cause of this tear is mobility of the flap (wound margin) adjacent to the potential regenerative site [20]. During the healing of periodontal wounds, there is the presence of multiple specialized cell types and attachment complexes, stromal–cellular interactions, diverse microbial flora, and avascular tooth surfaces that complicate the process of periodontal regeneration [21]. More predictable outcomes following GTR procedures will be achieved as the principles involved in the periodontal wound healing process are better understood.

Techniques used for regeneration

Root surface conditioning

Root surface conditioning with tetracycline or citric acid has been used as a part of regenerative procedures [22,23]. Root surface conditioning was originally suggested because of the ability of acid to modify the root surface by "detoxifying" it [24]. Root surface conditioning also showed that collagen fibrils were exposed within the cementum or dentin matrix [25]. Although animal studies demonstrated new connective tissue attachment following acid demineralization, histologic evaluation in human clinical trials demonstrated limited connective tissue attachment and limited regeneration following citric acid demineralization [26–28]. Recent studies showed that using ETDA, which has a less acidic pH, may also expose collagen fibers and thus promote cell attachment without having a damaging effect on the surrounding tissues [29]. Results from clinical trials using any type of root conditioning agent indicate no additional improvement in clinical conditions [27,30]. A recent meta-analysis systematic review confirmed that the use of citric acid, tetracycline, or EDTA to modify the root surface provides no clinically significant benefit of regeneration in patients with chronic periodontitis [31].

Coronally positioned (advanced) flaps

The periosteum is viewed as having regenerative potential due to its rich structure in osteoprogenitor cells [32]. The regenerative potential is thought to result from a combination of the cellular activity of the periosteum and a barrier-type effect by the repositioned periosteum. When coronally positioned flaps are used to treat mandibular class II furcation defects, the position of the flap margin is away from the critical healing area (the furcation site) and secured [33]. An approximate mean of 50% to 65% (by volume) bone fill in class II mandibular furcation defects has been reported in studies that performed re-entry surgeries [32]. It is necessary to test a larger number of patients with a longer follow-up period to fully evaluate this technique.

Bone replacement grafts

Bone replacement grafts include autografts, allografts, xenografts, and alloplasts. Bone replacement grafts are the most widely used treatment options for the correction of periodontal osseous defects [34]. It has been proved that bone replacement grafts provide clinical improvements in periodontal osseous defects compared with surgical debridement alone. For the treatment of intrabony defects, bone grafts have been found to increase bone level, reduce crestal bone loss, increase clinical attachment level, and reduce probing pocket depths compared with open flap debridement procedures [34]. Their benefits for the use of furcation defects remains to be determined.

Extra- and intraoral donor sites for autogenous bone grafts

Due to their osteogenic potential, autogenous bone grafts of extra- and intraoral sources have been used in periodontal therapy. Iliac grafts have been used fresh or frozen. Successful bone fill has been demonstrated using iliac cancellous bone with marrow in furcations, dehiscences, and intra-osseous defects of various morphologies [35,36]. One common complication is root resorption when using fresh grafts [35]. Iliac grafts have had only limited use because of the difficulty in obtaining the graft material, mor-bidity, and the possibility of root resorption.

The maxillary tuberosity or a healing extraction site is typically the donor choice for intraoral cancellous bone with marrow grafts. Intraosseous defects grafted with intraoral bone have demonstrated bone fill equal to that obtained with iliac grafts [37–40]. A mean bone fill range of 1.2 to 3.4 mm (filling greater than 50% of the initial defect) has been reported with intraoral grafts [38,40]. Other techniques report bone fill using cortical bone chips [39] and osseous coagulum or bone blend–type grafts [37]. Studies report histologic evidence of regeneration and new connective tissue at-tachment and the presence of a long junctional epithelium following these procedures [41,42].

Allogenic bone grafts

Allografts involve bone taken from one human for transplantation to another. Iliac cancellous bone and marrow, freeze-dried bone allograft (FDBA), and decalcified FDBA are the types of bone allografts widely available from commercial tissue banks. Grafts are taken from cadaver bone and typically freeze-dried and treated to prevent disease transmission. Typically, frozen iliac allografts are not used due to the need for extensive cross-matching to decrease the likelihood of graft rejection and disease transmission.

Freeze-dried bone allograft. FDBA works primarily through osteoconduction. The graft does not activate bone growth but acts like a scaffold for natural bone to grow into. Eventually the graft is resorbed and replace by new bone. Freeze-drying the bone decreases the antigenicity of the allograft. Radiographically, FDBA appears radiopaque because it is not demineralized. When using FDBA to treat periodontal defects, trials indicate bone fill ranging from 1.3 to 2.6 mm [43,44]. Using a combination of FDBA with tetracycline has also shown promise in the treatment of defects resulting from juvenile periodontitis [45,46].

Demineralized freeze-dried bone allografts. Urist [47] showed that demineralized FDBA (DFDBA) was osteoinductive (Table 1). DFDBA is believed to induce bone formation due to the influence of bone-inductive proteins called bone morphogenetic proteins (BMPs) exposed during the demineralization process. DFDBA is therefore thought to be osteoinductive and osteoconductive.

DFDBA has demonstrated periodontal regeneration in controlled human histologic studies. Significantly more regeneration was achieved with DFDBA than in nongrafted controls [2,5]. Superior gains in bone fill with DFDBA compared with open-flap debridement have consistently been reported [34]. Human trials using DFDBA have demonstrated bone fill similar to that achieved with FDBA, ranging from 1.7 to 2.9 mm [44,48]. It has been observed in several re-entry studies that grafting with DFDBA yields equal or better results than other graft materials and is always superior to debridement alone when used for the correct indications [49].

Studies have demonstrated that preparation of allograft material can differ from one distributor to another and that the material may differ in its

Table 1
Comparison of freeze-dried bone allograft and demineralized freeze-dried bone allograft

FDBA	DFDBA
Not demineralized	Demineralized
Better space maintenance	More bone morphogenetic protein
Slower resorption rate	expression potential
compared with DFDBA	Possible osteoinduction
Osteoconductive	Osteoconductive
More radio-opaque	More radiolucent
Breakdown by way of foreign body reaction	Rapid resorption
Primary indication: bone augmentation	Primary indication: periodontal
associated with implant treatment	disease associated with natural tooth
(eg, guided bone regeneration, sinus grafting,	
ridge augmentation)	

biologic activity [50–52]. DFDBA may vary from batch to batch. Some studies suggest that the quantity of BMPs is too small to induce bone formation and that bone formation occurs by other processes. Commercial bone banks do not verify the specific amount of BMPs or the levels of inductive capacity in any graft material. The development of stricter bone bank standards that evaluate the potency of their preparations, including (1) using bones from individuals under a specific age, using bones from individuals free of bone diseases [53], or using fresh bone, and (2) developing assays that can test the inductive capacity of the material before sales [50], may lead to more consistent and reliable clinical results.

Human mineralized bone. Puros (Zimmer Dental, Carlsbad, California) is a new allograft of cancellous bone on the market. It is human bone that undergoes a tutoplast process involving (1) delipidization with acetone and ultrasound, (2) osmotic treatment, (3) oxidation with hydrogen peroxide to destroy unwanted proteins, (4) solvent dehydration with acetone to preserve the collagenous fiber structure, and (5) low-dose gamma irradiation. Manufacturers believe that this new solvent preservation method preserves the trabecular pattern and mineral structure better than the freeze-drying process, thus being a more osteoconductive material. To date, no controlled clinical trials have compared Puros with other allografts (Table 2).

Grafton demineralized bone matrix (DBM). Grafton DBM (BioHorizons, Birmingham, Alabama) is processed from cadaver long bones by aseptically processing the bone to remove lipid, blood, and cellular components before it is frozen. Cortical bone is milled into elongated fibers of 0.5 mm in diameter or pulverized into particles of 100 to 500 μm. It is combined with a glycerol carrier to stabilize the proteins and improve the graft handling. It can be used in the flex form, as putty, or as matrix plugs (see Table 2) [54,55].

Alloplasts

Alloplastic materials are synthetic, inorganic, biocompatible, or bioactive bone graft substitutes. Alloplast materials are believed to promote bone healing through osteoconduction [6]. Currently, six types of alloplastic materials are commercially available: hydroxyapatite cement, nonporous hydroxyapatite, porous hydroxyapatite (replamineform), beta tricalcium

Table 2
Comparison of allografts

Allograft	Process	Protein	Mineral	Trabeculation	Remodeling
FDBA	Freeze-dried	Yes	Yes	No	Long
DFDBA (eg, Grafton)	Freeze-dried	Yes	No	No	Short
Human cancellous bone (eg, Puros)	Solvent	Yes	Yes	Yes	Short

phosphate, polymethylmethacrylate/hydroxyethylmethacrylate (PMMA/HEMA) calcium-layered polymer, and bioactive glass. Ideally, alloplast bone substitutes should have the following properties [56]: (1) biocompatibility, (2) minimal fibrotic reaction, (3) the ability to undergo remodeling and support new bone formation, (4) similar strength comparable to cortical/cancellous bone, and (5) similar modulus of elasticity comparable to bone to prevent fatigue fracture under cyclic loading.

Tricalcium phosphate and bioactive glass are absorbable. Porous and nonporous hydroxyapatite materials and PMMA/HEMA polymer are nonabsorbable. Grafted sites using nonporous and porous materials have shown significant clinical improvement compared with nongrafted controls and remained stable for a 5-year follow-up [57]. Defects grafted with tricalcium phosphate and PMMA/HEMA polymer have also shown significant clinical improvements compared with nongrafted controls [58,59].

Similar clinical results have been found when bone allografts and alloplasts are compared [60,61]. Histologically, however, alloplast grafts tend to heal encapsulated by connective tissue with minimal or no bone formation [62]. Some histologic evidence shows that a very limited amount of regeneration may be possible following PMMA/HEMA polymer grafts [63].

Bioactive glass is made from calcium salts, phosphate, sodium salts, and silicon [64,65]. Silicon forms a silica gel layer that promotes formation of a hydroxycarbonate-apatite layer. On this layer of hydroxycarbonate-apatite, osteoblasts are claimed to proliferate and form bone [66]. Mixed results have been reported in clinical studies evaluating bioactive glass particles [64,65,67]. Overall, histologic evaluation of bioactive glass shows limited regenerative potential, with minimal bone regeneration and no signs of new cementum or periodontal ligament [68].

Overall, the effect of alloplast material has been inconsistent [34]. It appears that alloplastic materials function as nonirritating fillers.

Xenografts

A xenograft (heterograft) is a graft taken from a donor of another species and is referred to as anorganic bone [6]. Proprietary processes are suggested to remove all cells and proteinaceous material. What is left behind is inert, absorbable bone scaffolding. It is on this scaffolding that revascularization, osteoblast migration, and woven bone formation supposedly occur [69]. Resorption of xenografts has been reported to occur very slowly [69].

To date, there are minimal clinical data supporting the use of xenografts in periodontal defects; only one study shows improvements in clinical parameters similar to DFDBA [70]. Positive clinical outcomes were reported when the combination of bovine hydroxyapatite and collagen membrane was used for the treatment of intrabony defects [71,72]. Signs of periodontal regeneration have been reported with xenografts [70,72]; however, most data support a bone fill or repair of bone for guided bone regeneration around implants, sinus lift procedures, and ridge augmentation [73,74]. Recently, concern about the risk of transmission of prion-mediated diseases from bovine-derived products has arisen [75]. It should be noted that prions have not been found in bone. The World Health Organization has labeled bone as type IV (no transmission) for prion diseases [76].

Guided cell repopulation/guided tissue regeneration

The concept of GTR is based on the exclusion of gingival connective tissue cells and prevention of epithelial downgrowth into the wound, thereby allowing cells with regenerative potential (PDL and bone cells) to enter the wound first. GTR has proved to be more effective than open-flap debridement in the gain of clinical attachment and probing depth reduction in the treatment of intrabony and furcation defects [77]. Absorbable and nonabsorbable membranes have been advocated and no differences have been detected among barrier types [77]. Because nonabsorbable membranes require a second surgical procedure for removal, biodegradable membranes are now commonly used [43].

Nonabsorbable membranes

The first nonabsorbable membrane available was made of expanded polytetrafluoroethylene. This membrane is composed of two parts: (1) a coronal collar with an open microstructure allowing ingrowth of connective tissue but preventing apical migration of the epithelium and (2) the remaining occlusive part that prevents the gingival tissue from interfering with the healing process at the root surface. Studies using expanded polytetrafluoroethylene to treat intraosseous defects show bone fill averaging approximately 3.0 to 5.0 mm with or without graft materials [30,78]. Results tend to vary depending on the type of defect treated. Three-wall defects typically respond the best [30,79].

Although nonabsorbable membranes are superior to open-flap debridement, they do not appear to be superior to DFDBA alone. No significant differences were found between sites treated with an expanded polytetrafluoroethylene membrane plus DFDBA versus allograft alone [80]. The use of DFDBA in combination with barrier membranes has questioned the value of adding bone graft materials for this type of defect [81]. For the treatment of mandibular class II furcation defects, significant clinical improvement has been shown [82]. The treatment of furcation defects with a combination of GTR barriers and bone replacement grafts appears to produce greater clinical improvements than GTR alone [83].

Absorbable membranes

Currently, polylactic acid and collagen membranes have reported clinical improvements comparable to nonabsorbable membranes [84–86]. The main advantage of absorbable membranes is that they do not require a second surgical procedure.

Collagen membranes are also effective in inhibiting epithelial migration and promoting new connective tissue attachment [85,87,88]. An advantage of collagen membranes is their hemostatic function of inducing platelet aggregation, which facilitates early clot formation and wound stabilization. Early clot formation and wound stabilization are considered essential for successful regeneration [89]. Collagen also possesses a chemotactic function for fibroblasts that aids in cell migration to promote primary wound closure [90]. When using bone replacement grafts and absorbable collagen membranes, clinical results are improved in furcations but not in intrabony defects [87,91].

Degradable polymers of polylactic acid, polyglycolic acid, or mixtures of both have had similar clinical results compared with other membranes [92–94]. Regeneration of periodontal tissues has been demonstrated [95]. Recently, a study comparing polylactic acid with polyglycolic acid, a type I collagen membrane in the treatment of intrabony defects, has reported similar clinical improvements for both membranes [96].

Biologic modifiers

Bone morphogenetic proteins

BMPs have unique properties in inducing ectopic bone formation [47] and new cementum formation. Several animal research studies reported improved regenerative results when BMP-2 and BMP-7 were used for the treatment of periodontal defects [97–99]. The first human study indicated that osteogenin combined with DFDBA significantly enhanced regeneration of a new attachment apparatus [100]. A higher incidence of ankylosis has been noted in animal studies [97]; however, this has not been observed in sites treated with BMP-7 [98]. Future research is needed to clearly understand the applicability of BMPs in periodontal regeneration.

Growth factors/cytokines

Transforming growth factor β, platelet-derived growth factor, insulin-like growth factor, and fibroblast growth factor act as mitogens or differential factors on regenerating periodontal tissues. Limited human clinical data are available. One human clinical trial using recombinant platelet-derived growth factor and insulin-like growth factor has shown promising results in intrabony defects and furcations [101]. Another study showed that the use of purified recombinant human platelet-derived growth factor BB mixed with bone allograft results in robust periodontal regeneration in class II furcations and in interproximal intrabony defects [102]. More studies are needed to fully evaluate the potential of growth factors for enhancing periodontal regeneration.

Other emerging materials (enamel matrix derivative, Pep-Gen p-15)

Enamel matrix derivative is a group of enamel matrix proteins isolated from developing porcine teeth [103–107]. It has recently been approved by the Food and Drug Administration for use in achieving periodontal regeneration in angular bony defects [107,108]. The freeze-dried protein extract is solubilized in a propylene glycol alginate carrier solution. This solution is then applied to debrided and root-conditioned periodontal intrabony defects [109]. Human case reports have reported inconsistent histologic evidence of regeneration [110–112]. A recent in vivo study showed that enamel matrix derivative was not an osteoinductive material but was osteoconductive (named osteopromotive by some) [113]. Although clinical trials of enamel matrix derivative have demonstrated significant improvements in probing measurements and radiographic evidence of bone fill, long-term benefits have not been established [114]. Enamel matrix derivative appears to offer some potential for regenerative therapy around natural teeth. To determine the long-term benefit of enamel matrix derivative, additional studies are needed.

Pep-Gen p-15 is another material recently introduced for periodontal regeneration. It is a putative collagen-binding peptide that uses a combination of an anorganic bovine-derived hydroxyapatite matrix and a synthetic 15–amino acid sequence type I collagen (P-15) [115]. P-15 is a collagen-derived cell-binding peptide that is reported to attract and bind fibroblasts and osteoblasts and to promote PDL fibroblast attachment to the anorganic bovine-derived hydroxyapatite matrix carrier [116,117]. Few clinical trials have reported greater regeneration compared with open-flap debridement, DFDBA, [115], or anorganic bovine-derived hydroxyapatite matrix alone [118,119]. Additional clinical and histologic data are needed to establish true periodontal regeneration using this material.

Factors that may influence regenerative therapy

The number of bony walls and the depth of the intrabony component are critical for positive GTR results (Box 1) [120]. Defects with 3-wall defects [30,79,121] and 4 mm or greater in depth [81] achieve the best results. Thin tissues have been found to show significantly less clinical improvement and percentage of root coverage [122].

The best results have been observed in healthy, nonsmoking patients demonstrating good plaque control and compliance with recommended oral hygiene measures [86]. The effects of bacterial contamination have been noted in studies reporting an inverse relationship between observed plaque contamination of retrieved membranes and clinical attachment gain [123].

Box 1. Indications and contraindications for guided tissue regeneration

Indications
- Narrow 2- or 3-wall infrabony defects
- Circumferential defects
- Class II molar furcations
- Recession defects

Contraindications
- Any medical condition contraindicating surgery
- Infection at defect site
- Poor oral hygiene
- Smoking (heavy)
- Tooth mobility >1 mm
- Defect <4 mm deep
- Width of attached gingiva at defect site ≤1 mm
- Thickness of attached gingiva at defect site ≤0.5 mm
- Furcations with short root trunks
- Generalized horizontal bone loss
- Advanced lesions with little remaining support
- Multiple defects

Data from Wang HL, Carroll WJ. Using absorbable collagen membranes for guided tissue regeneration, guided bone regeneration, and to treat gingival recession. Compend Contin Educ Dent 2000;21(5):399–406 [quiz: 414].

Smoking, poor plaque control, and premature exposure of the barrier have often resulted in poor regeneration outcomes [124,125].

Surgical principals for regenerative therapy

Clinical applications

Common clinical uses for periodontal regeneration include the treatment of furcations, intrabony defects, and recession defects.

Furcation defects

GTR procedures compared with open-flap debridement controls show more favorable gains in vertical probing attachment level, reductions in vertical probing depth, and improvement in horizontal open probing attachment measurements. The most favorable results are in class II mandibular furcations [77,82,85]. Less favorable results are found in

Table 3
Effect of various osseous grafts on defect fill and probing depth reduction

Graft	Defect fill (%)	Probing depth reduction (mm)
Autograph	75–80	2.5–3.0
Allograft	60–70	1.7–2.0
Synthetics (alloplast)	<50	1.0
Open-flap debridement	<50	2.0

Data from Murphy K, Gunsolley J. Guided tissue regeneration for the treatment of periodontal intrabony and furcation defects. A systematic review. Ann Periodontol 2003;8; 266–302.

mandibular and maxillary class III defects [7,126] and maxillary class II defects [127,128]. The best results are found using a combination of GTR and bone replacement grafts (91% overall improvement). Least favorable results are found with open-flap debridement (15% overall improvement). GTR procedures for furcation treatment should be limited to mandibular and some maxillary buccal class II furcation defects.

Intrabony defects

GTR procedures compared open-flap debridement controls result in significantly more favorable gains in clinical attachment level and probing depth reduction (Table 3) [77–79,87]. GTR is an effective treatment modality for the management of intrabony defects. No advantage has been found with the use of grafting materials in addition to membrane barrier in the treatment of intrabony defects [77]. Therefore, additional usage of bone graft in GTR for the treatment of intrabony defects is often unnecessary.

Gingival recession defects

GTR-based root coverage has an average of 76.4% (±11.3%) root coverage. In about 33.1% (±20.4%) of the treatments, 100% root coverage has been observed. Connective tissue grafting appears to be superior to GTR-based root coverage approaches [129]. Although GTR-based root coverage procedures are clinically effective in promoting root coverage, they are less predictable [130,131]. A critical factor is adequate flap thickness (≥ 0.8 mm in the defect area). With adequate flap thickness, there is a significant improvement in the percentage of root coverage (26.7% versus 95.9% in thin versus thick tissue, respectively) [131,132]. Therefore, case selection is critical for a positive outcome.

Technique

Suggestions for GTR placement are as follows (Figs. 1–3):

- Initial incision should be made away from the defect so that closure is not directly over the defect [133].

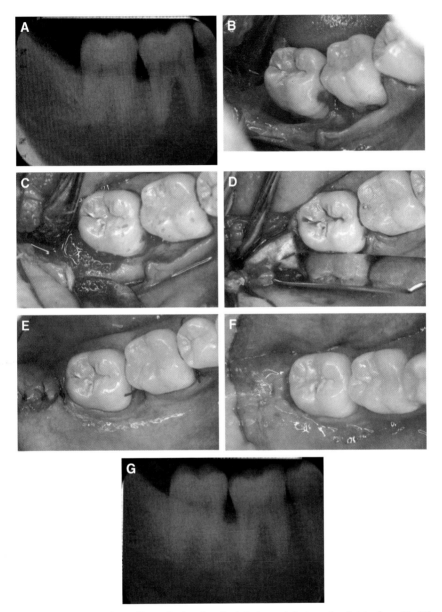

Fig. 1. (*A*) Preoperative radiograph showing the infrabony defect on the distal of no. 31. (*B*) The extent of the osseous defect (8 mm) after flap elevation. (*C*) Human mineralized allograft (Puros) placed. (*D*) Collagen membrane (BioMend, Zimmer Dental Inc., Carlsbad, California) in place. (*E*) Flap coronally repositioned and sutured with 5-0 Vicryl suture (Ethicon, Somerville, New Jersey). (*F*) Two weeks post surgery. (*G*) Postoperative radiograph at 1 year showing complete bone regeneration.

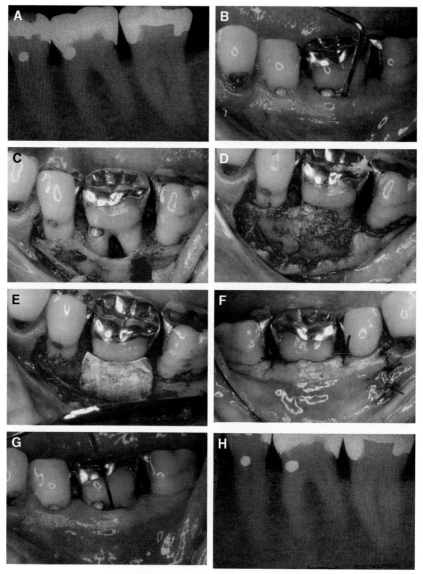

Fig. 2. (*A*) Preoperative radiograph suggesting furcation involvement on no. 19. (*B*) Intraoperative view of class II furcation with 6-mm probing pocket depth. (*C*) The extent of the furcation involvement shown after flap elevation. (*D*) Human mineralized allograft (Puros) placed. (*E*) Collagen membrane (BioMend) in place. (*F*) Flap coronally repositioned and sutured with 5-0 Vicryl suture. (*G*) One year postoperative clinical probing showing 3-mm probing pocket depth. (*H*) Postoperative radiograph at 1 year showing furcation bone fill.

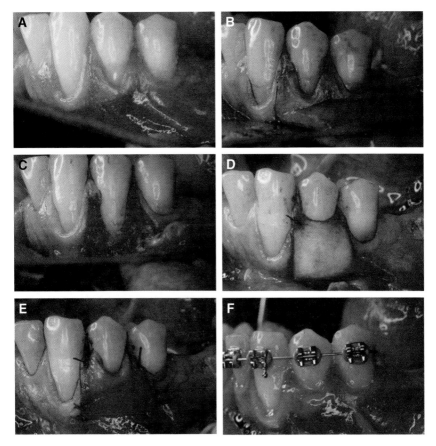

Fig. 3. (*A*) Preoperative view of a recession defect. (*B*) Initial incision (two diverging vertical releasing incisions). (*C*) Flap reflection. (*D*) Collagen membranes tacked to place with 5-0 gut suture. (*E*) Flap coronally repositioned and sutured with 5-0 silk suture. (*F*) Healing at 6 months post surgery showing 100% of root coverage.

- A full-thickness mucoperiosteal flap should be reflected 2 to 3 mm beyond the defect. Apical to the mucogingival junction, a partial-thickness flap is continued by blunt dissection to free the flap from tension [134].
- Granulation tissue is removed and curettes or burs are used to root plane and contour the exposed root surface [133,134].
- Where appropriate, interdental papillae are de-epithelialized with a blade or diamond bur to provide a bleeding tissue bed. Epithelium should also be removed from the inner surface of the flap with a sharp curette or diamond bur [120].
- The membrane should be trimmed so that it extends 2 to 3 mm beyond the margins of the defect in all directions. A trial membrane can serve as

a template for the final membrane. The membrane should be hydrated in sterile saline or sterile water for 5 to 10 minutes before use to improve handling [120].

- The flap should be trimmed if needed to achieve primary tension-free closure [120,134].
- Cortical perforations with a 1/2 round bur are made to create bleeding at the defect site to allow progenitor cells to egress from bone to the site [120,134].
- Graft material or biologic modifier is placed at the defect site to support the membrane [133].
- The membrane is adapted to the site and if stable, fixation is not necessary. If needed, pins, sutures, bone screws, or tacks can be used to achieve membrane stability [133].
- The suture site should be closed with Vicryl, expanded polytetrafluoro-ethylene, or silk sutures with passive tension [133]. Dressings should be used with caution because they may displace the graft material and collapse the membrane at the defect site.
- Postoperative care should consist of the following:

  - Antibiotic (amoxicillin) for a minimum of 10 days
  - Warm salt-water rinses for the first 2 to 3 weeks
  - Chlorhexidine gluconate 0.12% mouthrinse for the next 3 weeks
  - Sutures are removed at 10 to 14 days
  - Gentle brushing with a soft brush can resume at 3 weeks and flossing after 1 month
  - The surgical site is checked every 2 weeks for 2 months [120,133, 134]

Summary

Several options are available for GTR and grafting materials. Many critical factors are involved to achieve optimal results, such as case selection, flap management, patient management, technique, and graft selection. Clinicians need to be able to select the proper cases for the appropriate treatment and use the appropriate graft material when indicated. As new materials are developed such as BMPs, growth factors, and enamel matrix derivative, one must evaluate the literature critically and use these materials when properly indicated.

References

[1] Bowers GM, Chadroff B, Carnevale R, et al. Histologic evaluation of new attachment apparatus formation in humans. Part III. J Periodontol 1989;60(12):683–93.
[2] Bowers GM, Chadroff B, Carnevale R, et al. Histologic evaluation of new attachment apparatus formation in humans. Part II. J Periodontol 1989;60(12):675–82.

[3] Nyman S, Lindhe J, Karring T, et al. New attachment following surgical treatment of human periodontal disease. J Clin Periodontol 1982;9(4):290–6.

[4] Garrett S. Periodontal regeneration around natural teeth. Ann Periodontol 1996;1(1): 621–70.

[5] Bowers GM, Chadroff B, Carnevale R, et al. Histologic evaluation of new attachment apparatus formation in humans. Part I. J Periodontol 1989;60(12):664–74.

[6] Cohen RE, Mariotti A, Rethman M, et al. Glossary of periodontal terms. 4th edition. Chicago: The American Academy of Periodontology; 2001.

[7] Becker W, Becker BE, Berg L, et al. New attachment after treatment with root isolation procedures: report for treated Class III and Class II furcations and vertical osseous defects. Int J Periodontics Restorative Dent 1988;8(3):8–23.

[8] Becker W, Becker BE, Ochsenbein C, et al. A longitudinal study comparing scaling, osseous surgery and modified Widman procedures. Results after one year. J Periodontol 1988;59(6): 351–65.

[9] Kaldahl WB, Kalkwarf KL, Patil KD, et al. Long-term evaluation of periodontal therapy: I. Response to 4 therapeutic modalities. J Periodontol 1996;67(2):93–102.

[10] Pihlstrom BL, McHugh RB, Oliphant TH, et al. Comparison of surgical and nonsurgical treatment of periodontal disease. A review of current studies and additional results after 61/ 2 years. J Clin Periodontol 1983;10(5):524–41.

[11] Ramfjord SP, Caffesse RG, Morrison EC, et al. 4 modalities of periodontal treatment compared over 5 years. J Clin Periodontol 1987;14(8):445–52.

[12] Polson AM, Heijl LC. Osseous repair in infrabony periodontal defects. J Clin Periodontol 1978;5(1):13–23.

[13] Caton J, Nyman S. Histometric evaluation of periodontal surgery. I. The modified Widman flap procedure. J Clin Periodontol 1980;7(3):212–23.

[14] Caton J, Nyman S, Zander H. Histometric evaluation of periodontal surgery. II. Connective tissue attachment levels after four regenerative procedures. J Clin Periodontol 1980;7(3):224–31.

[15] Melcher AH. On the repair potential of periodontal tissues. J Periodontol 1976;47(5): 256–60.

[16] Caton JG, DeFuria EL, Polson AM, et al. Periodontal regeneration via selective cell repopulation. J Periodontol 1987;58(8):546–52.

[17] Nyman S, Gottlow J, Lindhe J, et al. New attachment formation by guided tissue regeneration. J Periodontal Res 1987;22(3):252–4.

[18] Wikesjo UM, Crigger M, Nilveus R, et al. Early healing events at the dentin-connective tissue interface. Light and transmission electron microscopy observations. J Periodontol 1991;62(1):5–14.

[19] Wikesjo UM, Nilveus RE, Selvig KA. Significance of early healing events on periodontal repair: a review. J Periodontol 1992;63(3):158–65.

[20] Egelberg J. Regeneration and repair of periodontal tissues. J Periodontal Res 1987;22(3): 233–42.

[21] McCulloch CA. Basic considerations in periodontal wound healing to achieve re-generation. Periodontol 2000 1993;1(1):16–25.

[22] Register AA, Burdick FA. Accelerated reattachment with cementogenesis to dentin, demineralized in situ. I. Optimum range. J Periodontol 1975;46(11):646–55.

[23] Register AA, Burdick FA. Accelerated reattachment with cementogenesis to dentin, demineralized in situ. II. Defect repair. J Periodontol 1976;47(9):497–505.

[24] Daly CG. Anti-bacterial effect of citric acid treatment of periodontally diseased root surfaces in vitro. J Clin Periodontol 1982;9(5):386–92.

[25] Garrett JS, Crigger M, Egelberg J. Effects of citric acid on diseased root surfaces. J Periodontal Res 1978;13(2):155–63.

[26] Crigger M, Bogle G, Nilveus R, et al. The effect of topical citric acid application on the healing of experimental furcation defects in dogs. J Periodontal Res 1978;13(6):538–49.

[27] Kersten BG, Chamberlain AD, Khorsandi S, et al. Healing of the intrabony periodontal lesion following root conditioning with citric acid and wound closure including an expanded PTFE membrane. J Periodontol 1992;63(11):876–82.

[28] Stahl SS, Froum SJ, Kushner L. Healing responses of human intraosseous lesions following the use of debridement, grafting and citric acid root treatment. II. Clinical and histologic observations: one year postsurgery. J Periodontol 1983;54(6):325–38.

[29] Blomlof J, Blomlof L, Lindskog S. Effect of different concentrations of EDTA on smear removal and collagen exposure in periodontitis-affected root surfaces. J Clin Periodontol 1997;24(8):534–7.

[30] Handelsman M, Davarpanah M, Celletti R. Guided tissue regeneration with and without citric acid treatment in vertical osseous defects. Int J Periodontics Restorative Dent 1991; 11(5):350–63.

[31] Mariott A. Efficacy of clinical root surface modifiers in the treatment of periodontal disease. A systematic review. Ann Periodontol 2003;8:205–26.

[32] Gantes B, Martin M, Garrett S, et al. Treatment of periodontal furcation defects. (II). Bone regeneration in mandibular class II defects. J Clin Periodontol 1988;15(4):232–9.

[33] Martin M, Gantes B, Garrett S, et al. Treatment of periodontal furcation defects. (I). Review of the literature and description of a regenerative surgical technique. J Clin Periodontol 1988;15(4):227–31.

[34] Reynolds M, Aichelmann-Reidy W, Branch-Mays G. The efficacy of bone replacement grafts in the treatment of periodontal osseous defects. A systematic review. Ann Periodontol 2003;1:227–65.

[35] Dragoo MR, Sullivan HC. A clinical and histological evaluation of autogenous iliac bone grafts in humans. I. Wound healing 2 to 8 months. J Periodontol 1973;44(10):599–613.

[36] Schallhorn RG, Hiatt WH, Boyce W. Iliac transplants in periodontal therapy. J Periodontol 1970;41(10):566–80.

[37] Froum SJ, Ortiz M, Witkin RT, et al. Osseous autografts. III. Comparison of osseous coagulum-bone blend implants with open curetage. J Periodontol 1976;47(5):287–94.

[38] Hiatt WH, Schallhorn RG. Intraoral transplants of cancellous bone and marrow in periodontal lesions. J Periodontol 1973;44(4):194–208.

[39] Nabers C, O'Leary T. Autogenous bone transplants in the treatment of osseous defects. J Periodontol 1965;36:5–14.

[40] Rosenberg MM. Free osseous tissue autografts as a predictable procedure. J Periodontol 1971;42(4):195–209.

[41] Listgarten MA, Rosenberg MM. Histological study of repair following new attachment procedures in human periodontal lesions. J Periodontol 1979;50(7):333–44.

[42] Moskow BS, Karsh F, Stein SD. Histological assessment of autogenous bone graft. A case report and critical evaluation. J Periodontol 1979;50(6):291–300.

[43] Blumenthal N, Steinberg J. The use of collagen membrane barriers in conjunction with combined demineralized bone-collagen gel implants in human infrabony defects. J Periodontol 1990;61(6):319–27.

[44] Rummelhart JM, Mellonig JT, Gray JL, et al. A comparison of freeze-dried bone allograft and demineralized freeze-dried bone allograft in human periodontal osseous defects. J Periodontol 1989;60(12):655–63.

[45] Evans GH, Yukna RA, Sepe WW, et al. Effect of various graft materials with tetracycline in localized juvenile periodontitis. J Periodontol 1989;60(9):491–7.

[46] Mabry TW, Yukna RA, Sepe WW. Freeze-dried bone allografts combined with tetracycline in the treatment of juvenile periodontitis. J Periodontol 1985;56(2):74–81.

[47] Urist MR. Bone: formation by autoinduction. Science 1965;150(698):893–9.

[48] Mellonig JT. Decalcified freeze-dried bone allograft as an implant material in human periodontal defects. Int J Periodontics Restorative Dent 1984;4(6):40–55.

[49] Mellonig JT. Bone allografts in periodontal therapy. Clin Orthop 1996;324:116–25.

[50] Schwartz Z, Mellonig JT, Carnes DL Jr, et al. Ability of commercial demineralized freeze-dried bone allograft to induce new bone formation. J Periodontol 1996;67(9):918–26.

[51] Shigeyama Y, D'Errico JA, Stone R, et al. Commercially-prepared allograft material has biological activity in vitro. J Periodontol 1995;66(6):478–87.

[52] Somerman MJ. Is there a role for DFDBA in periodontal regenerative therapy? J Periodontol 1996;67(9):946–8.

[53] Schwartz Z, Somers A, Mellonig JT, et al. Ability of commercial demineralized freeze-dried bone allograft to induce new bone formation is dependent on donor age but not gender. J Periodontol 1998;69(4):470–8.

[54] Callan DP, Salkeld SL, Scarborough N. Histologic analysis of implant sites after grafting with demineralized bone matrix putty and sheets. Implant Dent 2000;9(1):36–44.

[55] Zubillaga G, Von Hagen S, Simon BI, et al. Changes in alveolar bone height and width following post-extraction ridge augmentation using a fixed bioabsorbable membrane and demineralized freeze-dried bone osteoinductive graft. J Periodontol 2003;74(7):965–75.

[56] Moore WR, Graves SE, Bain GI. Synthetic bone graft substitutes. Aust N Z J Surg 2001;71(6):354–61.

[57] Yukna RA, Mayer ET, Amos SM. 5-year evaluation of durapatite ceramic alloplastic implants in periodontal osseous defects. J Periodontol 1989;60(10):544–51.

[58] Yukna RA. HTR polymer grafts in human periodontal osseous defects. I. 6-month clinical results. J Periodontol 1990;61(10):633–42.

[59] Yukna RA. Clinical evaluation of HTR polymer bone replacement grafts in human mandibular Class II molar furcations. J Periodontol 1994;65(4):342–9.

[60] Barnett JD, Mellonig JT, Gray JL, et al. Comparison of freeze-dried bone allograft and porous hydroxylapatite in human periodontal defects. J Periodontol 1989;60(5):231–7.

[61] Bowen JA, Mellonig JT, Gray JL, et al. Comparison of decalcified freeze-dried bone allograft and porous particulate hydroxyapatite in human periodontal osseous defects. J Periodontol 1989;60(12):647–54.

[62] Stahl SS, Froum S. Histological evaluation of human intraosseous healing responses to the placement of tricalcium phosphate ceramic implants. I. Three to eight months. J Periodontol 1986;57(4):211–7.

[63] Stahl SS, Froum SJ, Tarnow D. Human clinical and histologic responses to the placement of HTR polymer particles in 11 intrabony lesions. J Periodontol 1990;61(5):269–74.

[64] Froum SJ, Weinberg MA, Tarnow D. Comparison of bioactive glass synthetic bone graft particles and open debridement in the treatment of human periodontal defects. A clinical study. J Periodontol 1998;69(6):698–709.

[65] Ong MM, Eber RM, Korsnes MI, et al. Evaluation of a bioactive glass alloplast in treating periodontal intrabony defects. J Periodontol 1998;69(12):1346–54.

[66] Hench LL, Wilson J. Surface-active biomaterials. Science 1984;226(4675):630–6.

[67] Lovelace TB, Mellonig JT, Meffert RM, et al. Clinical evaluation of bioactive glass in the treatment of periodontal osseous defects in humans. J Periodontol 1998;69(9):1027–35.

[68] Nevins ML, Camelo M, Nevins M, et al. Human histologic evaluation of bioactive ceramic in the treatment of periodontal osseous defects. Int J Periodontics Restorative Dent 2000;20(5):458–67.

[69] Spector M. Anorganic bovine bone and ceramic analogs of bone mineral as implants to facilitate bone regeneration. Clin Plast Surg 1994;21(3):437–44.

[70] Mellonig JT. Human histologic evaluation of a bovine-derived bone xenograft in the treatment of periodontal osseous defects. Int J Periodontics Restorative Dent 2000;20(1):19–29.

[71] Camelo M, Nevins M, Lynch S. Periodontal regeneration with an autogenerous bone-Bio-Oss composite graft and a Bio-Gide membrane. Int J Periodontics Restorative Dent 2001;21:109–19.

[72] Nevins M, Camelo M, Lynch S. Evaluation of periodontal regeneration following grafting intrabony defects treated with bio-oss collagen: a human histologic report. Int J Periodontics Restorative Dent 2003;23:9–17.

[73] Hallman M, Lundgren S, Sennerby L. Histologic analysis of clinical biopsies taken 6 months and 3 years after maxillary sinus floor augmentation with 80% bovine hydroxyapatite and 20% autogenous bone mixed with fibrin glue. Clin Implant Dent Relat Res 2001;3(2):87–96.

[74] Hurzeler MB, Quinones CR, Kirsch A, et al. Maxillary sinus augmentation using different grafting materials and dental implants in monkeys. Part I. Evaluation of anorganic bovine-derived bone matrix. Clin Oral Implants Res 1997;8(6):476–86.

[75] Sogal A, Tofe AJ. Risk assessment of bovine spongiform encephalopathy transmission through bone graft material derived from bovine bone used for dental applications. J Periodontol 1999;70(9):1053–63.

[76] Asher DM, Padilla AM, Pocchiari M. WHO Consultation on Diagnostic Procedures for Transmissible Spongiform Encephalopathies: need for reference reagents and reference panels. Geneva, Switzerland, 22–23 March 1999. Biologicals 1999;27(3):265–72.

[77] Murphy K, Gunsolley J. Guided tissue regeneration for the treatment of periodontal intrabony and furcation defects. A systematic review. Ann Periodontol 2003;8:266–302.

[78] Cortellini P, Pini Prato G, Tonetti MS. Periodontal regeneration of human infrabony defects. II. Re-entry procedures and bone measures. J Periodontol 1993;64(4):261–8.

[79] Becker W, Becker BE. Treatment of mandibular 3-wall intrabony defects by flap debridement and expanded polytetrafluoroethylene barrier membranes. Long-term evaluation of 32 treated patients. J Periodontol 1993;64(Suppl 11):1138–44.

[80] Guillemin MR, Mellonig JT, Brunsvold MA. Healing in periodontal defects treated by decalcified freeze-dried bone allografts in combination with ePTFE membranes (I). Clinical and scanning electron microscope analysis. J Clin Periodontol 1993;20(7):528–36.

[81] Laurell L, Gottlow J, Zybutz M, et al. Treatment of intrabony defects by different surgical procedures. A literature review. J Periodontol 1998;69(3):303–13.

[82] Pontoriero R, Lindhe J, Nyman S, et al. Guided tissue regeneration in degree II furcation-involved mandibular molars. A clinical study. J Clin Periodontol 1988;15(4):247–54.

[83] Evans GH, Yukna RA, Gardiner DL, et al. Frequency of furcation closure with regenerative periodontal therapy. J West Soc Periodontol Periodontal Abstr 1996;44(4):101–9.

[84] Vernino AR, Jones FL, Holt RA, et al. Evaluation of the potential of a polylactic acid barrier for correction of periodontal defects in baboons: a clinical and histologic study. Int J Periodontics Restorative Dent 1995;15(1):84–101.

[85] Wang HL, O'Neal RB, Thomas CL, et al. Evaluation of an absorbable collagen membrane in treating Class II furcation defects. J Periodontol 1994;65(11):1029–36.

[86] Wang HL, MacNeil RL. Guided tissue regeneration. Absorbable barriers. Dent Clin N Am 1998;42(3):505–22.

[87] Chen CC, Wang HL, Smith F, et al. Evaluation of a collagen membrane with and without bone grafts in treating periodontal intrabony defects. J Periodontol 1995;66(10):838–47.

[88] Wang HL, O'Neal RB, MacNeil LM. Regenerative treatment of periodontal defects utilizing a bioresorbable collagen membrane. Pract Periodontics Aesthet Dent 1995;7(5): 59–66 [quiz: 68].

[89] Steinberg AD, LeBreton G, Willey R, et al. Extravascular clot formation and platelet activation on variously treated root surfaces. J Periodontol 1986;57(8):516–22.

[90] Postlethwaite AE, Seyer JM, Kang AH. Chemotactic attraction of human fibroblasts to type I, II, and III collagens and collagen-derived peptides. Proc Natl Acad Sci U S A 1978; 75(2):871–5.

[91] Bunyaratavej P, Wang HL. Collagen membranes: a review. J Periodontol 2001;72(2): 215–29.

[92] Caton J, Greenstein G, Zappa U. Synthetic bioabsorbable barrier for regeneration in human periodontal defects. J Periodontol 1994;65(11):1037–45.

[93] Vernino AR, Ringeisen TA, Wang HL, et al. Use of biodegradable polylactic acid barrier materials in the treatment of grade II periodontal furcation defects in humans—part I: a multicenter investigative clinical study. Int J Periodontics Restorative Dent 1998;18(6): 572–85.

[94] Vernino AR, Wang HL, Rapley J, et al. The use of biodegradable polylactic acid barrier materials in the treatment of grade II periodontal furcation defects in humans—part II: a multicenter investigative surgical study. Int J Periodontics Restorative Dent 1999;19(1): 56–65.

[95] Robert PM, Frank RM. Periodontal guided tissue regeneration with a new resorbable polylactic acid membrane. J Periodontol 1994;65(5):414–22.

[96] Mattson JS, Gallagher SJ, Jabro MH. The use of 2 bioabsorbable barrier membranes in the treatment of interproximal intrabony periodontal defects. J Periodontol 1999;70(5): 510–7.

[97] Ripamonti U, Reddi AH. Tissue engineering, morphogenesis, and regeneration of the periodontal tissues by bone morphogenetic proteins. Crit Rev Oral Biol Med 1997;8(2): 154–63.

[98] Giannobile WV, Ryan S, Shih MS, et al. Recombinant human osteogenic protein-1 (OP-1) stimulates periodontal wound healing in class III furcation defects. J Periodontol 1998; 69(2):129–37.

[99] Sigurdsson TJ, Tatakis DN, Lee MB, et al. Periodontal regenerative potential of space-providing expanded polytetrafluoroethylene membranes and recombinant human bone morphogenetic proteins. J Periodontol 1995;66(6):511–21.

[100] Bowers G, Felton F, Middleton C, et al. Histologic comparison of regeneration in human intrabony defects when osteogenin is combined with demineralized freeze-dried bone allograft and with purified bovine collagen. J Periodontol 1991;62(11):690–702.

[101] Howell TH, Fiorellini JP, Paquette DW, et al. A phase I/II clinical trial to evaluate a combination of recombinant human platelet-derived growth factor-BB and recombinant human insulin- like growth factor-I in patients with periodontal disease. J Periodontol 1997;68(12):1186–93.

[102] Nevins M, Camelo M, Nevins ML, et al. Periodontal regeneration in humans using recombinant human platelet-derived growth factor-BB (rhPDGF-BB) and allogenic bone. J Periodontol 2003;74(9):1282–92.

[103] Cattaneo V, Rota C, Silvestri M, et al. Effect of enamel matrix derivative on human periodontal fibroblasts: proliferation, morphology and root surface colonization. An in vitro study. J Periodontal Res 2003;38(6):568–74.

[104] Donos N, Glavind L, Karring T, et al. Clinical evaluation of an enamel matrix derivative in the treatment of mandibular degree II furcation involvement: a 36-month case series. Int J Periodontics Restorative Dent 2003;23(5):507–12.

[105] Cochran DL, Jones A, Heijl L, et al. Periodontal regeneration with a combination of enamel matrix proteins and autogenous bone grafting. J Periodontol 2003;74(9): 1269–81.

[106] McGuire MK, Cochran DL. Evaluation of human recession defects treated with coronally advanced flaps and either enamel matrix derivative or connective tissue. Part 2: histological evaluation. J Periodontol 2003;74(8):1126–35.

[107] McGuire MK, Nunn M. Evaluation of human recession defects treated with coronally advanced flaps and either enamel matrix derivative or connective tissue. Part 1: comparison of clinical parameters. J Periodontol 2003;74(8):1110–25.

[108] Sculean A, Chiantella GC, Miliauskaite A, et al. Four-year results following treatment of intrabony periodontal defects with an enamel matrix protein derivative: a report of 46 cases. Int J Periodontics Restorative Dent 2003;23(4):345–51.

[109] Sculean A, Reich E, Chiantella GC, et al. Treatment of intrabony periodontal defects with an enamel matrix protein derivative (Emdogain): a report of 32 cases. Int J Periodontics Restorative Dent 1999;19(2):157–63.

[110] Parodi R, Liuzzo G, Patrucco P, et al. Use of Emdogain in the treatment of deep intrabony defects: 12-month clinical results. Histologic and radiographic evaluation. Int J Periodontics Restorative Dent 2000;20(6):584–95.

[111] Francetti L, Del Fabbro M, Basso M, et al. Enamel matrix proteins in the treatment of intra-bony defects. A prospective 24-month clinical trial. J Clin Periodontol 2004;31(1): 52–9.

[112] Parodi R, Santarelli GA, Gasparetto B. Treatment of intrabony pockets with Emdogain: results at 36 months. Int J Periodontics Restorative Dent 2004;24(1):57–63.

[113] Boyan BD, Weesner TC, Lohmann CH, et al. Porcine fetal enamel matrix derivative enhances bone formation induced by demineralized freeze dried bone allograft in vivo. J Periodontol 2000;71(8):1278–86.

[114] Giannobile W, Somerman M. Growth and amelogenin-like factors in periodontal wound healing. A systematic review. Ann Periodontol 2003;8:193–204.

[115] Yukna RA, Callan DP, Krauser JT, et al. Multi-center clinical evaluation of combination anorganic bovine-derived hydroxyapatite matrix (ABM)/cell binding peptide (P-15) as a bone replacement graft material in human periodontal osseous defects. 6-month results. J Periodontol 1998;69(6):655–63.

[116] Qian JJ, Bhatnagar RS. Enhanced cell attachment to anorganic bone mineral in the presence of a synthetic peptide related to collagen. J Biomed Mater Res 1996;31(4):545–54.

[117] Bhatnagar RS, Qian JJ, Wedrychowska A, et al. Design of biomimetic habitats for tissue engineering with P-15, a synthetic peptide analogue of collagen. Tissue Eng 1999;5(1): 53–65.

[118] Yukna RA, Krauser JT, Callan DP, et al. Multi-center clinical comparison of combination anorganic bovine-derived hydroxyapatite matrix (ABM)/cell binding peptide (P-15) and ABM in human periodontal osseous defects. 6-month results. J Periodontol 2000;71(11): 1671–9.

[119] Yukna RA, Krauser JT, Callan DP, et al. Thirty-six month follow-up of 25 patients treated with combination anorganic bovine-derived hydroxyapatite matrix (ABM)/cell-binding peptide (P-15) bone replacement grafts in human infrabony defects. I. Clinical findings. J Periodontol 2002;73(1):123–8.

[120] Wang HL, Carroll WJ. Using absorbable collagen membranes for guided tissue regeneration, guided bone regeneration, and to treat gingival recession. Compend Contin Educ Dent 2000;21(5):399–406 [quiz: 414].

[121] Selvig KA, Kersten BG, Wikesjo UM. Surgical treatment of intrabony periodontal defects using expanded polytetrafluoroethylene barrier membranes: influence of defect configuration on healing response. J Periodontol 1993;64(8):730–3.

[122] Anderegg CR, Metzler DG, Nicoll BK. Gingiva thickness in guided tissue regeneration and associated recession at facial furcation defects. J Periodontol 1995;66(5):397–402.

[123] Selvig KA, Kersten BG, Chamberlain AD, et al. Regenerative surgery of intrabony periodontal defects using ePTFE barrier membranes: scanning electron microscopic evaluation of retrieved membranes versus clinical healing. J Periodontol 1992;63(12): 974–8.

[124] Machtei EE, Cho MI, Dunford R, et al. Clinical, microbiological, and histological factors which influence the success of regenerative periodontal therapy. J Periodontol 1994;65(2): 154–61.

[125] Tonetti MS, Pini-Prato G, Cortellini P. Effect of cigarette smoking on periodontal healing following GTR in infrabony defects. A preliminary retrospective study. J Clin Periodontol 1995;22(3):229–34.

[126] Pontoriero R, Lindhe J. Guided tissue regeneration in the treatment of degree III furcation defects in maxillary molars. J Clin Periodontol 1995;22(10):810–2.

[127] Metzler DG, Seamons BC, Mellonig JT, et al. Clinical evaluation of guided tissue regeneration in the treatment of maxillary class II molar furcation invasions. J Periodontol 1991;62(6):353–60.

[128] Pontoriero R, Lindhe J. Guided tissue regeneration in the treatment of degree II furcations in maxillary molars. J Clin Periodontol 1995;22(10):756–63.

[129] Oates T, Robinson M, Gunsolley J. Surgical therapies for the treatment of gingival recession. A systematic review. Ann Periodontol 2003;8:303–20.

[130] al-Hamdan K, Eber R, Sarment D, et al. Guided tissue regeneration–based root coverage: meta-analysis. J Periodontol 2003;74:1520–33.

[131] Harris RJ. A comparison of 2 root coverage techniques: guided tissue regeneration with a bioabsorbable matrix style membrane versus a connective tissue graft combined with a coronally positioned pedicle graft without vertical incisions. Results of a series of consecutive cases. J Periodontol 1998;69(12):1426–34.

[132] Baldi C, Pini-Prato G, Pagliaro U, et al. Coronally advanced flap procedure for root coverage. Is flap thickness a relevant predictor to achieve root coverage? A 19-case series. J Periodontol 1999;70(9):1077–84.

[133] Wang HL, Carroll MJ. Guided bone regeneration using bone grafts and collagen membranes. Quintessence Int 2001;32(7):504–15.

[134] Wang HL, Al-Shammari KF. Guided tissue regeneration-based root coverage utilizing collagen membranes: technique and case reports. Quintessence Int 2002;33(10):715–21.

ELSEVIER
SAUNDERS

Dent Clin N Am 49 (2005) 661–676

THE DENTAL
CLINICS
OF NORTH AMERICA

Peri-implantitis

Björn Klinge, DDS, Odont Dr[a],*,
Margareta Hultin, DDS, Odont Dr[a],
Tord Berglundh, DDS, Odont Dr[b]

[a]Karolinska Institutet, Institute of Odontology, Department of Periodontology,
P.O. Box 4064, SE-141 04 Huddinge, Sweden
[b]Göteborg University, The Sahlgrenska Academy, Faculty of Odontology,
Department of Periodontology, P.O. Box 450, SE-405 30 Göteborg, Sweden

At the turn of the millennium, marketing estimates indicated that over 2 million dental implants are installed annually, and this number is expected to rise further over the next few years. It is evident that the installation of oral implants is a routine procedure in the reconstruction of fully or partially edentulous individuals. Like natural teeth, the artificial abutments penetrate the oral mucosa and reach the contaminated oral cavity. When challenged by bacteria within the biofilms formed on implant surfaces, the peri-implant tissue response seems to follow patterns similar to those of the periodontal tissues in a susceptible host [1–3]. Documentation of implant therapy has so far included only exceptional reports on the destructive lesions around implants [4–6]. A systematic review of the incidence of biologic implant complications reported that data on peri-implantitis were provided in only 35% to 45% of the included studies on overdentures, fixed complete dentures, and fixed partial dentures [7]. One factor that may have influenced the detection of peri-implantitis is the historical dogma that probing around implants should be avoided. Another possible reason may be the rare occurrence of peri-implantitis in studies of short-term duration; observation periods exceeding 5 years may be required to detect tissue destruction around implants [8].

Peri-implantitis is defined as an inflammatory reaction with the loss of supporting bone in the tissues surrounding a functioning implant [9]. The overall frequency of peri-implantitis was reported to be 5% to 8% for selected implant systems [7]. A site-specific infection comparable to chronic

* Corresponding author.
E-mail address: bjorn.klinge@ofa.ki.se (B. Klinge).

periodontitis, possibly related to implant design and surface characteristics, may have caused the difference in prevalence of peri-implantitis in the various implant systems. Data on the transmission of periopathogenic microorganisms from the periodontal pocket to the peri-implant region have been presented [10]. In a study of partially edentulous patients, van Steenberghe et al [11] found a higher number of late fixture losses in patients with larger amounts of plaque accumulation.

In some studies, implant loss has clustered in a small subset of patients, which may indicate the existence of a high-risk group for implant failure. Other studies, however, have taken the opposite view. Prospective longitudinal data show that the incidence and the prevalence of radiographic bone loss vary among patients. An association between periodontal and peri-implant conditions has been reported. The higher the full-mouth clinical probing pocket depth and the greater the full-mouth attachment loss, the higher the attachment loss is to be expected around implants in the susceptible patient. In individuals with a history of chronic periodontitis, the incidence of peri-implantitis was four to five times higher than in individuals with no history of periodontitis [1]. Longitudinal bone loss around implants was correlated to previous experience of reduced periodontal bone support. Thus, periodontitis-susceptible subjects may show increased implant failure rate and marginal bone loss [12]. Smoking has also been reported to significantly correlate to marginal bone loss around implants [1].

Soft tissue around implants

The soft tissue surrounding healthy osseointegrated dental implants shares anatomic and functional features with the gingiva around teeth. The microstructure has been described in dog models and in human tissues. The outer surface of the peri-implant mucosa is lined by a stratified keratinized oral epithelium that is continuous with a junctional epithelium attached to the titanium surface by a basal lamina and by hemidesmosomes. The 2-mm long nonkeratinized junctional epithelium is only a few cell layers thick in the apical portion and separated from the alveolar bone by 1 to 2 mm of collagen-rich connective tissue. This 3- to 4-mm "biological barrier," formed irrespective of the original mucosal thickness, protects the zone of osseointegration from factors released from plaque and the oral cavity [13] (Fig. 1).

Unlike the gingiva around teeth, the connective tissue compartment between the junctional epithelium and the alveolar bone consists of a scarlike connective tissue, almost devoid of vascular structures, with greater amounts of collagen and fewer fibroblasts [14]. The fibroblast-rich barrier next to the titanium surface has a high cell turnover, and fibroblasts may play an important role in establishing and maintaining the mucosal seal.

In animal models and in humans, the inflammatory infiltrate in peri-implant tissue and the response to plaque accumulation have been described. As in gingivitis around natural teeth, an inflammatory infiltrate forms in the

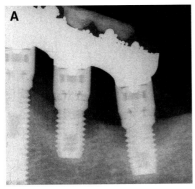
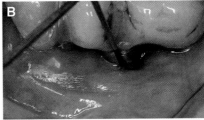

Fig. 1. (*A*) Radiograph from two implants exhibiting peri-implantitis, with crater- or saucer-shaped defects formed in the left side of the mandible. (*B*) Probing assessment (8 mm) at one of the implants with peri-implantitis. Note the bleeding and suppuration following probing.

connective tissue in response to microbial colonization of the titanium surface [15]. The infiltrate represents the local host response to bacterial accumulation and proliferates in an apical direction when the time for plaque accumulation is prolonged. The peri-implant mucosa is similar to the gingiva around teeth as regards function and host response to infection [16]. An inflammatory cell infiltrate of equal size and composition has been found in clinically healthy tissues of gingiva and in peri-implant mucosa [17]. Results from immunohistochemical and morphologic analyses show that inflammatory cells (eg, neutrophils, lymphocytes, macrophages, and plasma cells) are present. Functional adaptation of the junctional epithelium occurs, although its origin differs from that around the teeth (Fig. 2).

Periodontitis and tooth loss

Epidemiologic studies show that although the incidence of periodontitis increases with age, only a limited number of persons develop the more severe forms. Several studies report that 5% to 10% of the adult population has severe disease, which is unaffected by oral hygiene habits. This prevalence is similar in various parts of the world. In addition, the number of persons developing severe periodontitis appears to be consistent over time [18].

Periodontitis and other reasons for tooth extraction have been studied in various populations. Caries is the main reason for tooth extractions in persons up to 40 years of age. Above the age of 40 years, periodontitis accounts for about 30% to 35% of tooth extractions and caries and caries-related reasons account for 50% of tooth extractions. In older age groups, however, tooth extractions are performed equally due to periodontitis and caries. In general, the main risk factors for tooth loss include age, smoking, socioeconomic behavioral traits, and periodontitis scores. It therefore seems

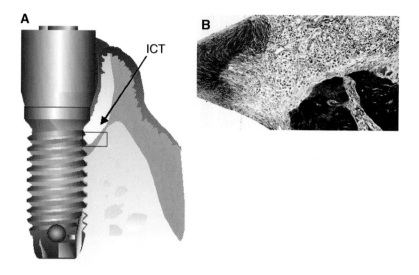

Fig. 2. (*A*) Schematic illustration of a peri-implantitis lesion. Note the apical extension of the inflammatory cell infiltrate (ICT). (*B*) Histologic section from an experimental peri-implantitis lesion illustrating the outlined area in *A*. Note the inflammatory cells close to the bone and the osteoclasts on the bone surface.

reasonable to assume that in partially edentulous patients, 30% to 40% of those given dental implants have lost their teeth due to periodontitis.

Microbiology of the peri-implant area

The transmucosal abutment of osseointegrated dental implants serves as a surface for bacterial colonization of microbial biofilms. Like the gingival crevice around the natural tooth, the peri-implant mucosa, which covers the alveolar bone, is closely adapted to the implant. Microbial colonization and the ensuing inflammatory reactions in the peri-implant tissues might be analogous to key events in the pathogenesis of periodontitis. In partially edentulous subjects, the developing microbiota around implants closely resembles the microflora of naturally remaining teeth [19,20]. A history of periodontitis and the presence of putative periodontal pathogens are factors that can influence the condition of peri-implant tissues in partially edentulous subjects. Quirynen and Listgarten [21] used phase-contrast microscopy to evaluate the impact of periodontitis around remaining teeth and probing depth around the implants on the composition of the peri-implant subgingival flora in partially edentulous subjects. The investigators found that the subgingival microflora around implants harbored increased spirochetes and motile rods compared with teeth present in the same jaw. Samples from deep peri-implant pockets (≥ 4 mm) in the residual dentition of patients with chronic or refractory periodontitis showed significantly higher proportions of spirochetes and motile rods than samples from periodontally healthy patients with comparable probing pocket depths.

Papaioannou et al [22], also using phase-contrast microscopy and DNA probes, determined the prevalence of putative periodontal pathogens in partially edentulous and edentulous patients with a history of periodontal disease. The microbiologic profiles were similar around teeth and dental implants of equal pocket depth, which may indicate that pockets around teeth can serve as a reservoir for putative periodontal pathogens. This finding was confirmed in several studies on partially edentulous patients [23]. As early as 1 month after implantation, putative periodontal pathogens were detected around the implants of partially edentulous patients [19].

Implant failures due to infection are characterized by a complex peri-implant microbiota resembling that of adult periodontitis. In edentulous subjects, *Actinobacillus actinomycetemcomitans* and *Porphyromonas gingivalis* are not as frequently associated with peri-implant infection as in dentate subjects [4]. Danser et al [24] reported that after total extraction in patients with severe periodontitis, *Porphyromonas gingivalis* could no longer be detected on the mucosal surface of edentulous patients. Furthermore, *A actinomycetemcomitans* and *Porphyromonas gingivalis* could not be isolated at the peri-implant pockets in these patients after insertion of implants [25].

In addition to the dark-pigmented, gram-negative anaerobic rods, other bacterial species are associated with peri-implant infections (eg, *Bacteroides forsythus, Fusobacterium nucleatum, Campylobacter, Peptostreptococcus micros* and *Prevotella intermedia*) [26]. Organisms that are less frequently associated with periodontitis, such as *Staphylococcus* spp, enterics, and *Candida* spp, have also been found in peri-implant infections [27,28]. Longitudinal data on implants in partially edentulous persons with a history of periodontal disease, however, have shown no association between periodontal pathogens and loss of attachment at implants after 36 months of function [19,29]. This finding corresponds to the situation observed in periodontitis: putative periodontal pathogens can also be detected in apparently healthy periodontal pockets and at sites with no periodontal progression. Thus, it has been suggested that the pathogens in peri-implant infections propagate from the periodontopathic bacteria of natural teeth into the saliva and become transmitted to the vicinity of implants [10].

Inflammation leading to tissue destruction

Inflammation is a complex reaction of the body in response to an infectious agent, antigen challenge, or injury. An accumulation of microbes at the peri-implant/mucosal margin is followed by a local inflammatory response. Within 10 to 20 days of plaque accumulation on teeth, clinical signs of inflammation can be seen. Even during early stages of inflammation, considerable tissue damage occurs. As reported in dogs, the collagen content of the inflammatory lesion in the gingival of teeth decreases by approximately

30% after 28 days of undisturbed plaque accumulation [30]. Thus, the cells in the inflammatory lesion cause considerable tissue damage in their effort to combat the invading microorganisms. Accumulation of plaque in the gingival crevice aggravates the inflammatory reaction over time, and consequently, irreversible tissue destruction occurs. Degradation of connective tissue is followed by epithelial migration and bone resorption, which marks the borderline between gingivitis/mucositis and periodontitis/peri-implantitis.

Periodontitis–peri-implantitis relation

Periodontitis is one of the main causes of tooth loss in adults. It can therefore be assumed that a great number of patients receiving dental implants have a history of periodontal disease. When replacing lost teeth with implants, it is important and necessary to determine whether a history of periodontitis will affect the prognosis and maintenance of implants. First, do patients with periodontal disease lose more implants in the early healing period, and second, is the long-term prognosis and maintenance of implants affected?

In the available literature concerning implant treatment of periodontally compromised patients, case reports show that implants are lost in those with severe forms of periodontitis [5,6]. Clustering of implant losses in certain individuals has been suggested to indicate systemic or host-related factors of importance for fixture losses [31]; however, early failure rates of implants in patients treated for periodontitis are similar to those in partly edentulous patients in general [29,32].

Few studies have evaluated attachment loss and marginal bone loss around implants in patients treated for periodontitis. In a retrospective study of periodontally treated patients receiving implants, Ellegaard et al [32] reported that the incidence of bone loss during the 5 years after implantation increased in 45% of all implants displaying marginal bone loss of 1.5 mm or more.

In another 5-year retrospective radiographic study, the outcome of implant therapy in relation to experience of periodontal tissue destruction was evaluated in 97 partially edentulous subjects. Hardt et al [12] defined two groups of subjects ("Perio" and "Non-Perio") with regard to an age-related bone loss score at teeth. The study reported that early failures of implants were more frequent in the Perio group than in the Non-Perio group. Furthermore, the proportion of subjects who had >2 mm bone loss at implant sites during the 5-year study period was significantly larger in the Perio group than in the Non-Perio group. It was concluded that longitudinal bone loss around implants was correlated with previous experience of periodontal bone loss.

In contrast, Wennström et al [33] performed a 5-year prospective study and reported the existence of few implant losses and relatively small amounts of marginal bone loss in a group of periodontally susceptive subjects. The conflicting outcomes of implant therapy in periodontally compromised subjects reported in the studies by Wennström et al [33] compared with

Ellegaard et al [32] and Hardt et al [12] may be related to differences in maintenance programs (such as the frequency of recall visits).

In a recent study, Karoussis et al [1] compared the failure, success, and complication rates of patients who lost their teeth due to periodontitis or other reasons. The group with a history of chronic periodontitis had a significantly higher incidence of peri-implantitis (28.6%) than the group with no history of periodontitis (5.8%).

Peri-implantitis

Peri-implantitis is defined as an inflammatory reaction, with the loss of supporting bone in the tissues surrounding a functioning implant [9]. It has also been described as "a site-specific infection yielding many features in common with chronic adult periodontitis" [4] or "an inflammatory, bacterial-driven destruction of the implant-supporting apparatus" [34]. The view that microorganisms play a major role in the development of peri-implantitis is supported by several clinical findings. A cause-related effect between plaque accumulation and peri-implant mucositis has been shown in animals and humans [15,35]. Moreover, the microbial colonization of implants follows the same pattern as that described around teeth [19,36]. During peri-implant breakdown, a complex microbiota is established, closely resembling that found in adult periodontitis [4]. When peri-implant tissue breakdown is induced by placing plaque-retentive ligatures submarginally in animals, a shift in the microflora occurs [36,37].

Rosenberg et al [38] divided patients with failing implants into two groups: suspected infection and trauma (overload). In the trauma group, patients had no pain or suppuration and the failed implants had a microbiologic profile similar to that found at healthy implant sites. In the infected group, however, implants were colonized by microbiota similar to that found in periodontitis.

Most information on the histopathologic features of peri-implantitis lesions has been obtained from experimental studies in dogs and monkeys [39–42]. In the experimental models used, plaque formation was allowed and ligatures were placed in a submarginal position around the neck of implants. The ligatures were removed when the ensuing inflammatory response in the peri-implant tissues had mediated advanced bone destruction. Histologic analysis of the biopsy material revealed the presence of large inflammatory lesions in the peri-implant mucosa and that these lesions extended to the alveolar bone. Lindhe et al [39] suggested that peri-implant tissues, in contrast to periodontal tissues, have a limited capacity to resolve progressive, plaque-associated lesions. Few reports exist on peri-implant tissues at failed implant sites in humans. Although some documentation reveals the presence of inflammatory lesions in the peri-implant mucosa [43,44], other reports claim that inflammatory cell infiltrates were virtually absent [45]. In a recent study on the histopathologic features of human peri-implantitis [46], it was reported that harvested soft tissue specimens harbored large inflammatory cell infiltrates that extended to a position apical of a pocket epithelium. Furthermore, about 60% of the lesions were occupied by inflammatory cells, among which plasma cells dominated. The investigators also reported that there were numerous polymorphonuclear cells in the connective tissue areas adjacent to the pocket epithelium and in the perivascular compartments in more central areas of the inflammatory cell infiltrate. Similar observations were made in a study on the immunohistochemical characteristics of human peri-implantitis lesions [47]. This study reported that peri-implantitis lesions consistently exhibited elastase-positive cells (ie, polymorphonuclear cells) in the central portions of the infiltrate. The findings concerning polymorpho-nuclear cells in human peri-implantitis lesions are also consistent with results from studies on crevicular fluid at implants with peri-implantitis [8,48].

Smoking

Several epidemiologic studies have shown the negative influence of smoking on periodontal status [49]. Its role as a risk factor for periodontal disease progression has recently been confirmed [50], and current data suggest that smokers have at least a threefold increased risk of developing periodontitis [51].

The possible relationship between smoking and implant failures has been evaluated in several retrospective and prospective clinical studies [52]. In a retrospective analysis of the outcome of 2194 implants placed in 540 subjects, Bain and Moy [53] reported that a significantly greater percentage of implant failures occurred in smokers than in nonsmokers. Smokers had an overall failure rate of 11.3%, whereas only 4.8% of the implants placed in nonsmokers failed. Gorman et al [54] found that implant failures were twice as common in smokers as in nonsmokers at second-stage surgery. In general, it can be concluded that smoking has a negative effect on implant survival, especially during the early healing period after implant installation.

The effect of smoking on marginal bone loss has also been evaluated. Cigarette smoking was associated with significantly greater marginal bone loss at implants used in the treatment of edentulous mandibles [55]. The 10- and 15-year follow-up reports on this group of edentulous patients showed that bone loss, although limited, was related to several factors, among which smoking and oral hygiene were the most important.

Haas et al [56] compared the association between smoking and peri-implantitis in 107 smokers compared with 314 nonsmokers. Smokers had higher bleeding scores, more signs of clinical inflammation, deeper probing pocket depth, and more radiographic bone loss around implants than nonsmokers. The investigators further stated that the effect of smoking on the condition of peri-implant tissues was more pronounced in the maxilla than in the mandible.

Clinical appearance of peri-implantitis

Peri-implantitis lesions are often asymptomatic and usually detected at routine recall appointments. Careful probing around teeth and implants should be routine procedures included at these check-up appointments. The validity of probing around implants to properly detect peri-implant lesions has previously been questioned, although this dogma needs to be reassessed. Increased clinical probing pocket depth, often accompanied by bleeding and sometimes suppuration, is an indicator of pathology in peri-implant tissues. A common clinical problem regarding probing at implants is accessibility (ie, the design of the bridgework may interfere with the probing procedure). In this context, it is important to realize that peri-implant defects normally encompass the full circumference of the implant; therefore, it may be sufficient to probe only solitary sites at any given implant when there is obstruction by the prostheses. Based on the findings of the clinical examination, radiographs of the selected areas may be proposed. In peri-implantitis, a bony defect develops around single or multiple implants. The radiographic appearance is often in the shape of a saucer or rounded beaker and, as stated earlier, the lesion most often extends the full circumference of the implant.

Peri-implant lesions may develop after several years. In biomedicine, a "safety zone" of 5 years has often been misinterpreted to denote safe survival or no further risk for disease progression. In periodontitis, tissue destruction seems to be a relatively slow process; consequently, a function time exceeding 5 years for implants may be required to detect destructive peri-implantitis sites. Regular check-up visits and life-long supportive therapy is an absolute necessity for the implant patient.

Treatment of peri-implantitis

According to the best available evidence, traditional periodontal infection control including plaque control regimens and mechanical instrumentation of the affected areas possessing surgical flap access should be performed. It is essential to inform the patient about the need for effective oral hygiene procedures (particularly around implants), and the patient should be carefully instructed in the proper use of necessary additional oral hygiene aids. Oral hygiene procedures should be trained under professional supervision (Figs. 3–8).

A systematic review of the studies done on anti-infective therapy for the treatment of peri-implantitis reported that many different treatment regimens were used [57,58]. Type of antibiotic, dosage, duration, and time for initiation of antibiotic treatment were different for all studies. Leonhardt et al [59] reported 5-year outcomes following the treatment of peri-implantitis in humans. Implants that demonstrated marginal bone loss (>3 threads compared with baseline measurements at 1 year on intraoral radiographs), bleeding on probing, and suppuration from the sulci were

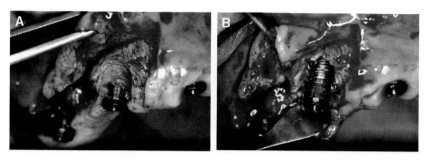

Fig. 3. (*A*) Peri-implant lesion in the anterior maxillary region. A surgical procedure with a full-thickness flap was performed to expose the affected area. (*B*) Mechanical instrumentation was performed to remove inflamed tissues (similar to conventional periodontal surgery). Implant surface was cleaned using EDTA solution.

included. Subgingival bacterial samples were collected for each individual and cultured. Surgical exposure of the lesions was performed, and the affected implants were cleaned using hydrogen peroxide. Systemic antibiotics were administered according to a susceptibility test of target bacteria. The applied surgical and antimicrobial treatment strategy was successful in less than 60% of the treated implants during the 5-year follow-up. Despite treatment and re-treatment of peri-implantitis–affected areas, additional loss of supporting bone was found in up to 40% of the advanced peri-implant lesions.

New data support the need for treatment of peri-implant lesions. Spontaneous progression of experimentally induced peri-implantitis was reported by Zitzmann el al [60]. Additional bone loss occurred in most of the implant sites following ligature removal in this experimental model. The reason why some peri-implantitis lesions were associated with extensive bone loss and others with only minor bone loss is currently not understood. Differences between implant sites regarding the subgingival biofilm or the

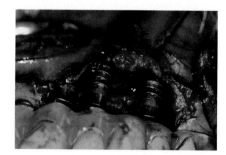

Fig. 4. Peri-implant lesion in the anterior maxillary region 4 years after implant surgery. Inflamed tissue has been removed.

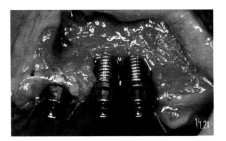

Fig. 5. Peri-implant lesion in the anterior maxillary region 3 years after implant surgery. The area has been instrumented and inflamed tissue removed. Note the circumferential appearance of the bone destruction.

quality of the inflammatory response to the infection may be factors of importance.

In a prospective, randomized controlled clinical trial, Wennström et al [33] studied the outcome of restorative therapy in periodontitis-susceptible patients who, following basic periodontal therapy, had been restored with

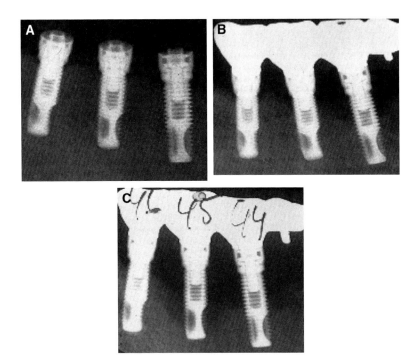

Fig. 6. (A) Implants inserted in the lower right mandible. (B) In the same patient 9 months later, an early peri-implant lesion can be detected around the right implant. (C) In the same patient an additional 22 months later, severe peri-implant tissue destruction can be seen, especially around the middle and right implants.

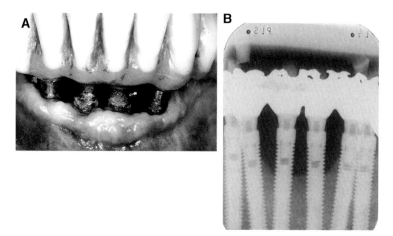

Fig. 7. (*A*) Patient has neglected oral hygiene at anterior mandibular implants for 5 years. (*B*) Radiograph of the anterior region in the same patient.

implants. The amount of peri-implant bone loss that occurred during a 5-year observation period was small in general but more pronounced in the maxilla than in the mandible. A further analysis also revealed that the amount of bone loss that occurred in smokers during the 5-year interval was more pronounced than the corresponding change in nonsmokers.

This finding is also interesting in the light of a recent observation by Airila-Månsson et al [61]. In their study on periodontitis subjects over a 17-year period, it was found that marginal bone loss was most severe in the maxillary molar region. In addition, smokers in this study showed more severe marginal bone loss over time.

Thresholds for peri-implantitis and standardized internationally accepted criteria for the definition of success are lacking. Relying on purely clinical

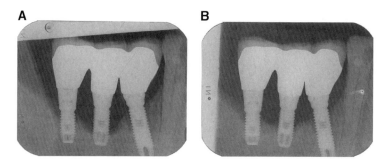

Fig. 8. (*A*) Peri-implant lesion in lower right mandibular region 5 years following placement of implants. Surgical infection control procedures were performed, including flap procedure, mechanical implant instrumentation, and postoperative antibiotics. (*B*) Radiograph of ongoing bone healing 5 months after surgical intervention.

parameters instead of combining clinical and radiographic assessments may over-rate the success [62]. To arrive at an agreement on how to evaluate the outcome of implant treatment in longitudinal studies, complications such as peri-implantitis should always be reported.

Summary

Peri-implant lesions may develop after several years. Patients who have lost their teeth due to periodontal disease seem to be at greater risk. Although several anti-infective treatment strategies have demonstrated beneficial clinical effects in humans (eg, resolution of inflammation, decrease in probing depth, and gain of bone in the defects), there is insufficient evidence to support a specific treatment protocol. Available studies on the treatment of peri-implantitis have included only a small number of subjects, and in general, the study periods have been relatively short. To date, there is no reliable evidence that suggests which interventions could be the most effective for treating peri-implantitis [3,57,58]. This is not to say, however, that currently used interventions are not effective.

References

[1] Karoussis IK, Salvi GE, Heitz-Mayfield LJA, et al. Long-term implant prognosis in patients with and without a history of chronic periodontitis: a 10 year prospective cohort study of the ITI dental implant system. Clin Oral Impl Res 2003;14:129–39.

[2] Hultin M, Factors affecting peri-implant tissue reactions [thesis]. Stockholm (Sweden): Karolinska Institutet; 2001. Available at: http://diss.kib.ki.se/2001/91-628-4761-9.

[3] Esposito M, Wothington HV, Coulthard P. Interventions for replacing missing teeth: treatment of periimplantitis. Cochrane Database Syst Rev 2004;4 CD004970.

[4] Mombelli A, van Oosten MA, Schurch E Jr, et al. The microbiota associated with successful or failing osseointegrated titanium implants. Oral Microbiol Immunol 1987;2:145–51.

[5] Malmström HS, Fritz ME, Timmis DP, et al. Osseo-integrated implant treatment of a patient with rapidly progressive periodontitis. A case report. J Periodontol 1990;61:300–4.

[6] Fardal O, Johannessen AC, Olsen I. Severe, rapidly progressing peri-implantitis. J Clin Periodontol 1999;26:313–7.

[7] Berglundh T, Persson L, Klinge B. A systematic review of the incidence of biological and technical complications in implant dentistry reported in prospective longitudinal studies of at least 5 years. J Clin Periodontol 2002;29(Suppl 3):197–212.

[8] Hultin M, Gustafsson A, Hallström H, et al. Microbiological findings and host response in patients with peri-implantitis. Clin Oral Impl Res 2002;13:349–58.

[9] Albrektsson T, Isidor F. Concensus report of session IV. In: Lang NP, Karring T, editors. Proceedings of the 1st European Workshop on Periodontology. London: Quintessence Publishing; 1994. p. 365–9.

[10] Sumida S, Ishihara K, Kishi M, et al. Transmission of periodontal disease–associated bacteria from teeth to osseointegrated implant regions. Int J Oral Maxillofac Implants 2002; 17:696–702.

[11] van Steenberghe D, Klinge B, Lindén U, et al. Periodontal indices around natural and titanium abutments: a longitudinal multicenter study. J Periodontol 1993;64:538–41.

[12] Hardt CRE, Gröndahl K, Lekholm U, et al. Outcome of implant therapy in relation to experienced loss of periodontal bone support. ClinOral Impl Res 2003;13:488–94.

[13] Berglundh T, Lindhe J. Dimension of the periimplant mucosa. Biological width revisited. J Clin Periodontol 1996;23:971–3.

[14] Berglundh T, Lindhe J, Jonsson K, et al. The topography of the vascular systems in the periodontal and peri-implant tissues in the dog. J Clin Periodontol 1994;21:189–93.

[15] Berglundh T, Lindhe J, Marinello C, et al. Soft tissue reaction to de novo plaque formation on implants and teeth. An experimental study in the dog. Clin Oral Implants Res 1992;3:1–8.

[16] Zitzmann NU, Berglundh T, Marinello C, et al. Experimental peri-implant mucositis in man. J Clin Periodontol 2001;28:517–23.

[17] Liljenberg B, Gualini F, Berglundh T, et al. Composition of plaque-associated lesions in the gingiva and the peri-implant mucosa in partially edentulous subjects. J Clin Periodontol 1997;24:119–23.

[18] Hugoson A, Norderyd O, Slotte C, et al. Distribution of periodontal disease in a Swedish adult population 1973, 1983 and 1993. J Clin Periodontol 1998;25:542–8.

[19] Leonhardt A, Adolfsson B, Lekholm U, et al. A longitudinal microbiological study on osseointegrated titanium implants in partially edentulous patients. Clin Oral Implants Res 1993;4:113–20.

[20] Mombelli A, Marxer M, Gaberthuel T, et al. The microbiota of osseointegrated implants in patients with a history of periodontal disease. J Clin Periodontol 1995;22:124–30.

[21] Quirynen M, Listgarten M. The distribution of bacterial morphotypes around natural teeth and titanium implants ad modum Brånemark. Clin Oral Implants Res 1990;1:8–13.

[22] Papaioannou W, Quirynen M, Van Steenberghe D. The influence of periodontitis on the subgingival flora around implants in partially edentulous patients. Clin Oral Implants Res 1996;7:405–9.

[23] van Winkelhoff AJ, Goene RJ, Folmer T. Early colonization of dental implants by putative periodontal pathogens in partially edentulous patients. Clin Oral Implants Res 2000;11:511–20.

[24] Danser MM, van Winkelhoff AJ, de Graaff J, et al. Putative periodontal pathogens colonizing oral mucous membranes in denture-wearing subjects with a past history of periodontitis. J Clin Periodontol 1995;22:854–9.

[25] Danser MM, van Winkelhoff AJ, van der Velden U. Periodontal bacteria colonizing oral mucous membranes in edentulous patients wearing dental implants. J Periodontol 1997;68:209–16.

[26] Tanner A, Maiden MF, Lee K, et al. Dental implant infections. Clin Infect Dis 1997;25(Suppl 2):S213–7.

[27] Slots J, Rams TE. New views on periodontal microbiota in special patient categories. J Clin Periodontol 1991;18:411–20.

[28] Leonhardt Å, Renvert S, Dahlén G. Microbial findings at failing implants. Clin Oral Implants Res 1999;10:339–45.

[29] Sbordone L, Barone A, Ciaglia RN, et al. Longitudinal study of dental implants in a periodontally compromised population. J Periodontol 1999;70:1322–9.

[30] Lindhe J, Rylander H. Experimental gingivitis in young dogs. Scand J Dent Res 1975;83:314–26.

[31] Weyant RJ, Burt BA. An assessment of survival rates and within-patient clustering of failures for endosseous oral implants. J Dent Res 1993;72:2–8.

[32] Ellegaard B, Baelum V, Karring T. Implant therapy in periodontally compromised patients. Clin Oral Implants Res 1997;8:180–8.

[33] Wennström JL, Ekestubbe A, Gröndahl K, et al. Oral rehabilitation with implant-supported fixed partial dentures in periodontitis-susceptible subjects. J Clin Periodontol 2004;31:713–24.

[34] Tonetti M. Peri-implantitis: biological considerations. J Parodontol Implantol Orale 1996;15:284–96.

[35] Pontoriero R, Tonelli MP, Carnevale G, et al. Experimentally induced peri-implant mucositis. A clinical study in humans. Clin Oral Implants Res 1994;5:254–9.

[36] Leonhardt Å, Berglundh T, Ericsson I, et al. Putative periodontal pathogens on titanium implants and teeth in experimental gingivitis and periodontitis in beagle dogs. Clin Oral Implants Res 1992;3:112–9.

[37] Lang NP, Brägger U, Walther D, et al. Ligature-induced peri-implant infection in cynomolgus monkeys. I. Clinical and radiographic findings. Clin Oral Implants Res 1993;4: 2–11.

[38] Rosenberg ES, Torosian JP, Slots J. Microbial differences in 2 clinically distinct types of failures of osseointegrated implants. Clin Oral Implants Res 1991;2:135–44.

[39] Lindhe J, Berglundh T, Ericsson I, et al. Experimental breakdown of peri-implant and periodontal tissues. A study in the beagle dog. Clin Oral Implants Res 1992;3:9–16.

[40] Lang NP, Brägger U, Walther D, et al. Ligature-induced peri-implant infection in cynomolgus monkeys. I. Clinical and radiographic findings. Clin Oral Implants Res 1993;4: 2–11.

[41] Schou S, Holmstrup P, Stoltze K, et al. Ligature-induced marginal inflammation around osseointegrated implants and ankylosed teeth. Clin Oral Implants Res 1993;4: 12–22.

[42] Marinello CP, Berglundh T, Ericsson I, et al. Resolution of ligature-induced peri-implantitis lesions in the dog. J Clin Periodontol 1995;22:475–9.

[43] Sanz M, Alandez J, Lazaro P, et al. Histo-pathologic characteristics of peri-implant soft tissues in Branemark implants with 2 distinct clinical and radiological patterns. Clin Oral Implants Res 1991;2:128–34.

[44] Piattelli A, Scarano A, Piattelli M. Histologic observations on 230 retrived dental implants: 8 years experience (1989–1996). J Periodontol 1998;69:178–84.

[45] Esposito M, Thomsen P, Ericson L, et al. Histopathologic observations on late oral implant failures. Clin Implant Dent Relat Res 2000;2:18–32.

[46] Berglundh T, Gislason O, Lekholm U, et al. Histopathological observations of human periimplant lesions. J Clin Periodontol 2004;31:341–7.

[47] Gualini F, Berglundh T. Immunohistochemical characteristics of inflammatory lesions at implants. J Clin Periodontol 2003;30:14–8.

[48] Plagnat D, Giannopoulou C, Carrel A, et al. Elastase, α-2-macroglobulin and alkaline phosphatase in crevicular fluid from implants with and without periimplantitis. Clin Oral Implants Res 2002;13:227–33.

[49] Bergström J, Eliasson S, Preber H. Cigarette smoking and periodontal bone loss. J Periodontol 1991;62:242–6.

[50] Norderyd O, Hugoson A, Grusovin G. Risk of severe periodontal disease in a Swedish adult population. A longitudinal study. J Clin Periodontol 1999;26:608–15.

[51] Papapanou PN. Periodontal diseases: epidemiology. Ann Periodontol 1996;1:1–36.

[52] De Bruyn H, Collaert B. The effect of smoking on early implant failure. Clin Oral Implants Res 1994;5:260–4.

[53] Bain CA, Moy PK. The association between the failure of dental implants and cigarette smoking. Int J Oral Maxillofac Implants 1993;8:609–15.

[54] Gorman LM, Lambert PM, Morris HF, et al. The effect of smoking on implant survival at second-stage surgery: DICRG Interim Report No. 5. Dental Implant Clinical Research Group. Implant Dent 1994;3:165–8.

[55] Carlsson GE, Lindquist L, Jemt T. Long-term marginal periimplant bone loss in edentulous patients. Int J Prosthodontics 2000;13:295–302.

[56] Haas R, Haimbock W, Mailath G, et al. The relationship of smoking on peri-implant tissue: a retrospective study. J Prosthet Dent 1996;76:592–6.

[57] Klinge B, Gustafsson A, Berglundh T. A systematic review of the effect of anti-infective therapy in the treatment of peri-implantitis. J Clin Periodontol 2002; 29(Suppl 3):213–25.

[58] Roos-Jansåker A-M, Renvert S, Egelberg J. Treatment of peri-implant infections: a literature review. J Clin Periodontol 2003;30:467–85.
[59] Leonhardt Å, Dahlén G, Renvert S. Five-year clinical, microbiological, and radiological outcome following treatment of peri-implantitis in man. J Periodontol 2003;74:1415–22.
[60] Zitzmann NU, Berglundh T, Ericsson I, et al. Spontaneous progression of experimentally induced periimplantitis. J Clin Periodontol 2004;31:845–9.
[61] Airila-Månsson S, Söder B, Klinge B. Bone height changes in individuals with periodontal disease—a 17-year prospective longitudinal study. J Clin Periodontol, in press.
[62] Karoussis IK, Müller S, Salvi GE, et al. Association between periodontal and peri-implant conditions: a 10 year prospective study. Clin Oral Impl Res 2004;15:1–7.

ELSEVIER
SAUNDERS

Dent Clin N Am 49 (2005) 677–694

THE DENTAL
CLINICS
OF NORTH AMERICA

Future Treatment and Diagnostic Strategies for Periodontal Diseases

Howard C. Tenenbaum, DDS, PhD, FRCD(C)[a],
Henri Tenenbaum, DDS, PhD, HDR(F)[b],
Ron Zohar, DDS, PhD, FRCD(C)[c],*

[a]Discipline of Periodontology, Faculty of Dentistry, University of Toronto, 124 Edward Street,
Suite 349C, Toronto, Ontario, Canada M5G 1G6
[b]Department of Periodontology, Dental Faculty, University Louis Pasteur, Strasbourg, France
[c]Disciplines of Periodontology and Biomaterials, Faculty of Dentistry, University of Toronto,
124 Edward Street, Suite 464A, Toronto, Ontario, Canada M5G 1G6

Treatment of periodontal diseases has undergone a series of changes—perhaps not quite a revolution—over the past 20 years [1–6]. The goal of treatment has always been to regenerate lost periodontal tissues, but clinicians have had to "settle" for treatments that lead to disease cessation and healing if not outright regeneration. That said, there are newer treatment strategies that may become available over time that will allow clinicians to achieve limited or more robust regeneration of the periodontium. Because of the absence of reliable methods for regeneration, new approaches to disease control are also being pursued that will benefit those suffering chronic periodontal diseases [7,8]. In addition to novel therapeutics, there has been increasing focus on the development of more sensitive and specific diagnostic tests for periodontal diseases [9–11]. It is hoped that such tests will allow the clinician to determine whether a patient has active disease and what sort of attachment loss might be expected if the patient were not treated. In addition, by developing newer diagnostic tests, it will also be possible to focus therapy more on the disease process. Using collagenase levels as an example, if a diagnostic test shows this to be elevated [9], in addition to treating the microbial trigger, one might also attempt to regulate (reduce) collagenase levels or activity to prevent further tissue degradation.

* Corresponding author.
E-mail address: ron.zohar@utoronto.ca (R. Zohar).

Periodontal disease diagnosis

Periodontal diseases are probably one of the most common bacterial infections in humans. It has become evident that only a few of the several hundred species of microorganisms within the gingival crevice and the periodontal pocket play a significant role in initiation and progression of the disease [10,12]. Thus, such pathogens at low levels should be considered as part of the normal oral flora. The notion of a "critical mass" of these periodontal pathogens has recently been introduced because of their presence in healthy gingival sites, albeit in low numbers [13]. The inflammatory and degradative processes associated with chronic periodontitis are likely induced by a critical mass of different pathogens, thereby leading to tissue destruction, possibly by way of three different pathways:

1. Pathogens may directly release proteolytic enzymes that degrade periodontal structures without the intervention of host cells.
2. Pathogens may elaborate products such as toxins, enzymes, and lipopolysaccharide that may trigger host cell populations to express degradative enzymes.
3. Pathogens may stimulate an immune response resulting in release of proinflammatory cytokines such as interleukin (IL)-1, IL-6, and tumor necrosis factor α [14].

The components of the periodontal tissue extracellular matrix, especially collagens, appear to be the main target of degradation in periodontal diseases. Among host proteases degrading the extracellular matrix, matrix metalloproteinases (MMPs) seem to be highly associated with tissue destruction and remodeling events in periodontal diseases.

Regarding the balance between pathogens and host responses, reliable diagnostic tests should focus on three main objectives:

1. Determine the presence and the proportions of pathogens in diseased sites or in susceptible patients.
2. Identify factors that indicate the first steps of disease activity in apparently healthy sites that may appear clinically normal.
3. Detect patients in whom the host response is unable to balance pathogen aggressiveness or diagnose the degree of genetic predisposition at an early age when periodontal destruction has not yet developed.

To achieve these goals, microbiologic testing, analysis of disease activity, and genetic analyses have been proposed to identify patients at increased risk for periodontal disease [15].

Microbiologic testing

Periodontal diseases are considered a mixed infection. It has never been possible to prove that specific bacteria directly cause periodontal disease according to Koch's postulates. In consequence, the ideal that a single causative agent of the disease would be identified and a rapid chairside test would be used to assess the bacterial risk has never been reached.

To be considered true periodontal pathogens, bacteria should fulfill the following criteria [16]:

- They must occur at higher numbers in disease-active lesions compared with healthy or disease-inactive sites.
- Their elimination should lead to arrest of disease progression.
- They should express virulence factors relevant to the disease process.
- They should evoke a specific immune host response.
- They should be able to induce similar periodontal destruction in relevant animal models.

Several types of microbiologic tests have been developed and are available on the market.

First, it must be noted that the information generated by microbiologic analysis of a sample collected from a periodontal pocket is highly dependent on sampling technique. Two methods can be used to collect subgingival plaque samples: curettes and paper points. Both methods require careful removal of supragingival plaque to avoid contamination.

It has been shown that it is possible to remove 60% to 90% of the bacteria populating a diseased pocket with the use of a curette, whereas only about 6% to 41% of bacteria are sampled with the use of a paper point [17,18]. Moreover, with the latter method, it has been suggested that most of the sampled bacterial mass is from the outer layers of the subgingival biofilm; however, the inner layers may contain the more-pathogenic species [19].

The following microbiologic tests have been proposed:

Microscopic identification

This method is limited to the determination of the relative proportion of coccal and the more-pathogenic, filamentous-shaped bacteria [20]. This technique cannot be used to help in selection of an antimicrobial therapeutic agent if desired or to predict recurrence of the disease. In fact, bacteria thought to be periodontal pathogens cannot be identified or distinguished by microscopic assessment alone. The monitoring of plaque maturation does not give value over conventional clinical evaluation for the assessment of therapeutic efficacy; hence, as a chairside diagnostic system, the cost-to-benefit ratio is essentially negative.

Cultures

Bacterial culture is still considered the "gold standard" against which other microbiologic identification methods must be compared. It is a quantitative method and most cultivable microorganisms can be identified.

Nevertheless, the technique has limitations such as (1) the inability to detect noncultivable organisms such as spirochetes; (2) high cost; (3) the short time required for transportation to the culture laboratory before cells die and cannot be cultured (24–48 hours); and (4) a prolonged period before results are obtained.

Enzymatic assays

Although enzymatic assays permit detection of bacteria that possess trypsinlike enzymes, other pathogenic bacteria that do not produce such enzymes are not detected. Two tests have been developed: the BANA test (PerioScan; Oral B, Redwood, California) [21] and the PerioCheck test (Sunstar, Osaka, Japan) [22].

Both of these tests can be done at chairside and are interpreted or rated by the use of color intensity scores. For the BANA test, trypsinlike enzymes from *Tannerella forsythensis*, *Treponema denticola*, and *Porphyromonas gingivalis* hydrolyze the substrate *N*-benzoyl-DL-arginine-2-naphthylamide, thereby producing a blue-black color, the intensity of which is proportional to the total amount of the three bacteria [23,24].

The PerioCheck test differs from the BANA test in that a different substrate is used. Neither test can be used to distinguish between the relative proportions of the three bacteria and, of course, cannot identify the presence of other potential pathogens that do not produce trypsinlike enzymes.

Given these issues, their utility in diagnosis is limited due to a low reliability to predict clinical disease progression [22].

Immunoassays

Detection of immunoglobulin against bacterial antigens present in serum by the use of immunoassays (ELISA, agglutination assays, immunofluorescence) requires the development of polyclonal or monoclonal antibodies that recognize specific lymphocyte epitopes [25–28].

The advantages of immunoassays are (1) the detection of specific virulence factors of given bacteria; (2) the investigation of the specific role of protein (eg, cytolethal distending toxin CdT from *Actinobacillus actinomycetemcomitans*); and (3) their low cost for large-scale studies.

It is unfortunate that there are also the following disadvantages: (1) local sampling cannot be done, so site-specific disease parameters cannot be assessed; and (2) immunoassays cannot be used to determine bacterial virulence.

Nucleic acid probes

DNA extracts from samples of pocket-derived bacteria can be hybridized with so-called "anti-sense DNA probes" [29]. When these probes are also labeled with an enzyme such as alkaline phosphatase, they can be detected using enzyme-staining assays, thus indicating the presence of DNA from specific bacteria. The probe sequences may be derived from (1) whole genomic DNA; (2) randomly cloned sequences of nucleic acids from target bacteria (greater risk of false-positive reactions than whole genomic probes); and (3) synthetic oligonucleotides that hybridize to 16S ribosomal RNA-DNA sequences that contain highly conserved and extreme heterogeneous sequences that make them ideal for distinction of species [30].

Nucleic acid probes have other interesting advantages including easy sampling and transport (viability of bacteria is not a requirement), rapid analysis, high sensitivity and specificity, and the ability to detect a wide spectrum of bacterial species including the detection of noncultivable organisms. Despite these strengths, currently available molecular techniques cannot be used to assess antibiotic sensitivity or bacterial virulence. To address this problem, however, a variation of standard molecular identification was suggested in 1994 by Socransky et al [31] who described "Checkerboard" DNA-DNA hybridization analysis that may permit some inferences as to pathogenicity.

Polymerase chain reaction

Polymerase chain reaction is a molecular biologic method that allows for high-yield replication of DNA. Therefore, it allows for the synthesis of a vast number of copies of even the smallest samples of bacterial DNA [32]. A modification of the original polymerase chain reaction method, real-time polymerase chain reaction, permits not only detection of specific bacteria but also quantification. Polymerase chain reaction is generally considered reliable when used in combination with synthetic 16S ribosomal RNA probes, which are highly specific to given species.

Biosensors

Metabolites (eg, volatile sulfur compounds) from pathogenic bacteria can be detected by various physical methods [33,34]. Various pathogenic bacteria (*Treponema denticola, Porphyromonas gingivalis, Prevotella intermedia*, and *Tannerella forsythis*) can reduce sulphates, thereby producing significant levels S, HS, H_2S, and CH_3SH by degradation of serum proteins, cysteine, and methionine. A sulfide sensor, Perio 2000 (Diamond General Corp., Ann Arbor, Michigan) can measure levels of these compounds and report them as scores ranging from 0 to 5 in increments of 0.5. A score of 0 represents undetectable S ($<10^{-7}$ M sulfide), whereas a score of 5 represents a concentration of 10^{-2} M sulfide. This chairside technique can be used repeatedly on the same sites and produces results rapidly. This test, however, is nonspecific and only semiquantitative, and its usefulness is limited by the fact that not all pathogenic bacteria produce sulfides. Because the detectable species are highly pathogenic, however, the detection of high sulfide levels could indicate that this site is at higher risk of disease activity

and attendant attachment loss [34]. This indication could lead to earlier treatment and prevention of tissue loss. Furthermore, although it is
conceivable that sulfide levels could be used to assess efficacy of treatment,
this methodology still needs to be validated by clinical trials.

Currently, no single diagnostic approach can be used to provide enough
information for the clinician to make a diagnosis that would necessarily be
different from one derived from clinical assessment. Similarly, treatment
decisions, apart from the need for adjunctive antibacterial therapy or
perhaps MMP regulation (see later discussion), are not necessarily
influenced by currently available testing methods. In this regard, the
following questions remain unanswered:

1. Was a specific bacterial species present when the disease was initiated (is
   there a causal relationship)?
2. Were the bacteria present at the site after the disease occurred (is there
   an opportunistic relationship)?

Perhaps in the future, more attention should be paid to identification of
common virulence factors (especially pathogen-associated molecular patterns) and how these virulence factors regulate the responses of different
host cells like keratinocytes, Langerhans cells, dendritic cells, and macrophages [16].

Analysis of disease activity

Salivary and gingival crevicular fluid enzymes and other proteins have the
potential to be useful markers of disease progression. Presently, more than
65 gingival crevicular fluid components have been examined and identified
as potential markers of disease progression. These components fall into
three general categories:

1. Host-derived enzymes such as MMPs and their inhibitors
2. Inflammatory mediators and host response modifiers such as cytokines
3. Tissue breakdown products such as glycosaminoglycans, osteonectin,
   osteopontin, and laminin

A major problem with measurement of enzymes is that it is often difficult
to distinguish those associated with gingivitis and periodontitis sites from
active and inactive disease sites. Enzymes like the collagenases (MMP-1,
MMP-3, MMP-8, and MMP-13), elastase, and gelatinases (MMP-2 and
MMP-9) may be significantly elevated in the presence of existing disease, but
measurement of their levels to predict future destruction remains unclear
(such as the test for aspartate aminotransferase [AST]) [35,36]. Hence,
virtually all enzyme tests evaluated to date have demonstrated fairly high
rates of false-positive findings (ie, although a test is "positive," there may
still not be any disease activity and therefore no disease progression). The
same can be said about assays for inflammatory mediators.

The most promising gingival crevicular fluid markers of disease progression are probably host breakdown products (as opposed to the enzymes that breakdown host tissues). Among these products, chondroitin-4-sulfate (a cartilage- and bone-specific glycosaminoglycan) [37,38], pyridinoline cross-links of the carboxyterminal telopeptide of type I collagen, and RankL (receptor activator for NF-xB ligand) are potential markers of bone and connective tissue destruction [39,40].

Genetic analyses

The etiology of periodontal disease is multifactorial and thus influenced by genetics (ie, the host) and the environment [41]. With regard to genetics, studies have revealed that most forms of periodontal disease are likely associated with multiple modifying genes (the disease is said to be polygenic). For example, in Papillon-Lefèvre syndrome and in generalized forms of prepubertal periodontitis, Hart et al [42] identified and localized a modified gene on chromosome 11 that caused a decrease in cathepsin C activity. The same decrease in cathepsin C activity has been demonstrated in severe chronic periodontitis [43]. Other studies have focused on IL-1 gene polymorphism leading to the development of the periodontitis susceptibility trait test [44]. The periodontitis susceptibility trait test is the only genetic susceptibility test for severe periodontitis that is commercially available. The periodontitis susceptibility trait test evaluates the simultaneous occurrence of allele 2 at the IL-1A +4845 and IL-1B +3954 loci. A patient with allele 2 at both these loci is considered genotype positive and therefore more susceptible to develop severe periodontitis.

Although genetic tests might be used to identify a predisposition to disease (even before disease development) [45], treatment approaches and outcomes will still be influenced by environmental and behavioral factors whether or not the individual is genetically susceptible to periodontal disease. Moreover, genetic testing gives no information on disease activity or susceptibility.

Although great strides are being made with respect to the development of diagnostic tests, there remains a great need for well-designed long-term longitudinal investigations and controlled clinical treatment studies.

Periodontal diseases—novel therapeutics

Regenerative treatment

From a historical perspective, regeneration of periodontal tissues lost as a result of periodontitis has been an elusive goal despite the development of widely available regenerative surgical techniques. Such approaches have involved the use of bone grafts to replace lost bone; however, bone is but one component of the connective tissues composing the periodontium. Inasmuch as bone loss has been considered one of the major sequelae of periodontitis and is the most striking radiographic feature of periodontally diseased tissues, the use of bone grafting treatments has been popular. Critical analyses of clinical, histologic, and radiographic data, however, suggest that although correction of bone defects can be demonstrated [46,47], the regeneration of a new attachment apparatus following bone grafting including new bone, cementum, and a functionally oriented periodontal ligament does not generally occur except at the very base of the periodontal defect. Because bone grafting has been shown to have limited effectiveness with respect to regeneration of lost periodontium, other approaches have been developed that ostensibly would exploit the biologic principles that describe cellular domains [48]. If specific cell types occupy specific domains to the exclusion of other cell types, then the creation of an environment that would preferentially select for cells that might regenerate the periodontal ligament would provide for reliable regenerative treatment outcomes. To accomplish this, investigators have developed an array of membrane technologies. These treatments require the insertion of a membrane over a periodontal defect to, in effect, "exclude" epithelial cells from the previously diseased root surface, thereby permitting upward migration of periodontal ligament cells or their precursors. A variety of membrane materials has been developed, including some that had to be removed from the surgically treated site weeks or months later and some that were resorbable and could be left in place. Initial reports regarding the use of these membranes (a technique called guided tissue regeneration) were positive, but over the longer-term, it became apparent that apart from the use of guided tissue regeneration to regenerate bone (called guided bone regeneration) about implants or in other osseous sites requiring augmentation, periodontal regeneration could still not be expected to occur reliably [47] (Zohar and Tenenbaum, submitted for publication, 2005).

Enamel matrix derivatives

Taking advantage of developmental biologic studies of the periodontal attachment apparatus, it was noted that before development of cementum and new periodontal ligament, enamel matrix proteins are deposited directly onto dentine surfaces [49,50]. This observation led investigators to hypothesize that enamel matrix proteins might play an important role in the signaling for and recruitment of cells required for production of a normal tooth attachment apparatus. This observation further led to the notion that if such proteins could be purified or otherwise harvested, then they might prove useful in regenerative therapy. In this regard, it was thought that by adding such proteins to a previously diseased or exposed tooth root surface, they might signal a recapitulation of the embryologic developmental sequence, leading to the creation of a new gomphosis. As a result, there is now a growing body of evidence based on randomized controlled trials [4,51] that enamel matrix proteins can be used for limited regeneration of the periodontium. In addition, further studies have demonstrated that these proteins may prove useful in periodontal plastics and root coverage procedures, thereby reducing or eliminating the need for the harvesting of connective tissue [51,52]. As the mechanisms underlying enamel matrix derivative effects are understood more precisely, it is likely that other related extracts or even purified proteins will become a part of the routine armamentarium of periodontists in the future when regenerative therapy is required.

Bisphosphonates to inhibit bone loss

The bisphosphonates are a class of drugs related to pyrophosphate [53]. Unlike pyrophosphate, which can be degraded by alkaline phosphatase [54] and pyrophosphatase, the bisphosphonates are resistant to degradation and have a high affinity for mineralized tissue [55]. One of the most important uses of bisphosphonates relates to their ability to inhibit bone resorption, presumably by direct or indirect inhibition of osteoclast cell activity [53]. This property could prove useful in the development of future therapeutic approaches to the prevention of periodontal bone loss [53,56] and possibly bone-supported implants [57,58]. In addition, it has been shown that local application of bisphosphonates reduces the bone loss that occurs following periodontal flap surgery [59]. In addition, given their affinity for mineralized tissues such as bone, the bisphosphonates, when tagged with a radionuclide such as technetium 99m, can also be used for diagnostic purposes. In this regard, the bisphosphonates would "home" to areas of bone that are undergoing active remodeling. Hence, the bisphosphonates would target or be concentrated in areas in which periodontal bone loss is about to occur or in other areas with increased remodeling in which bone loss may occur. Radioactively tagged bisphosphonates can be detected using various radiologic imaging methods and can be localized to sites where bone loss may occur. In fact, in using these methods, it is possible to identify sites within the periodontium in which bone loss will occur even before radiographic changes have occurred. Thus, although not discussed in detail previously, it is possible that these drugs could prove useful in the future not only for prevention of bone loss but also (from a diagnostic perspective) to identify areas where bone loss may occur much earlier than might be possible radiographically [60].

Bisphosphonates may stimulate bone formation

In addition to their ability to inhibit bone formation, it is also known that at certain concentrations, bisphosphonates inhibit mineralization [61]. This particular effect was thought to be essentially deleterious, and in fact, second- and third-generation bisphosphonates were developed to increase their ability to inhibit bone resorption so that they could be used in lower doses and not interfere with mineralization [62]. This approach has proved to be effective, particularly for management of osteoporosis [62]; however, recent studies have suggested that inhibition of mineralization might be useful so long as it is a transitory phenomenon. In relation to this, it has been demonstrated that bone matrix (osteoid) formation is inversely proportional to mineralization [63]. When mineralization is inhibited using the first-generation bisphosphonate etidronate (HEBP), osteoid formation has been shown to double in vivo and in vitro [56,61,64]. When the HEBP is continually present, more osteoid forms but is poorly mineralized. Alternatively, when HEBP treatment (in culture or in vivo) is stopped, the newly formed "excess" osteoid mineralizes and, as demonstrated in cell culture, the mineral is even more dense than control. This property of HEBP could be exploited to stimulate new bone formation in the periodontium and elsewhere. It could prove useful for acceleration of osseointegration about implants; however, the dosage regime in this model has not been clearly worked out. HEBP treatment has also been shown to induce the periodontal ligament to produce high levels of the bone protein bone sialoprotein and to induce the ligament to produce bone tissue. Thus, it is possible that judicious local application or systemic administration of HEBP or similar agents could prove useful for regeneration of lost bone in implant or other sites and for the acceleration of endosseous implant integration in the future.

Antimicrobial therapy

Local delivery systems

It has been well established that most forms of periodontitis are related to chronic infection with periodontal pathogens [15] (usually gram-negative anaerobic species [34]). As a result, there has been an extensive amount of investigation related to the development of effective antimicrobial regimes for treatment of chronic, refractory, or other forms or periodontitis. Indeed, double-blind placebo-controlled randomized trials have demonstrated that antimicrobial treatment is an extremely useful adjunct for treatment of periodontitis [10,65]. Before the advent of antimicrobial therapy, so-called "refractory periodontitis" (eg, periodontitis demonstrating a downhill or extreme downhill course [65a]) might constitute about 20% of all cases. This figure, however, is now in the 5% range because it has been shown that the previously difficult-to-treat cases, or cases that do not respond well to conventional periodontal treatments, can be managed or improved with the use of antimicrobials [57,66]. That said, the use of systemic antimicrobial medications to treat a local infection has drawbacks including, for example, gastrointestinal side effects such as pseudomembranous colitis, allergic reaction [67], superinfection with commensal organisms, or development of resistant organisms. Therefore, there have been a number of attempts to develop locally delivered antimicrobials to infected periodontal pockets [57]. The antimicrobials have included metronidazole in an ointment form (Elyzol), chlorohexidine (Periochip), and doxycycline in a fiber form (Actisite) or in a polymeric delivery system (Atridox) [66]. These locally delivered antimicrobials, and in particular Atridox, have been demonstrated to be efficacious in the treatment of localized periodontal pockets. On average, Atridox, for example, seems to be equally as effective as scaling and root planing but is more difficult to administer for generalized disease than for treatment of localized defects. This type of drug delivery system should definitely be considered for treatment of refractory periodontal pockets, infected implant sites, and possibly even in surgical sites. This approach may be particularly useful in the future for treatment of recall patients who present with localized sites showing recurrent disease.

Photodynamic therapy

Although local delivery of an agent such as doxycycline can be useful, the use of self-polymerizing gels can be difficult when considering treatment of generalized periodontitis. Moreover, it has been demonstrated that full-mouth "decontamination" may lead to better short-term and possibly longer-term outcomes when managing periodontal diseases compared with staged decontamination approaches [68]. Agents delivered in gel or fiber form, however, cannot readily be delivered to periodontal pockets within the whole mouth and certainly cannot be used in the eradication of periodontal pathogens from nondental oral surfaces (eg, cheeks, tongue, and tonsil bed in addition to periodontal pockets). In addition, although the antimicrobials mentioned previously are delivered in high concentrations to minimize bacterial resistance, this does not preclude the possibility that resistant bacteria will be selected following treatment.

To address these problems, other approaches for antimicrobial therapy for periodontitis have been investigated, including an approach known as photodynamic therapy. Photodynamic therapy essentially involves the use of light-activated drugs to kill periodontal pathogens. This therapeutic tool was initially investigated for treatment of malignancy because chemotherapeutic drugs could be given to patients systemically in an essentially inert form and then activated by administering light (usually laser) at the site of a tumor, thereby killing tumor cells without making a patient ill from chemotherapy [69]. Photodynamic therapy has also been used successfully for the management of macular degeneration [70]. Recently, it has been demonstrated that toluidine blue, when activated by laser light, can be used to kill periodontal pathogens [71]. Hence, it was postulated that toluidine blue or other photoactivated drugs could be used to treat periodontitis, presumably by laser activating such chemicals after they have been instilled within periodontal pockets. The problem with this approach, however, is that it would be necessary to irradiate every single pocket following lavage with the photoreactive agent, and full-mouth decontamination would be equally as difficult as suggested earlier for locally delivered antimicrobials [72].

Clinical trials focusing on the use of laser-activated drugs are underway for treatment of periodontitis. Future trials will likely take advantage of broad-spectrum light, thereby permitting more effective elimination of periodontal pathogenic bacteria that are resident in the oral cavity as a whole. This approach could lead to more robust treatment responses and would serve as a useful adjunct for management of periodontal infection in conjunction with conventional therapy. This treatment would also prove useful for periodontal maintenance, during periodontal surgery, and in periodontal management of infected endosseous implant surfaces.

Inhibition of matrix degradation

As discussed previously with respect to diagnostic tests, matrix degradation is a major hallmark and even a predictor of bone and periodontal attachment loss. Hence, there have been major efforts devoted to the development of treatment approaches that interfere with or completely block matrix degradation. The bisphosphonates, previously addressed in relation to their ability to inhibit bone resorption, do not inhibit destruction of connective tissue matrices, although the authors' laboratory has some evidence suggesting that HEBP might interfere with MMP activity [72a]. Most investigation in this area has focused on the use of tetracycline and its derivatives for prevention of connective tissue (even hard connective tissue) destruction mediated by MMPs. To this end, it has been suggested that given that MMPs are elevated in the presence of periodontitis, particularly in persons with diabetes mellitus, a major goal of therapy would be to reduce MMP activity. In addition to tetracycline's antimicrobial actions, it has the ability to inhibit MMP activity [57,73,74]. This nonantimicrobial action of MMP inhibition has also been demonstrated with the tetracycline derivative doxycycline [66]. When administered in doses that are nonantibacterial, doxycycline has been shown to prevent periodontal breakdown due to its ability to inhibit MMP enzyme activity [57]. Tetracycline's anti-colagenolytic activity has given rise to the development and use of Periostat (CollaGenex Pharmaceuticals, Inc., Newtown, Pennsylvania), a form of low-dose doxycycline for management of periodontitis. Low-dose doxycycline may prove useful in the management of refractory periodontal diseases or other forms of chronic periodontitis that for various reasons cannot be managed with conventional therapy. For instance, patients who are medically compromised and who cannot tolerate conventional in-office treatment could benefit from low-dose doxycycline. In the authors' experience, low-dose doxycycline has proved to be very helpful in management of periodontitis in a large hospital-based population of young and old patients. Despite its effectiveness, it does not appear that low-dose doxycycline would be a first-line choice of conventional periodontal therapy, but it definitely shows promise in management of difficult-to-treat patients or difficult-to-manage forms of periodontitis. Furthermore, it is probable that drugs designed to inhibit MMP or other proteinase activity will be developed further to be more specific in targeting proteinases of interest (eg, MMP-8 in the case of periodontitis). It is possible that certain proteins or peptides related to decorin [75] will become therapeutic adjuncts. Decorin binds to collagen and may prevent its degradation, which could be an interesting approach to management of periodontal breakdown because in this case, MMP activity would not be inhibited, but the drug's effects would be through alteration of the substrates.

Management of periodontal diseases in smokers

It clearly has been demonstrated that individuals who smoke cigarettes are at greater risk for the development of periodontitis, have more severe periodontitis, and do not respond to treatment of periodontitis as well as those who do not smoke [8,10,76]. This finding was thought to be a lifestyle issue (eg, poor oral hygiene), but a number of studies have shown that compared with nonsmokers, smokers do not necessarily have more bacterial plaque and their plaque is not populated by more periodontal pathogens. Therefore, there must be constituents of cigarette smoke that trigger or act as cofactors to initiation and progression of periodontitis. For obvious reasons, nicotine has received much attention in the literature and, indeed, it has the ability to cause a number of changes in the immune system and in the vasculature that could lead to exacerbation of periodontal disease risk and severity [77–79]. In addition, there are hundreds of other potentially toxic compounds in cigarette smoke that likely damage periodontal tissues. The authors' research group has focused on a particular class of agents found in high levels in cigarette smoke and in the environment: aryl hydrocarbons [80]. The most prevalent aryl hydrocarbons in cigarette smoke are benzo-α-pyrene and dimethyl benzanthracene [81]. Benzo-α-pyrene in particular has been shown to directly inhibit osteoblast differentiation [80]. To carry out further studies, the authors used a prototypical aryl hydrocarbon (dioxin) to study the effects of these agents on bone tissues and bone cells. These studies confirmed that aryl hydrocarbons inhibit osteoblast differentiation and bone production. Moreover, they interfere with osteoclast cell formation (Tenenbaum et al, unpublished data), an action that leads to overall reductions in bone remodeling, which could exacerbate periodontal diseases. Moreover, the authors' laboratory demonstrated that the aryl hydrocarbon benzo-α-pyrene acts in a synergistic manner with lipopolysaccharide from one of the periodontal pathogens described earlier (*Porphyromonas gingivalis*) in blocking bone cell differentiation and function [80]. These deleterious effects were shown to be mediated through the aryl hydrocarbon receptor (a cytosolic receptor). Of importance, the authors identified an agent commonly found in red wine, resveratrol, which is an aryl hydrocarbon receptor antagonist that inhibits the effects of aryl hydrocarbons. Hence, it may be possible in the future to use agents such as resveratrol or synthetic and more powerful analogs to ameliorate some of the effects of smoking on the periodontium and other tissues. Certainly, smoking cessation is the ultimate goal, but this has not proved to be as effective as its proponents would like. Thus, other approaches such as the inhibition of aryl hydrocarbon effects should be considered, especially because these agents are found in high levels within the environment, not only in cigarette smoke. It is with this in mind that a clinical trial focusing on the use of resveratrol to manage periodontitis in smokers is now underway.

Summary

It can be inferred from the foregoing that new technologies have been developed or are in development that could be used to enhance the ability to predict, diagnose, and treat periodontitis. Not all of these technologies will bear fruit; however, those that do will provide clinicians of the twenty-first century with more effective means of detection, prevention, and treatment of periodontitis than are currently available. Hence, periodontists and dentists will take on the role of physicians dedicated to the prevention and treatment of oral diseases and rely less on mechanical or nonbiologically based treatment modalities.

References

[1] Nyman S, Lindhe J, Karring T, et al. New attachment following surgical treatment of human periodontal disease. J Clin Periodontol 1982;9(4):290–6.

[2] Sanders JJ, Sepe WW, Bowers GM, et al. Clinical evaluation of freeze-dried bone allografts in periodontal osseous defects. Part III. Composite freeze-dried bone allografts with and without autogenous bone grafts. J Periodontol 1983;54(1):1–8.

[3] Axelsson P, Nystrom B, Lindhe J. The long-term effect of a plaque control program on tooth mortality, caries and periodontal disease in adults. Results after 30 years of maintenance. J Clin Periodontol 2004;31(9):749–57.

[4] Kalpidis CD, Ruben M. Treatment of intrabony periodontal defects with enamel matrix derivative: a literature review. J Periodontol 2002;73(11):1360–76.

[5] Nakashima M, Reddi AH. The application of bone morphogenetic proteins to dental tissue engineering. Nat Biotechnol 2003;21(9):1025–32.

[6] Nevins M, Camelo M, Nevins ML, et al. Periodontal regeneration in humans using recombinant human platelet-derived growth factor-BB (rhPDGF-BB) and allogenic bone. J Periodontol 2003;74(9):1282–92.

[7] Cobb CM. Clinical significance of non-surgical periodontal therapy: an evidence-based perspective of scaling and root planing. J Clin Periodontol 2002;29(Suppl 2):6–16.

[8] Albandar JM. Global risk factors and risk indicators for periodontal diseases. Periodontol 2000 2000;29:177–206.

[9] Mancini S, Romanelli R, Laschinger CA, et al. Assessment of a novel screening test for neutrophil collagenase activity in the diagnosis of periodontal diseases. J Periodontol 1999;70(11):1292–302.

[10] Maupome G, Pretty IA, Hannigan E, et al. A closer look at diagnosis in clinical dental practice: part 4. Effectiveness of nonradiographic diagnostic procedures and devices in dental practice. J Can Dent Assoc 2004;70(7):470–4.

[11] Moseley R, Stewart JE, Stephens RJ, et al. Extracellular matrix metabolites as potential biomarkers of disease activity in wound fluid: lessons learned from other inflammatory diseases? Br J Dermatol 2004;150(3):401–13.

[12] Dahan M, Nawrocki B, Elkaim R, et al. Expression of matrix metalloproteinases in healthy and diseased human gingiva. J Clin Periodontol 2001;28(2):128–36.

[13] Li J, Helmerhorst EJ, Leone CW, et al. Identification of early microbial colonizers in human dental biofilm. J Appl Microbiol 2004;97(6):1311–8.

[14] Seymour GJ, Gemmell E. Cytokines in periodontal disease: where to from here? Acta Odontol Scand 2001;59(3):167–73.

[15] Michalek SM, Katz J, Childers NK, et al. Microbial/host interactions: mechanisms involved in host responses to microbial antigens. Immunol Res 2002;26(1–3):223–34.

[16] Ezzo J, Cutler CW. Microorganisms as risk indicators for periodontal disease. Periodontol 2000 2000;32:24–35.

[17] Socransky SS, Haffajee AD. Dental biofilms: difficult therapeutic targets. Periodontol 2000 2000;28:12–55.

[18] Van Winkelhoff AJ, Loos BG, Van Der Reijden WA, et al. Porphyromonas gingivalis, Bacteroides forsythus and other putative periodontal pathogens in subjects with and without periodontal destruction. J Clin Periodontol 2002;29(11):1023–8.

[19] Tanner AC, Goodson JM. Sampling of microorganisms associated with periodontal disease. Oral Microbiol Immunol 1986;1(1):15–22.

[20] Offenbacher S, Odle B, van Dyke T. The microbial morphotypes associated with periodontal health and adult periodontitis: composition and distribution. J Clin Periodontol 1985;12(9):736–49.

[21] Loesche WJ, Giordano J, Hujoel PP. The utility of the BANA test for monitoring anaerobic infections due to spirochetes (Treponema denticola) in periodontal disease. J Dent Res 1990;69(10):1696–702.

[22] Hemmings KW, Griffiths GS, Bulman JS. Detection of neutral protease (Periocheck) and BANA hydrolase (Perioscan) compared with traditional clinical methods of diagnosis and monitoring of chronic inflammatory periodontal disease. J Clin Periodontol 1997;24(2):110–4.

[23] Bretz WA, Lopatin DE, Loesche WJ. Benzoyl-arginine naphthylamide (BANA) hydrolysis by Treponema denticola and/or Bacteroides gingivalis in periodontal plaques. Oral Microbiol Immunol 1990;5(5):275–9.

[24] Lopez NJ, Socransky SS, Da Silva I, et al. Subgingival microbiota of Chilean patients with chronic periodontitis. J Periodontol 2004;75(5):717–25.

[25] Snyder B, Ryerson CC, Corona H, et al. Analytical performance of an immunologic-based periodontal bacterial test for simultaneous detection and differentiation of Actinobacillus actinomycetemcomitans, Porphyromonas gingivalis, and Prevotella intermedia. J Periodontol 1996;67(5):497–505.

[26] Papapanou N, Neiderud AM, Sandros J, et al. Checkerboard assessments of serum antibodies to oral microbiota as surrogate markers of clinical periodontal status. J Clin Periodontol 2001;28(1):103–6.

[27] Pussinen J, Vilkuna-Rautiainen T, Alfthan G, et al. Multiserotype enzyme-linked immunosorbent assay as a diagnostic aid for periodontitis in large-scale studies. J Clin Microbiol 2002;40(2):512–8.

[28] O'Brien-Simpson NM, Veith D, Dashper SG, et al. Antigens of bacteria associated with periodontitis. Periodontol 2000 2000;35:101–34.

[29] Conrads G. DNA probes and primers in dental practice. Clin Infect Dis 2002;35(Suppl 1): S72–7.

[30] Tenenbaum H, Elkaim R, Cuisinier F, et al. Prevalence of six periodontal pathogens detected by DNA probe method in HIV vs non-HIV periodontitis. Oral Dis 1997; 3(Suppl 1):S153–5.

[31] Socransky SS, Smith C, Martin L, et al. "Checkerboard" DNA-DNA hybridization. Biotechniques 1994;17(4):788–92.

[32] Asai Y, Jinno T, Igarashi H, et al. Detection and quantification of oral treponemes in subgingival plaque by real-time PCR. J Clin Microbiol 2002;40(9):3334–40.

[33] Boopathy R, Robichaux M, LaFont D, et al. Activity of sulfate-reducing bacteria in human periodontal pocket. Can J Microbiol 2002;48(12):1099–103.

[34] Torresyap G, Haffajee AD, Uzel NG, et al. Relationship between periodontal pocket sulfide levels and subgingival species. J Clin Periodontol 2003;30(11):1003–10.

[35] Atici K, Yamalik N, Eratalay K, et al. Analysis of gingival crevicular fluid intra-cytoplasmic enzyme activity in patients with adult periodontitis and rapidly progressive periodontitis. A longitudinal study model with periodontal treatment. J Periodontol 1998; 69(10):1155–63.

[36] Yucekal-Tuncer B, Uygur C, Firatli E. Gingival crevicular fluid levels of aspartate amino transferase, sulfide ions and N-benzoyl-DL-arginine-2-naphthylamide in diabetic patients with chronic periodontitis. J Clin Periodontol 2003;30(12):1053–60.

[37] Smith AJ, Wade W, Addy M, et al. The relationship between microbial factors and gingival crevicular fluid glycosaminoglycans in human adult periodontitis. Arch Oral Biol 1997;42(1):89–92.

[38] Waddington RJ, Langley MS, Guida L, et al. Relationship of sulphated glycosamino-glycans in human gingival crevicular fluid with active periodontal disease. J Periodontal Res 1996;31(3):168–70.

[39] Al-Shammari KF, Giannobile WV, Aldredge WA, et al. Effect of non-surgical periodon-tal therapy on C-telopeptide pyridinoline cross-links (ICTP) and interleukin-1 levels. J Periodontol 2001;72(8):1045–51.

[40] Mogi M, Otogoto J, Ota N, et al. Differential expression of RANKL and osteoprotegerin in gingival crevicular fluid of patients with periodontitis. J Dent Res 2004;83(2):166–9.

[41] Genco RJ. Current view of risk factors for periodontal diseases. J Periodontol 1996; 67(Suppl 10):1041–9.

[42] Hart TC, Hart S, Bowden DW, et al. Mutations of the cathepsin C gene are responsible for Papillon-Lefevre syndrome. J Med Genet 1999;36(12):881–7.

[43] Soell M, Elkaim R, Tenenbaum H. Cathepsin C, matrix metalloproteinases, and their tissue inhibitors in gingiva and gingival crevicular fluid from periodontitis-affected patients. J Dent Res 2002;81(3):174–8.

[44] Mark LL, Haffajee AD, Socransky SS, et al. Effect of the interleukin-1 genotype on monocyte IL-1beta expression in subjects with adult periodontitis. J Periodontal Res 2000; 35(3):172–7.

[45] Papapanou N, Abron A, Verbitsky M, et al. Gene expression signatures in chronic and aggressive periodontitis: a pilot study. Eur J Oral Sci 2004;112(3):216–23.

[46] Bowers GM, Chadroff B, Carnevale R, et al. Histologic evaluation of new attachment apparatus formation in humans. Part III. J Periodontol 1989;60(12):683–93.

[47] Froum SJ, Gomez C, Breault MR. Current concepts of periodontal regeneration. A review of the literature. N Y State Dent J 2002;68(9):14–22.

[48] Melcher AH. On the repair potential of periodontal tissues. J Periodontol 1976;47(5): 256–60.

[49] Esposito M, Coulthard P, Worthington HV. Enamel matrix derivative (Emdogain) for periodontal tissue regeneration in intrabony defects. Cochrane Database Syst Rev 2003;2 CD003875.

[50] Wennstrom JL, Lindhe J. Some effects of enamel matrix proteins on wound healing in the dento-gingival region. J Clin Periodontol 2002;29(1):9–14.
[51] Caffesse RG, de la Rosa M, Mota LF. Regeneration of soft and hard tissue periodontal defects. Am J Dent 2002;15(5):339–45.
[52] Karring T. Regenerative periodontal therapy. J Int Acad Periodontol 2000;2(4): 101–9.
[53] Tenenbaum HC, Shelemay A, Girard B, et al. Bisphosphonates and periodontics: potential applications for regulation of bone mass in the periodontium and other therapeutic/diagnostic uses. J Periodontol 2002;73(7):813–22.
[54] Ryan LM. The ank gene story. Arthritis Res 2001;3(2):77–9 [Epub 2000 Dec 19].
[55] Shinozaki T, Pritzker K. Regulation of alkaline phosphatase: implications for calcium pyrophosphate dihydrate crystal dissolution and other alkaline phosphatase functions. J Rheumatol 1996;23(4):677–83.
[56] Lekic I, Rubbino F, Krasnoshtein S, et al. Bisphosphonate modulates proliferation and differentiation of rat periodontal ligament cells during wound healing. Anat Rec 1997; 247(3):329–40.
[57] Reddy MS, Geurs NC, Gunsolley JC. Periodontal host modulation with antiproteinase, anti-inflammatory, and bone-sparing agents. A systematic review. Ann Periodontol 2003; 8(1):12–37.
[58] Sela J, Gross UM, Kohavi D, et al. Primary mineralization at the surfaces of implants. Crit Rev Oral Biol Med 2000;11(4):423–36.
[59] Yaffe A, Fine N, Alt I, et al. The effect of bisphosphonate on alveolar bone resorption following mucoperiosteal flap surgery in the mandible of rats. J Periodontol 1995;66(11): 999–1003.
[60] Armitage GC. Diagnosis of periodontal diseases. J Periodontol 2003;74(8):1237–47.
[61] D'Aoust P, McCulloch CA, Tenenbaum HC, et al. Etidronate (HEBP) promotes osteoblast differentiation and wound closure in rat calvaria. Cell Tissue Res 2000;302(3): 353–63.
[62] Rodan GA. Mechanisms of action of bisphosphonates. Annu Rev Pharmacol Toxicol 1998;38:375–88.
[63] Lian JB, Stein GS. Concepts of osteoblast growth and differentiation: basis for modulation of bone cell development and tissue formation. Crit Rev Oral Biol Med 1992;3(3):269–305.
[64] Yaffe A, Golomb G, Breuer E, et al. The effect of topical delivery of novel bisacylphosphonates in reducing alveolar bone loss in the rat model. J Periodontol 2000;71(10):1607–12.
[65] Tenovuo J. Antimicrobial function of human saliva—how important is it for oral health? Acta Odontol Scand 1998;56(5):250–6.
[65a] Hirschfeld L, Wasserman B. A long-term survey of tooth loss in 600 treated periodontal patients. J Periodontol 1978;49(5):225–37.
[66] Niederman R, Abdelshehid G, Goodson JM. Periodontal therapy using local delivery of antimicrobial agents. Dent Clin N Am 2002;46(4):665–77 viii.
[67] Karlowsky J, Ferguson J, Zhanel G. A review of commonly prescribed oral antibiotics in general dentistry. J Can Dent Assoc 1993;59(3):292–300.
[68] De Soete M, Mongardini C, Peuwels M, et al. One-stage full-mouth disinfection. Long-term microbiological results analyzed by checkerboard DNA-DNA hybridization. J Periodontol 2001;72(3):374–82.
[69] Xue LY, Chiu SM, Oleinick NL. Staurosporine-induced death of MCF-7 human breast cancer cells: a distinction between caspase-3-dependent steps of apoptosis and the critical lethal lesions. Exp Cell Res 2003;283(2):135–45.
[70] Beck RW. Photodynamic therapy for age-related macular degeneration. Am J Ophthalmol 2004;138(3):513 [author reply: 513–4].

[71] Wilson M. Lethal photosensitisation of oral bacteria and its potential application in the photodynamic therapy of oral infections. Photochem Photobiol Sci 2004;3(5):412–8 [Epub 2004 Feb 05].

[72] Koshy G, Corbet EF, Ishikawa I. A full-mouth disinfection approach to nonsurgical periodontal therapy—prevention of reinfection from bacterial reservoirs. Periodontol 2000 2000;36:166–78.

[72a] Goziotis A, Sukhu B, Torontali M, et al. Effects of bisphosphonates APD and HEBP on bone metabolism in vitro. Bone 1995;16:17S–27S.

[73] Golub LM, Lee HM, Ryan ME, et al. Tetracyclines inhibit connective tissue breakdown by multiple non-antimicrobial mechanisms. Adv Dent Res 1998;12(2):12–26.

[74] Zohar R, Nemcovsky CE, Kebudi E, et al. Tetracycline impregnation delays collagen membrane degradation in vivo. J Periodontol 2004;75(8):1096–101.

[75] Bhide VM, Smith L, Overall CM, et al. Use of a fluorogenic septapeptide matrix metalloproteinase assay to assess responses to periodontal treatment. J Periodontol 2000; 71(5):690–700.

[76] Quirynen M, De Soete M, van Steenberghe D. Infectious risks for oral implants: a review of the literature. Clin Oral Implants Res 2002;13(1):1–19.

[77] Genco RJ, Loe H. The role of systemic conditions and disorders in periodontal disease. Periodontol 2000 2000;2:98–116.

[78] Grossi S. Smoking and stress: common denominators for periodontal disease, heart disease, and diabetes mellitus. Compend Contin Educ Dent 2000;30(Suppl):31–9 [quiz: 66].

[79] Kinane DF, Chestnutt IG. Smoking and periodontal disease. Crit Rev Oral Biol Med 2000;11(3):356–65.

[80] Andreou V, D'Addario M, Zohar R, et al. Inhibition of osteogenesis in vitro by a cigarette smoke-associated hydrocarbon combined with *Porphyromonas gingivalis* lipopolysaccharide: reversal by resveratrol. J Periodontol 2004;75(7):939–48.

[81] Singh SU, Casper RF, Fritz C, et al. Inhibition of dioxin effects on bone formation in vitro by a newly described aryl hydrocarbon receptor antagonist, resveratrol. J Endocrinol 2000;167(1):183–95.

ELSEVIER
SAUNDERS

Dent Clin N Am 49 (2005) 695–699

THE DENTAL
CLINICS
OF NORTH AMERICA

Index

Note: Page numbers of article titles are in **boldface** type.

A

Allogenic bone grafts, for periodontal regeneration, 640–641

Alloplasts, for periodontal regeneration, 642–643

Antibiotics, in periodontal disease, 618–622

Antimicrobials, locally applied, 618–622
    systemic, 622–623

Antiseptics, periodontal disease and, 616–618

Arestin, 621–622

Atherosclerosis, periodontal disease associated with, 535–537

Atridox, 620–621

Autogenous bone grafts, for periodontal regeneration, 640

B

B cells, and periodontitis, 506

Bacterial cultures, in periodontal disease, 679–680

Biofilm-associated bacteria, antimicrobial resistance and, 494
    bacterial antigens and virulence factors in, 495
    cell-cell communication in, 494
    extracellular proteolytic enzymes and, 497
    fimbriae in, 496–497
    gene transfer in, 494
    heat shock proteins and, 495–496
    lipopolysaccharide, 495
    regulation of gene expression in, 494

Biomarkers, host response and inflammatory mediators as, 555–557

Biotin, 600

Bisphosphonates, in periodontal disease, 685–686

Bone allograft, demineralized freeze-dried, for periodontal regeneration, 641–642
    freeze-dried, for periodontal regeneration, 641

Bone grafts, allogenic, in periodontal regeneration, 640–641
    autogenous, in periodontal regeneration, 640
    human mineralized, for periodontal regeneration, 642
    replacement, for periodontal regeneration, 640–642

Bone matrix, demineralized, Grafton, for periodontal regeneration, 642

Bone morphogenetic proteins, for periodontal regeneration, 645

Bone-specific markers, of tissue destruction, for periodontal diagnosis, 557–558

C

Calcium, in body, 602, 605

Carbohydrates, role in nutrition, 596–597

Cardiovascular disease, periodontal disease associated with, 535–537

Chewing stick, 608

Chlorhexidine, 585, 617

Chromium, functions of, 604

Coenzyme Q_{10}, 607

Collagen, type 1, pyridinoline cross-linked carboxyterminal telopeptide of, 558–560

Copper, sources of, 604

D

Demineralized freeze-dried bone allograft, for periodontal regeneration, 641–642

Dental plaque. See *Plaque.*

doi:10.1016/S0011-8532(05)00050-9

dental.theclinics.com

Changing Your Address?

Make sure your subscription changes too! When you notify us of your new
address, you can help make our job easier by including an exact copy of your
Clinics label number with your old address (see illustration below.) This
number identifies you to our computer system and will speed the processing of
your address change. Please be sure this label number accompanies your old
address and your corrected address—you can send an old Clinics label with
your number on it or just copy it exactly and send it to the address listed below.

We appreciate your help in our attempt to give you continuous coverage.
Thank you.

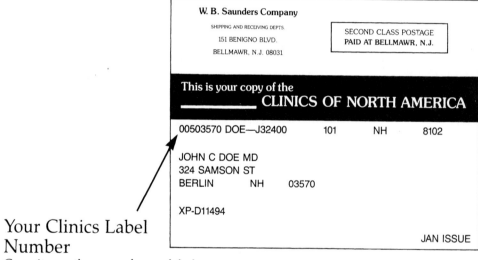

W. B. Saunders Company

SHIPPING AND RECEIVING DEPTS.
151 BENIGNO BLVD.
BELLMAWR, N.J. 08031

SECOND CLASS POSTAGE
PAID AT BELLMAWR, N.J.

This is your copy of the

CLINICS OF NORTH AMERICA

00503570 DOE—J32400   101   NH   8102

JOHN C DOE MD
324 SAMSON ST
BERLIN   NH   03570

XP-D11494

JAN ISSUE

Your Clinics Label Number

Copy it exactly or send your label
along with your address to:
W.B. Saunders Company, Customer Service
Orlando, FL 32887-4800
Call Toll Free 1-800-654-2452

Please allow four to six weeks for delivery of new subscriptions and for
processing address changes.

Order your subscription today. Simply complete and detach this card and drop it in the mail to receive the best clinical information in your field.

Please Print:

Name _____

Address_____

City_____ State _____ ZIP _____

Method of Payment

❑ Check (payable to **Elsevier**; add the applicable sales tax for your area)

❑ VISA ❑ MasterCard ❑ AmEx ❑ Bill me

Card number _____ Exp. date _____

Signature _____

Staple this to your purchase order to expedite delivery

❑ **Adolescent Medicine Clinics**
  ❑ Individual $95
  ❑ Institutions $133
  ❑ *In-training $48

❑ **Anesthesiology**
  ❑ Individual $175
  ❑ Institutions $270
  ❑ *In-training $88

❑ **Cardiology**
  ❑ Individual $170
  ❑ Institutions $266
  ❑ *In-training $85

❑ **Chest Medicine**
  ❑ Individual $185
  ❑ Institutions $285

❑ **Child and Adolescent Psychiatry**
  ❑ Individual $175
  ❑ Institutions $265
  ❑ *In-training $88

❑ **Critical Care**
  ❑ Individual $165
  ❑ Institutions $266
  ❑ *In-training $83

❑ **Dental**
  ❑ Individual $150
  ❑ Institutions $242

❑ **Emergency Medicine**
  ❑ Individual $170
  ❑ Institutions $263
  ❑ *In-training $85
  ❑ Send CME info

❑ **Facial Plastic Surgery**
  ❑ Individual $199
  ❑ Institutions $300

❑ **Foot and Ankle**
  Individual $160
  Institutions $232

❑ **Gastroenterology**
  ❑ Individual $190
  ❑ Institutions $276

❑ **Gastrointestinal Endoscopy**
  ❑ Individual $190
  ❑ Institutions $276

❑ **Hand**
  ❑ Individual $205
  ❑ Institutions $319

❑ **Heart Failure (NEW in 2005!)**
  ❑ Individual $99
  ❑ Institutions $149
  ❑ *In-training $49

❑ **Hematology/ Oncology**
  ❑ Individual $210
  ❑ Institutions $315

❑ **Immunology & Allergy**
  ❑ Individual $165
  ❑ Institutions $266

❑ **Infectious Disease**
  ❑ Individual $165
  ❑ Institutions $272

❑ **Clinics in Liver Disease**
  ❑ Individual $165
  ❑ Institutions $234

❑ **Medical**
  ❑ Individual $140
  ❑ Institutions $244
  ❑ *In-training $70
  ❑ Send CME info

❑ **MRI**
  ❑ Individual $190
  ❑ Institutions $290
  ❑ *In-training $95
  ❑ Send CME info

❑ **Neuroimaging**
  ❑ Individual $190
  ❑ Institutions $290
  ❑ *In-training $95
  ❑ Send CME info

❑ **Neurologic**
  ❑ Individual $175
  ❑ Institutions $275

❑ **Obstetrics & Gynecology**
  ❑ Individual $175
  ❑ Institutions $288

❑ **Occupational and Environmental Medicine**
  ❑ Individual $120
  ❑ Institutions $166
  ❑ *In-training $60

❑ **Ophthalmology**
  ❑ Individual $190
  ❑ Institutions $325

❑ **Oral & Maxillofacial Surgery**
  ❑ Individual $180
  ❑ Institutions $280
  ❑ *In-training $90

❑ **Orthopedic**
  ❑ Individual $180
  ❑ Institutions $295
  ❑ *In-training $90

❑ **Otolaryngologic**
  ❑ Individual $199
  ❑ Institutions $350

❑ **Pediatric**
  ❑ Individual $135
  ❑ Institutions $246
  ❑ *In-training $68
  ❑ Send CME info

❑ **Perinatology**
  ❑ Individual $155
  ❑ Institutions $237
  ❑ *In-training $78
  ❑ Send CME info

❑ **Plastic Surgery**
  ❑ Individual $245
  ❑ Institutions $370

❑ **Podiatric Medicine & Surgery**
  ❑ Individual $170
  ❑ Institutions $266

❑ **Primary Care**
  ❑ Individual $135
  ❑ Institutions $223

❑ **Psychiatric**
  ❑ Individual $170
  ❑ Institutions $288

❑ **Radiologic**
  ❑ Individual $220
  ❑ Institutions $331
  ❑ *In-training $110
  ❑ Send CME info

❑ **Sports Medicine**
  ❑ Individual $180
  ❑ Institutions $277

❑ **Surgical**
  ❑ Individual $190
  ❑ Institutions $299
  ❑ *In-training $95

❑ **Thoracic Surgery (formerly Chest Surgery)**
  ❑ Individual $175
  ❑ Institutions $255
  ❑ *In-training $88

❑ **Urologic**
  ❑ Individual $195
  ❑ Institutions $307
  ❑ *In-training $98
  ❑ Send CME info

BUSINESS REPLY MAIL

FIRST-CLASS MAIL   PERMIT NO 7135   ORLANDO FL

POSTAGE WILL BE PAID BY ADDRESSEE

PERIODICALS ORDER FULFILLMENT DEPT
ELSEVIER
6277 SEA HARBOR DR
ORLANDO FL 32821-9816